RIGHT HEMISPHERE COMMUNICATION DISORDERS: THEORY AND MANAGEMENT

Clinical Competence Series

Series Editor
Robert T. Wertz, Ph.D.

Right Hemisphere Communication Disorders: Theory
and Management
Connie A. Tompkins, Ph.D., CCC-SLP

Manual of Voice Treatment: Pediatrics Through Geriatrics
Moya Andrews, Ed.D.

Videoendoscopy: From Velopharynx to Larynx
Michael P. Karnell, Ph.D.

Prosody Management of Communication Disorders
Patricia M. Hargrove, Ph.D., and Nancy S. McGarr, Ph.D.

Clinical Manual of Laryngectomy and Head and Neck
Cancer Rehabilitation
Janina K. Casper, Ph.D., and Raymond H. Colton, Ph.D.

Source Book for Medical Speech Pathology
Lee Ann C. Golper, Ph.D., CCC-SLP

RIGHT HEMISPHERE COMMUNICATION DISORDERS: THEORY AND MANAGEMENT

Connie A. Tompkins, Ph.D., CCC-SLP
Associate Professor,
Communication Science and Disorders
Department of Communication
University of Pittsburgh
Pittsburgh, Pennsylvania

SINGULAR PUBLISHING GROUP, INC
SAN DIEGO, CALIFORNIA

Published by Singular Publishing Group, Inc.
4284 41st Street
San Diego, California 92105-1197

©1995 by Singular Publishing Group, Inc.

Typeset in 10/12 Times by So Cal Graphics
Printed in the United States of America by BookCrafters

Library of Congress Cataloging-in-Publication Data

Tompkins, Connie Ann.
    Right hemisphere communication disorders: theory and management/
Connie Tompkins
        p. cm.—(Clinical competence series)
    Includes bibliographical references and index.
    ISBN 1-56593-176-9
        1. Communicative disorders.   2. Brain damage—Complications.
    3. Cerebral hemispheres.   I. Title.   II. Series.
        [DNLM: 1. Communicative Disorders—therapy.   2. Brain—physiology.
    3. Dominance, Cerebral.   WL 340 T662r 1994]
    RC423.T55 1994 1995
    616.85'52—dc20
    DNLM/DLC
    for Library of Congress   94-28509
                                                                    CIP

CONTENTS

FOREWORD

com•pe•tence (kom'pə təns)   n.   The state or quality
of being properly or well qualified; capable.

Clinicians crave competence. They pursue it through education and experience, through emulation and innovation. Some are more successful than others in attaining what they seek. This book, **Right Hemisphere Communication Disorders: Theory and Management**, by Dr. Connie A. Tompkins is one of several in the Singular Clinical Competence Series. It is designed to move each of us further along the path that leads to clinical competence. Dr. Tompkins covers the variety of symptoms that may be present subsequent to right hemisphere brain damage. She provides the theory that guides appraisal and management. Most of all, she cautions we should not assume we know what we do not. Dr. Tompkins is a skilled investigator and a competent clinician. Her book conveys what makes her that way. She knows that no principle or technique is true or useful until it has been tested; that tests do not diagnose, and treatment programs do not treat—clinicians do. Indeed, we are fortunate to have colleagues like Connie Tompkins to tell us where we are and to indicate the direction that will lead us to where we want to be. Your attention to what she provides indicates your competence and your effort to improve it, because competent clinicians seek competence as much for what it demands as for what it promises.

Robert T. Wertz, Ph.D.
Series Editor

PREFACE

Several years ago, when Terry Wertz asked me write a book on the management of communication disorders associated with right hemisphere brain damage in adults, my initial response was that such an effort was premature. Although there has been an acceleration of basic research on right hemisphere function and dysfunction in the past dozen years or so, the accumulated evidence remains rudimentary, and few clinical applications to right hemisphere communication disorders have been suggested, much less evaluated. "But," Terry persisted, "it is not premature to establish some direction." Persuaded by his argument, I began to write this book.

The resulting text reflects the still embryonic nature of research and practice with this clinical population. The book is put forward as a vehicle to help readers ascertain what we do and do not know at the present time about right hemisphere communication disorders and the processes presumed to underlie them; to illustrate how to generate hypotheses about evaluation and management based on theory, data, logic, and patients' communicative needs; and to charge clinicians to become critical evaluators of both the literature that contributes to these hypotheses, and their own treatment plans and procedures. I have provided many practical suggestions, as well, to guide clinical planning and process, but I have leavened them liberally with cautions that are intended to keep readers thinking, questioning, and examining their beliefs and assumptions.

The title of the book emphasizes "theory" along with "management," because I believe that the two are crucially intertwined. Digesting theoretical information may be difficult for some, but theory should define what we do in treatment. At a general level, our theory of a disorder will influence how we approach it. For example, if we believe that some right hemisphere communication deficits are manifestations of attentional or perceptual impairments, we may want to assess and treat those underlying problems, while measuring the impact on the communicative symptoms. At a more specific level, empirically supported theories of cognitive and communicative function are invaluable guides to developing assessment and treatment techniques that reflect what is known (or at least reasonably believed) at any point in time about the component processes and skills involved in thinking and communicating. Well-founded theory is essential to help us move beyond a low-level concern with *what* to do in our clinical interactions, to a focus on *why* specific approaches and tactics should be fruitful. It is imperative for clinicians to learn to derive clinical hypotheses and procedures from theoretical and empirical foundations. This problem-solving skill will assist them in modifying their approaches along with evolving theories and accumulating evidence, and, as a result, providing the most principled services possible to those most important consumers, our patients.

This book was written primarily for practicing clinicians, clinical scientists, and graduate students in communication science and disorders, and its foundations derive from cognitive psychology, psycholinguistics, and neuropsychology as well as speech-language pathology. Although the text focuses on symptoms and theories germane to right hemisphere function and dysfunction, the reader will find that many of the orientations and principles presented here are relevant more broadly for studying or working with adults who have neurologically based communication impairments. It is hoped that clinicians and clinical scientists from related fields (e.g., behavioral neurology, neuropsychology, occupational therapy) will find something of value in this material, as well.

The text was organized to make the information clear and accessible. For instance, I have tried to distill and exemplify theoretical material to make it understandable; and I have used extensive cross-referencing to help readers tie together related information from various parts of the book. A note on literature citations is in order here. Consistent with the design of the Clinical Competence Series, of which this book is a part, I limited the number of first-hand references that are cited in the text, and referenced a number of more general secondary sources. But I do not intend for this stylistic feature to imply that I consider the primary references to be unimportant; far from it. Just as the material I have presented here has passed through my filter, the content in other secondary sources reflects their authors' interpretations of primary reports. As another of the many "challenges to clinicians" that are set forward in this book, I strongly encourage readers to identify first-hand sources that are cited in the review papers, chapters, and other books referenced here, and then to read, evaluate, and extrapolate from the original works themselves.

Connie A. Tompkins, Ph.D.

ACKNOWLEDGMENTS

Over the several years that I worked on this book, many people have offered major encouragement and support that helped to make the undertaking less daunting. The Tompkins family, in particular, never had any doubts about my ability to see this project through, and their optimism and pride often helped to sustain my efforts. My colleagues and students at the University of Pittsburgh also expressed their support on a regular basis, even when my writing obligations lessened my participation in other professional commitments and interactions.

I would like to convey my gratitude to a number of specific people, as well, for their contributions to the project. The Clinical Competence Series editor, Terry Wertz, was always just a phone call away when I hit a roadblock or needed a boost in confidence, and he invariably managed to restore my enthusiasm. My dear friend and colleague Chris Dollaghan read every word of the earliest drafts, made her typical cogent comments, and generally buoyed my spirits with her genuine interest, good cheer, and encouraging words. Don Robin also inquired regularly and encouraged continually, along with reading diligently and critiquing generously portions of Chapters 1 and 2. In addition, Patrick Doyle, Mick McNeil, Carl Coelho and his graduate students, Penny Myers, Annette Baumgaertner, and Margaret Lehman made valuable comments and suggestions about earlier drafts of some of the other material in the book; though I hasten to acknowledge that any errors or oversights are wholly my own. Christine Gable and Kris Spencer assisted capably and cheerfully with essential background research and organizational and editing tasks. Christine Gable also wrote a terrific initial draft summarizing the published treatment literature on neglect (included in Chapter 7). Finally, I give special thanks to my husband, Richard Schulz, for his patience, humor, and continuing confidence in my work. We are both delighted that I will have evening and weekend time for something other than the book, and relieved that the portable computer and "book disk" will not be joining us on our next trip away from Pittsburgh.

Connie A. Tompkins, Ph.D.

For C.T.T., A.W.T., and B.T.C.

CHAPTER

1

Introduction to the Book and to the Population

I. NATURE, SCOPE, AND INTENT OF THIS BOOK

A. Right Hemisphere Communication Disorders: An Emerging Concern

Speech-language pathologists are reporting increasing numbers of adults with right hemisphere damage (RHD) in their caseloads. However, few practicing clinicians have been trained specifically to work with this population. At present, our clinical role is sketchy and underspecified, in part because there is little evidence to guide intervention decisions: when and if to treat, what and how to treat, whether our treatment brings about changes beyond those that would occur with natural recovery, and whether our treatment makes a difference in everyday functioning. But the literature relevant to the communicative abilities and deficits of RHD adults is accumulating rapidly. This book summarizes some of the available knowledge, raises some of the many remaining questions, and generates some potential directions for clinical assessment and intervention with RHD adults. It is also intended to motivate clinicians to take a more rigorous approach to designing and evaluating their own clinical procedures and interactions.

B. Focus of This Book

The book focuses on the consequences of relatively focal damage to the right hemisphere; the diffuse effects of dementing conditions or traumatic injuries, which in most cases involve the right hemisphere to some extent, will not be considered here. In addition, the book does not provide an exhaustive account of symptomatology or of supporting research, for which the reader is referred to other sources. Rather, it reviews selected communicative, perceptual/cognitive, and behavioral symptoms; addresses the presumed underlying nature of these symptoms where possible; and provides suggestions for appraisal/assessment and management, tied as closely as possible to current notions of underlying causes and everyday communicative needs. Along the way, the book identifies challenges to clinicians and researchers working with RHD persons, to help foster ways of thinking about, and working with, this population. Some of these challenges identify areas where more tools, information, or evidence are needed; others raise qualifiers, caveats, and complications in interpreting what we think we already know.

C. Overarching Clinical Themes

Four themes permeate the clinical material in this book:

1. We should consider a symptom's impact in planning assessment and management, focusing where possible on making a difference in daily life interactions;

2. We should attempt to discover where, and why, performance breaks down, melding this "process" analysis with functional concerns to guide management whenever possible;

3. We should involve patients and their significant others in the treatment process as soon and as much as possible, to maximize independence in daily life communication and problem solving;

4. We should try to determine whether a symptom or a performance deficit can be changed by speech-language intervention. There may not be a solution for all problems that exist, and we must be accountable enough to acknowledge this possibility.

II. EPIDEMIOLOGY, DEMOGRAPHICS, AND ETIOLOGY

A. Etiology

Right hemisphere damage has the same etiologies as left hemisphere damage. Strokes (ischemic/occlusive and hemorrhagic) are the leading cause of right hemisphere dysfunction, but relatively focal symptoms can be associated with tumors and some types of head trauma as well. Of course generalized neurological conditions such as Alzheimer's disease will compromise right hemisphere communicative functions, but the deficits will occur in the context of widespread and deteriorating perceptual, cognitive, and motor impairments.

B. An Epidemiologic Sketch

Cerebrovascular disease is distributed fairly equally between the right and left hemispheres of the brain. We know little about the epidemiology of right hemisphere damage per se, but perhaps we can extrapolate from the existing data about stroke in general.

1. The term "stroke" refers to a number of related disorders, characterized by the sudden onset of prominent and often persistent neurological deficit due to impaired circulation in the brain. Mlcoch and Metter (1994) summarize much of the relevant epidemiologic data. They note an annual incidence in North America of about 1–2 per 1,000 people; each year in the United States, stroke leaves more than 250,000 people with permanent disability. At any one time, about 6 out of 1,000 people are living with the consequences of stroke. For a population of 265 million, this translates to more than 1.5 million people at any given time. In has been estimated that, in today's dollars, stroke care costs run at least $5–10 billion per year (see Mlcoch & Metter, 1994).

2. The incidence of stroke increases dramatically with age (Table 1–1), so minor increases in the mean age of the population result in large increases in stroke incidence. However, the annual incidence of stroke has declined since the start of this century, due largely to improved public awareness and medical control of major risk factors such as hypertension, heart disease, diabetes, and smoking. Mlcoch and Metter (1994) report some evidence that stroke rates began increasing again in 1980; this upturn has been attributed to improved diagnosis resulting from the widespread use of computed tomography (CT) scanning.

Table 1–1. Incidence of stroke with age

Age	Rate per 1000
< 18	0.7
18–44	1.7
45–64	16.7
65–74	49.7
≥ 75	83.5

Source: National Center for Health Statistics. (1991). *National health survey* [DHHS Publication No. PHS 92-1509]. Hyattsville, MD: U.S. Department of Health and Human Services.

3. Stroke is the third leading cause of death among older persons, after heart disease and cancer. Deaths among stroke survivors are much higher than for the age-adjusted general population (see Mlcoch & Metter, 1994). For post-stroke patients who survive beyond 3 weeks, there is a 3-year mortality rate of about 46% (Marquardsen, 1969) as compared with 12% in the general population. About 80% of strokes are of thromboembolic (occlusive) etiology. The male-to-female ratio of stroke occurrence in all age ranges is about 3:2, but as people get older the sex difference begins to even out.

C. Which Right Hemisphere-Damaged Adults Exhibit Communication Disorders?

The incidence of communication disturbances in right brain-damaged patients has not been examined or classified systematically, leading to the critical question: Who among RHD patients will have communication deficits? A "best guess" from empirical data and clinical observation is that about half of RHD adults will have communication impairments. This is about the same as the proportion of unselected patients with left brain damage who have aphasia. As summarized by Joanette, Goulet, and Hannequin (1990), RHD adults whose communication is impaired tend to have less schooling than RHD patients without communication deficits; they also have a greater incidence of familial left-handedness, are more likely to have cortical than subcortical lesions, and are more likely to exhibit anosognosia (see definition in section III-E-1-e-(2), below). In addition, they tend to function with fewer cognitive resources as indexed by measures of attention and memory (Tompkins, 1990, 1991a; Tompkins, Boada, & McGarry, 1992; Tompkins, Bloise, Timko, & Baumgaertner, 1994).

III. PRESUMED LOCALIZATION AND NATURE OF SELECTED NEUROPSYCHOLOGICAL AND COGNITIVE FUNCTIONS

A. Types of Hemispheric Asymmetries

Both behavioral and biological asymmetries, or left versus right hemisphere differences, in brain function have been identified. We know much more about behavioral asymmetries, covered in some detail below, than we do about biological asymmetries.

B. Biological Hemispheric Asymmetries

Some biological asymmetries are anatomical in nature: for example, the Sylvian fissure tends to be longer in the left hemisphere than in the right. It has also been observed that there is a higher ratio of white matter (axons) to gray matter (nerve cell bodies) in the right than the left hemisphere (Gur et al., 1980). This interconnectedness has been proposed to predispose the right hemisphere to more diffuse information coding and activation than the left hemisphere. However, the relation of anatomical to behavioral asymmetries is unknown.

C. Biochemical Asymmetries

Similarly, very little is known about biochemical asymmetries and their influences on behavior. It has been suggested that the right hemisphere has greater concentrations of noradrenergic and serotonergic content than the left (Whitehead, 1991; Whyte, 1992). The noradrenergic system influences, among other things, the orienting of attention. Serotonin is active in counteracting feelings of depression and fear.

D. Behavioral Asymmetries

Behavioral asymmetries, inferred from neuropsychological testing, are believed to reflect cerebral lateralization of function. The discussion below summarizes some of the lateralized functions associated primarily with right hemisphere parietal, temporal, and frontal lobes (readers who want more information, or original reference citations, may consult Kolb & Whishaw, 1990, and McCarthy & Warrington, 1990). The right hemisphere circuitry for its role in attentional functions, emotional processes, and paralinguistic behavior (e.g., prosody) will be considered briefly with the review of these areas in Chapter 2.

E. Some Correlations Between Right Hemisphere Anatomy and Function

A few words of caution are in order about attributing specific skills and deficits to particular anatomical zones. First, the characterizations below are only as valid as the inferences drawn from performance on various neuropsychological or psychophysiological tests or procedures. But, perhaps more importantly, brain structures are richly interconnected; consequently, damage in a region that provides input to or modulates the function of another area may produce symptoms mimicking those associated with primary damage in the second region.

1. **Parietal lobe:** Anterior zones of the parietal lobes appear to be involved primarily with somatic sensations and perceptions, and posterior zones serve mainly sensory-integrative functions. In the right parietal lobe, cross-modal matching integrates somatic and visual sensory information to form percepts and to code spatial location of sensory information. The analysis of visual, auditory, and somatic input requires that information be integrated to determine what is being perceived and where it is coming from. Thus, parietal areas play a major role in recognizing abstract stimuli. Parietal regions are also important for manipulating spatial information about abstract (mental) stimuli. An example may make this function easiest to understand. When someone is asked to imagine a bicycle and to draw it from the perspective of the rider, he or she must manipulate the "mental representation" of the bicycle to draw it.

   a. Damage to these right parietal systems can result in difficulty appreciating complex visuospatial information, impaired recognition of objects in unfamiliar views, and various disorders of spatial orientation and processing (e.g., judging distances, finding one's way in space, assessing the orientation of lines, coding spatial locations, recognizing faces). When a disturbance of spatial integration affects the ability to see relationships between objects or things in space, a patient with right parietal damage may use spatial cues that are increasingly ego-centered, perceiving space in relation to his or her own body. Similar egocentric changes might be observed in higher cognitive functions, such as difficulties understanding things from others' points of view, although a definitive link has not been observed.

   b. Right parietal areas are implicated in various facets of attention as well.

(1) They are active, along with a number of other cortical areas, during sustained attention tasks. Narrowly defined, sustained attention involves the duration and consistency with which people can detect rare target stimuli or events in conditions that require continuous monitoring, or vigilance. More generally, sustained attention involves maintaining a consistent behavioral response under conditions of constant and active monitoring. The work of radar and sonar operators in wartime was a real-life activity that initiated interest in vigilance and sustained attention, as it was important that they detect infrequent targets rapidly and consistently. Some examples of experimental conditions that require vigilance include visual arrays in which individual points of light, somewhat like "stars," blink on and off in an unpredictable way, or auditory signals in which particular tones occur inconsistently along with other tones and tone sequences.

(2) Right parietal functions also participate in spatial selective attention for both visual fields. Selective attention is widely assumed to reflect system limitations. That is, our cognitive systems are limited in capacity or "energy," and thus can handle only so much information without becoming overloaded (but see Allport, 1989, for a competing point of view). On this view, attentional selectivity enables processing, allowing us to prioritize the relevant elements of an information source by focusing on them while ignoring or attenuating the strength of nontarget or competing information. Selective attention may operate by enhancing task-relevant signals, such as individual elements or groups of features associated with objects and events; this idea can be captured by several metaphors that have been proposed to describe the ways in which spatial selective attention works. One popular analogy for spatial selective attention describes an "attentional spotlight" that is aimed on the internal mental environment. Stimulus features that are contained within the spotlight's beam are highlighted as important for further mental activity (e.g., perception) and so receive processing priority. Features that fall close to the margins or outside of the beam are minimized or unavailable. Another metaphor describes a "zoom lens" function that widens or narrows an attentional focus as needed for the requirements of the task and situation. Initially, attention may be focused in a general way on the spatial position of an object or message. If this global focus does not provide sufficient information for the task at hand, attention may be zoomed in or refocused to identify specific elements of the object or message. The amount of attention committed to a spatial location appears to increase as well with task difficulty (e.g., demands for making subtle discriminations or processing degraded information or non-meaningful stimuli) and expectancies. In any case, selective attention is generally presumed to limit the amount of information that enters our cognitive systems, and to facilitate behavioral responding to attended stimuli.

Several subcomponents of spatial selective attending have been identified. In one prominent model (Posner, Walker, Friedrich, & Rafal, 1984, 1987), orienting attention to a particular location in space is accomplished through at least three component operations: disengaging from a current focus, shifting or moving the attentional focus, and engaging attention to the selected stimulus. These processes have been associated with covert mental activity (in contrast to observable behaviors or processes), as they can be inferred from performance on tasks even when eye position remains fixed. The "disengage" function, in particular, appears to be mediated by the parietal lobes, and has been suggested as one potential mechanism underlying hemispatial neglect (see definition in III-E-1-e, below). Selective attentional phenomena and processes are discussed further in Chapter 2.

c. To interpret the information conveyed by selectively-attended sensory signals, a memory system must hold onto that information long enough to allow for effective integration. Right parietal zones appear to house a working memory system for temporarily holding the mental representations (or abstract codings) of nonverbal material, such as the spatial location of sensory inputs.

d. Parietal cortex also contains one of several motor command systems in the brain. Parietal cortex receives signals of the position and movement of the body in space and functions to direct or guide movements toward behavioral goals. In particular, right parietal areas appear to provide input to direct movements for reproducing spatial properties of objects. Lesions can lead to constructional impairments (see below).

e. Major deficits associated with right parietal lobe damage are identified and defined below.

(1) hemispatial neglect: Hemispatial neglect is often discussed as if it is a single entity, but it is more likely a constellation of disorders of spatial exploration and selective attention. These impairments are manifest primarily in a directional bias for perception and action, in the absence of basic sensory or motor deficits such as visual field cuts or hemiparesis. Patients with neglect may fail to report, respond to, or orient towards stimuli contralateral to their brain lesions (although neglect can have ipsilateral consequences as well). Neglect can follow left hemisphere brain damage, but it occurs more frequently, lasts longer, and is generally more severe after RHD (e.g., Ratcliff, 1982).

Some patients will neglect auditory and tactile stimuli, but visual neglect has been documented most often and studied most extensively. Visual neglect typically involves some combination of the following behavioral signs: excluding detail from the left side when drawing an imagined object, such as a flower, from memory; making more errors of omission for response choices on the left side during language or psychological testing; omitting or misidentifying letters from the left side of words, or words from the left portion of a page, when reading; dressing or grooming only the right half of the body; bumping into doorframes or furniture on the left side of the body; and generally ignoring sensory stimulation on the left side of the body. However, as noted above, patients with visual neglect often have ipsilateral deficits as well. Visual neglect may or may not be accompanied by homonymous hemianopsia. It improves with time, but less so when it is initially severe or when it is associated with extensive premorbid cortical atrophy. Further, the directional bias in neglect can be modulated in various ways, through cues and body positioning; some of these are noted in Chapter 2 (Table 2–9).

Neurologists often diagnose neglect on the basis of a phenomenon called "extinction to double simultaneous stimulation" (or simply "extinction"). Patients who demonstrate extinction respond adequately to unilateral stimuli presented on either side of the body, but have difficulty reporting contralesional stimuli when stimulation is presented bilaterally.

Although extinction is widely used to diagnose neglect, the two should not be equated. Either can occur in the absence of the other, and extinction is more common than true neglect (Bradshaw, Pierson-Savage, & Nettleton, 1988).

Various forms of neglect appear to have attentional, representational, and/or intentional (action) components. Several potential attentional mechanisms are discussed briefly below. The representational nature of neglect symptoms is easiest to understand with an example. Patients with neglect who are asked to imagine familiar places and to describe them as if looking at them from different vantage points may omit details from the left side *for each imagined view;* thus, their mental frame of reference influences which details they omit. This suggests that they have knowledge of the relevant details, but have difficulty accessing or scanning a fully elaborated mental image, or representation, for performing the task.

The literature on the mechanisms of neglect is complex and confusing. Attentional/arousal theories of neglect predominate at present. Some attentional theories note difficulty directing attention to the neglected hemifield; however, Posner et al.'s (1984, 1987) proposal that parietal neglect is better characterized by difficulty disengaging from the intact field or current attentional focus (see also Morrow & Ratcliff, 1988), has gained popularity. The nature of Posner's paradigm, and some of its limitations, are described further in Chapter 2 (section III-D-8-b). Recently, Arguin and Bub (1993) argued that the deficit in neglect is one of attentional capture (like engagement) for contralesional stimuli, rather than disengagement. By the time this book is published, there will be many more contributions to this ongoing debate. On the basis of evidence assumed to reflect representational impairments, like that noted above, some aspects of parietal neglect have also been described as deficits in either the active mental representation of information from internal or external sources, or problems of inspecting those mental representations (or maps of space) for use in particular tasks, once they are constructed.

Two final points deserve mention here. First, it is important to note that neglect is not exclusively associated with the parietal lobe. Deficits of intention or action toward contralateral space are often linked to frontal lobe damage, and severe neglect has also been observed to follow damage to the insula, which is the polymodal integration cortex contained within the Sylvian fissure. Second, neglect affects vertical, as well as lateral dimensions of spatial exploration and response. Patients with neglect often make more errors in the lower quadrants when processing externally presented or imagined objects.

(2) **anosognosia:** Meaning "lack of knowledge of disease," the term "anosognosia" is used to indicate unawareness or denial of deficits. The anosognosic patient may deny the need for treatment; "disown" his own affected side; or insist that he is just about to go play a round of golf, when in fact he is unable to walk. In less severe forms, the person with anosognosia may merely be indifferent to the fact and severity of his disabilities. Anosognosia and neglect often co-occur.

(3) **topographical disability:** "Topographical disability" refers to confusion about location in space, which may involve difficulty drawing or reading maps or floorplans of well-known places (patient may distort directions, arrangement of landmarks, and distances); difficulty describing how to travel from one place to another; or getting lost. This impairment frequently occurs in combination with neglect and face recognition disorders and often follows bilateral brain damage.

(4) **geographic disorientation:** Patients with geographic disorientation can relate to their immediate surroundings (e.g., realize that they are in a hospital), but fail to conceive of their general location. They may believe that they are in other parts of the world, even in places that they have never visited. Geographic disorientation is dissociable from orientation for time, but frequently co-occurs with topographical disorientation.

(5) **constructional impairments:** This term refers to deficits in organizing complex actions in space, which cannot be accounted for by visual-perceptual or basic motor impairments. Constructional impairment, sometimes called constructional apraxia or visuo-constructive deficit, affects spatially directed movements that are under visual control, and may be manifest as difficulty in assembling components to form an object or a drawing. Commonly used tasks for assessing constructional impairment include combining

blocks to form designs or copying shapes and figures. Constructional impairment in RHD adults tends to be qualitatively different from that seen in left-hemisphere-damaged (LHD) adults. Disturbances of spatial relationships (e.g., fragmented or rotated drawings; piecemeal or altered relationships among components so that the whole picture is distorted) and neglect (e.g., left side of drawing incomplete or underdeveloped) are most commonly observed on constructional tasks after RHD. In contrast, LHD adults with constructional impairment may produce generally simpler drawings, with fewer lines and fewer details. Right parietal lesions may disturb drawing or constructional abilities because the frontal motor system receives inadequate sensory-spatial information to plan and execute the relevant movements.

2. **Temporal lobe:** Right temporal areas have been particularly implicated for receiving and interpreting nonverbal auditory sensations, for nonverbal learning and memory, and for assigning affective tone to sensory input.

   a. Temporal RHD has been associated with deficits in music processing, including difficulties discriminating time, loudness, timbre (differences in harmonic structure), and extracting and retaining pitch information in auditory short-term memory. However, it has also been suggested that left and right auditory cortices differ more generally in temporal resolution for sensory input. Left auditory cortex appears to be capable of fine temporal acuity and thus to be specialized for analyzing brief acoustic stimuli, while right auditory cortex may be suited to analyzing longer, less time-dependent acoustic stimuli.

   b. Right temporal damage has also been associated with a variety of deficits in nonverbal memory. The medial temporal lobe houses the hippocampus, a structure that contributes crucially to the consolidation and formation of nonverbal memories, particularly for spatial information in the right hemisphere. Right temporal lobectomy affects recognition and recall of a variety of materials, including complex visual figures, simple nonsense figures, faces, unfamiliar melodies, and tunes. Extent of right hippocampal removal correlates with degree of memory deficit on tests of diverse functions, including tactile maze learning, visual maze learning, facial recognition, spatial block span, spatial position, spatial association, spatial memory, and self-ordered recall of designs.

    c. Right temporal impairment may also disrupt the recognition, recall and interpretation of facial expressions and other subtle social signals such as vocal irony and emotional intonation. Some patients with right temporal damage have difficulties with voice recognition as well.

    d. Finally, right temporal damage has sometimes been associated with "poor contextual use" for interpreting nonverbal information. For example, when something anomalous is depicted in a stimulus (e.g., a monkey in a cage has an oil painting hanging on the wall), patients with right temporal excisions have evidenced difficulties in pointing out the oddity, even though they recognized and described all of the pictured elements.

3. Frontal lobe: With the exception of contralateral motor control and control of movement primarily related to nonverbal abilities, the laterality of function disturbed by frontal lesions is less striking than that observed from more posterior lesions (see Table 1–2). Regardless of the side of lesion, frontal brain damage can be associated with impairments enumerated below. Striking deficits in these areas may occur even when patients have intact IQs and good recognition memory. Kimberg and Farah (1993) have proposed a unified account of cognitive deficits following frontal brain damage, in which they attribute impairments on seemingly disparate tasks to a difficulty in maintaining associations between mental representations of goals, stored knowledge, and environmental stimulus attributes. Typical deficits include:

    a. difficulty with planning, problem solving, divergent thinking, and strategy formation, particularly where no routine or over-learned procedures are available;

    b. decreased behavioral spontaneity and initiation;

    c. distractibility;

    d. decreased ability to profit from cues to regulate or change behavior (e.g., using feedback to evaluate performance, solving problems according to rules, inferring rules from changes in tasks);

    e. perseveration, impaired response inhibition, and inflexible behavior;

    f. poor memory for the order of occurrence of events (temporal memory), for which of several events occurred more recently (recency memory), or for the source or context in which they learned or observed facts or events (source memory).

Table 1–2. Deficits that may be associated with right frontal damage

Impaired performance on block construction, design copying, and nonverbal design fluency tasks (which require the participant to draw as many designs as possible with a designated number of lines).

Impaired estimates of recency, frequency of occurrence, and source or temporal context for correctly recalled nonverbal stimuli/events.

Impaired performance on delayed response spatial memory tasks (but not for immediate spatial discrimination and recognition).

Impaired ability to profit from error signals and feedback in spatial and tactile learning or problem-solving tasks.

Difficulty developing strategies when no rote answer or routine procedure is available, as in cognitive estimation tasks (e.g., "How tall is the Empire State Building?" or "How much does this cost?").

Difficulty inhibiting dominant, or routine responses that conflict with goal-appropriate behavior (e.g., when a color term such as "blue" is printed in a different color of ink, such as red, and the task is to name the ink color ("red"), patients may have trouble inhibiting the dominant tendency to read the word "blue").

Decreased vigilance, or sustained attention for detecting rare signals (parietal regions also contribute).

Impaired "motor maps" or programs, for the distribution of scanning, orienting, and exploring in extrapersonal space.

Difficulty switching to a new motor program ("stuck-in-set" perseveration; Sandson & Albert, 1984).

Hemihypokinesia (hemiakinesia), or difficulty directing responses to the neglected side in the absence of gross motor deficit. Signs include decreased initiation and prolonged response times for movements toward contralateral hemispace, difficulty raising arm contralateral to the lesion when asked, and failure to orient eyes and head to contralateral stimuli. May be related to impairment of intentional mechanisms for preparatory stages of movement.

Transient symptoms typically associated with parietal neglect.

Social disinhibition, including pointless storytelling, liberal profanity, lack of tact and restraint, promiscuous sexual behavior, and general immaturity and lack of social graces.

F. Right Hemisphere Communicative Functions

Apart from the few conclusions reviewed above, there is precious little known about localization of communicative functions within the right hemisphere. It has been difficult to gather reliable and generalizable data, for a variety of reasons. Most investigations have been conducted using relatively small subject samples; when samples are fractionated to form subgroups based on lesion site, the number in each subgroup may be untenably reduced. The lesion data can be problematic as well. Investigators often face the practical necessity of studying patients from diverse hospitals, and each hospital may use a different radiologic protocol. In addition, patients' lesions generally do not respect anatomical borders, even those intended only to distinguish grossly between primarily anterior and posterior lesions.

G. Accounts of Cerebral Localization

One question about existing accounts of functional cerebral localization deserves mention here. That is, what is the appropriate metric for describing inter-hemispheric differences? The old dichotomy pitting verbal (left hemisphere) against nonverbal (right hemisphere) functions has been discredited. One other recent attribution, that the left hemisphere is an analytic processor and the right hemisphere processes holistically, or in a gestalt fashion, also does not hold up to close scrutiny. Both hemispheres appear to be capable of either type of processing, and the characterization is typically invoked after the fact, as it has been difficult to develop *a priori* performance expectations. Suggestions that the right hemisphere is more diffusely organized than the left also proliferate in the literature. This distinction was initially based on elementary sensorimotor testing. Recently, it has resurfaced as an explanation for performance dissociations on certain visual judgment tasks (Kosslyn, Chabris, Marsolek, & Koenig, 1991) and as a proposal about the nature of lexical-semantic coding in the two hemispheres (Beeman, 1993). This position will be hard to test for the higher cognitive domains, given potential problems of differential test sensitivity for left and right hemisphere function and differential severity of impairments after unilateral brain damage. Researchers interested in characterizing functional asymmetries must continue to search for independently motivated theories of cognitive behavior to test against them (Trope, Rozin, Nelson, & Gur, 1992).

IV. GENERALITY OF COMMUNICATIVE DISORDERS AFTER RHD

One of the most important things to remember about adults with RHD is one of the most important characteristics of any "category" of people they are quite heterogenous. Not all patients will have communicative impairments. Those who do will not have all symptoms, and individual patients will display different patterns of behavior. Complicating things further, it can be quite difficult to specify "disordered" status, because normative information is almost nonexistent for abilities and performances broken down by age, education, socioeconomic status, and cultural variables. It is part of the clinical challenge in working with brain-damaged individuals to identify the presence and absence of the deficits that result from neurologic insult, as well as those that are not necessarily due to the brain damage.

V. OTHER CHALLENGES TO CLINICIANS AND RESEARCHERS

A. Lack of Recovery Data

There are almost no data regarding recovery after RHD, either natural or assisted. So we do not know the amount and pattern of improvement to expect without our intervention; whether our treatments can accelerate, modify, or amplify natural neurological recovery processes; or whether various treatments effect meaningful changes.

B. Lack of Attention to Individual Differences

In many group studies, overall results are reported with no attempt to identify whether different patterns contributed to the averaged results. In interpreting and generalizing from group studies, we should remember that substantial numbers of subjects in a group may perform quite differently from the reported average.

C. Lack of Attention to Components of Impaired Performance

Relatedly, it is well known that different patients may attain identical scores for very different reasons. However, little work has been done to try to tease out component processes and skills that may contribute differentially to an overall impaired performance.

D. Methodological Limitations of Existing Research

Much of the published data base suffers from methodological limitations that may decrease our confidence in the reliability and generalizability of findings. Some of these include:

1. **Small sample sizes:** Group studies of small numbers of subjects may yield misleading or irreproducible findings, due in part to chance influences on the group composition.

2. **Sampling biases:** Subject characteristics affect the applicability or generalizability of results. For example, if only the most severely involved subjects are studied (e.g., those referred for rehabilitative services, those who have long-lasting or severe neglect, those who are still in the acute post-onset stage), the results may not characterize other, more mildly impaired persons.

3. **Lack of validated materials or appropriate control judgments:** This problem is similar to the lack of normative information, mentioned above. It is common to assess and study subjective phenomena like interpretations and inferences in RHD adults, but interpretations and inferences are not absolute. An examiner's expectation of the "correct" or "most likely" interpretation is frequently not borne out when appropriate non-brain-damaged subjects are asked to perform the task.

4. **Insufficient operationalization of variables:** When performance is monitored on characteristics that are not explicitly and clearly defined, it is not possible to determine whether we agree with the investigator's criteria, or whether a particular patient's behavior is the same as that reported. Criteria and definitions used to designate, for example, anosognosia, tangential speech, monotonous prosody, or flat affect, should be provided in detail.

5. **Questionable reliability of subjective judgments:** Designations such as those indicated above are often made using subjective judgments or ratings. Investigators should also demonstrate independent observer agreement on their judgments or ratings. Otherwise, the results may reflect an idiosyncratic, and unreplicable, interpretation.

6. **Lack of sound evaluation instruments:** There are few tests and procedures with adequate reliability and validity, but this problem is compounded in published research when an informal measure is designed for some purpose. Preliminary information is needed about various aspects of reliability and validity for these measures (see Chapter 3, section V-C).

E. Lack of Information About Underlying Processes

Finally, we lack models and data regarding underlying processes that may relate groups of symptoms, though work is currently focusing on this problem (see Chapter 2, section V). Plausible proposals about presumed underlying causes should help to guide treatment planning and to direct investigations of treatment effectiveness.

VI. Conclusion

This book was written in an attempt to provide some direction for those who study or work with right brain-damaged adults, while data and models that can guide our efforts are being collected, formulated, and tested. This first chapter has provided some basic foundations for the rest of the book. Subsequent chapters consider further what can go wrong after RHD, how we can check for behavioral strengths and weaknesses (approaches and procedures for appraisal and evaluation), and what we may have to offer clinically (the processes of estimating recovery and outcome, formulating treatment goals and strategies, delivering treatment and documenting its efficacy, and enhancing psychosocial adjustment).

CHAPTER

2

Review and Proposed Accounts of Selected Symptoms

I. CLINICAL CHALLENGES

When considering the litany of symptoms that can follow RHD, it is important to remember the caveats discussed below. With these cautions in mind, the remainder of this chapter reviews selected communicative, perceptual, cognitive, and behavioral symptoms that can follow RHD in adults and examines some of the current thinking about potential explanations of these symptoms.

A. Patient Heterogeneity

The variability among patients with RHD can create problems for interpreting the results of group studies of patient characteristics, especially when group patterns are not inspected for individual differences. When we look carefully, we usually find more than one pattern in group data. So, while a study may suggest that RHD patients have difficulty with a set of tasks, it is highly unlikely that every RHD adult will have those deficits. Also, those who do make errors may do so for different reasons (e.g., perceptual, attentional, memorial, etc). Clinically, we need to remember that it is doubtful that any patient will exhibit all of the problems discussed below, and that individual RHD patients will present with different combinations of symptoms and different levels of impairment in affected areas. We have to be aware of our tendency to bring to the appraisal a narrow set of expectations about what is "typical" in this population.

B. Symptom Co-occurrence

Relatedly, we do not yet know whether there are predictable sets of symptoms that routinely co-occur in subsets of RHD patients. For example, we have seen two patients with roughly similar damage on CT scans who presented very different profiles. One was emotionally animated, highly verbal, and had a "typically" tangential conversational style; yet he had little apparent difficulty sustaining attention or using and interpreting figurative language or inference. The other presented with "flattened affect," said little, and was occasionally concrete in interpreting nonliteral language; but her discourse was organized, relevant, and informative. The fact that little can be predicted or assumed when we meet a RHD adult can present a considerable challenge for planning a communicative appraisal and evaluation.

C. Lack of Norms for Pragmatic and Conversational Skills

There are almost no normative data for the "higher level" skills we usually evaluate and target after RHD. We do not know how aging, educational history, and cultural factors, to name a few, affect narrative or conversational styles, inferencing abilities, humor or nonliteral language interpretation, nonverbal behavior, and other communicative performances. This makes it difficult to attribute abnormality, to assign prognoses, and to select remediation targets.

D. Uncertainty About Recovery Course

Finally, we know little about the recovery course in various deficit areas. Some of our information about RHD patients' performance has been gathered during the very early post-stroke period, before symptoms have resolved or stabilized to provide an accurate picture of long-term difficulties. Therefore, some apparent contradictions in the literature about symptom prevalence or severity may be due to time-post-onset variables.

II. OVERVIEW OF COMMUNICATIVE SYMPTOMS

A. Pragmatics Domain

Many of the communicative consequences of RHD can be captured under the rubric of pragmatics. Pragmatics involves the relation between language behavior and the contexts in which it is used and interpreted. These contexts include external variables, such as the existing situation or preceding utterances, and internal factors, such as the participants' emotional states, intentions, and knowledge of the world. Some of the components of interest include prosody, emotional interpretation and response, speech act use and interpretation, figurative and implied meanings, sensitivity to situation and listener needs, humor appreciation, and other forms of inference. Those who wish more information than what is provided here may consult Joanette and colleagues (1990) for a summary and critical evaluation of much of what has been concluded in the area.

1. **Prosody.** Elements of speech melody, rate, stress, juncture, and duration have a pervasive influence on communication and are critical in speech production and perception. Prosodic influences cut across linguistic levels, providing cues to consonant voicing, syntactic clause boundaries, utterance form, semantic stress and novelty, and utterance intent. Several characterizations of hemispheric contributions to prosody are provided in Table 2–1.

   a. Impressionistically, some RHD adults have speech that is less varied intonationally than that of non-brain-damaged adults.

Table 2–1. Characterizations of hemispheric specialization for prosodic processing

Left Hemisphere	Right Hemisphere
Temporal utterance characteristics	Spectral characteristics
Rapidly changing acoustic events	Longer, less time-dependent stimuli
Linguistic utterance characteristics (e.g., lexical stress; vowel duration contrasts)	Emotional characteristics
Linguistic utterance characteristics	All aspects of prosody

That is, their voices may sound "flat" and monotonous. Reading voices of RHD adults have been rated as similar to those of depressed patients on a scale that ranged from "sad" to "excited," and in terms of tempo and pitch variation (House, Rowe, & Standen, 1987). RHD patients may produce less stress on individual words in sentences, and less emphatic stress, so that their productions take on a "monotone" quality. However, one report (Colsher, Cooper, & Graff-Radford, 1987) found that time postonset was related to perceived dysprosody, which suggests that early apparent deficits may diminish. It should be remembered as well that dysarthrias associated with RHD may be responsible for much of the perception of restricted intonational variability (see II-E, below).

b. On the other hand, some RHD adults sound hypermelodic. Acoustic evidence suggests that these individuals tend to have abnormally high mean fundamental frequency, together with high pitch variability (Colsher et al., 1987).

c. In general, whether linguistic or emotional prosody is the subject of concern, the evidence on prosodic production problems after RHD is mixed. Many studies have failed to replicate or have directly contradicted the findings of other studies; the conclusions of each study will depend in part on the mix of participating individuals with differing profiles. It should be remembered as well that prosodic production deficits are not particular to RHD patients.

d. RHD adults may demonstrate difficulties interpreting linguistic prosody as well, but much of the difficulty appears due to a perceptual impairment of prosodic decoding, apart from its linguistic nature (see Joanette et al., 1990). Adults with RHD may also respond less consistently to emotional tone or intonationally implied meanings in interactions with others, but again their prosodic comprehension disorders are not necessarily due to the emotional content of the message. In fact, their deficits in emotional prosodic comprehension have been associated with difficulty discriminating between filtered, nonemotional speech patterns (Tompkins & Flowers, 1985). A more purely perceptual component may underlie or contribute to both linguistic and emotional prosodic impairments. Some research indicates that RHD adults have more difficulty processing intonational, or fundamental frequency aspects of prosodic signals, than temporal or durational components (e.g., Robin, Tranel, & Damasio, 1990).

e. Before leaving this section, a position advanced by Ross and his associates (Ross, 1981, 1984a, 1984b; Ross, Harney, de Lacoste-

Utamsing, & Purdy, 1981) deserves some comment. Ross describes various difficulties with the expression, comprehension, and repetition of emotional prosody after RHD, and dubs these deficits "aprosodias." Ross describes a taxonomy of aprosodias determined by site of lesion in the right hemisphere. His classification scheme mirrors classical aphasia taxonomies; thus, for example, right frontoparietal damage is associated with a motor aprosodia, characterized by deficits in expression and repetition of emotional prosody but relatively good comprehension. Ross's characterization has attracted much attention in the neurology literature and has been cited uncritically in writings for speech-language pathologists as well. But the conclusions should be viewed with caution, as they were derived from observations of limited subject samples, using an unvalidated protocol, with unreported judgment reliability. Additionally, the proposed functional-anatomic correlations have not been observed by other researchers, and much work indicates that the neurologic correlates of emotional prosody disruption are more complex than this framework suggests (see Cooper & Klouda, 1987; Joanette et al., 1990).

2. **Emotion and nonverbal communication.** Emotional processing may vary depending on both the side and site of brain lesion. A great deal of evidence suggests that emotional behavior is mediated primarily by the right hemisphere (see, e.g., Tucker & Frederick, 1989, for review). Some research points to differential hemispheric specialization depending on stimulus valence, but the evidence is conflicting as to whether the right hemisphere is more important for processing negative emotions and the left hemisphere for positive emotions, or vice versa.

   a. Within the right hemisphere, frontal lesions tend to result in emotional disinhibition; for example, patients with frontal impairments may tell pointless stories with liberal profanity, even when others take exception. Patients with more posterior right hemisphere damage may minimize and rationalize their deficits and have difficulty assigning meaning to emotional stimuli.

   b. Some of the work on emotional interpretation points to problems in the way that RHD patients link a relatively intact appreciation of emotional material with decisions about situations and contexts. For example, patients may do well inferring the affect conveyed by sentences describing emotional situations (Tompkins & Flowers, 1985), but may falter when required to match their emotional inferences with specific pictures or settings (Cicone, Wapner, & Gardner, 1980). At the same time, some patients with RHD also have problems appreciating the visuospatial and acoustic/prosodic stimuli in which emotional messages are embedded, potentially leading to emotional misinterpretation (e.g., Blonder, Bowers, & Heilman, 1991). Some exhibit emotional interpretation deficits across modalities, including pictures, body language, facial and vocal expression, and complex nonredundant discourse units. Data on skin response, respiration, and heart rate indicate that some RHD patients are hypoaroused in the presence of emotional stimuli (e.g., Heilman,Watson, & Valenstein, 1985; Morrow, Vrtunski, Kim, & Boller, 1981). However, this hypoarousal does not necessarily co-occur with impaired emotional recognition (Zoccolotti, Scabini, & Violani, 1982), suggesting that autonomic and cognitive aspects of emotional processing can be separately impaired.

c. In terms of expression, many RHD patients show reduced nonverbal animation and coverbal behaviors relative to non-brain-damaged adults (Blonder, Burns, Bowers, Moore, & Heilman, 1993; Golper, Gordon, & Rau, 1984). Again, there are important exceptions; the patient mentioned previously for his disinhibited expression of humor was extremely animated. In fact, while some patients are nearly unresponsive to cartoons, others react with unrestrained hilarity. Either extreme has potential implications for interpersonal interactions. RHD adults can also be deficient in adhering to rules of social discourse involving eye contact, facial expression, spontaneous use of gesture, vocal inflection, and turn-taking.

3. **Speech acts.** Often, a speaker's intention differs from the literal meaning of his or her utterance. Consider the classic example of an indirect request, such as "Can you pass the salt?" The person asking the question expects an action, passing the salt, rather than a literal answer to the question. The "real" meaning conveyed by an utterance is known as a speech act. Other speech acts include asserting, directing, questioning, and warning.

a. Most of our knowledge about RHD adults' use and interpretation of speech acts has come from assessments of indirect commands and requests, and much of that work has focused on comprehension. Some RHD adults may have difficulty interpreting indirect requests, exhibiting a tendency to take them literally; such a patient may respond "Yes" to the question about the salt. Other patients are sensitive to the fact that such forms often solicit actions, but they appear to have difficulty judging the appropriateness of action responses in particular situations. For example, when asked to choose an appropriate response to a literal conversational question like "Can you play tennis?" RHD adults may think that a scene of a person demonstrating his tennis stroke in the living room depicts a perfectly fine response (Hirst, LeDoux, & Stein, 1984). Of course, as Joanette and colleagues (1990) note, difficulty in this instance may reflect a problem judging the plausibility of the depiction, rather than a problem interpreting the contextual appropriateness of the response. With verbal material, RHD patients may demonstrate less sensitivity to context overall than non-brain-damaged persons, but they do tend to select indirect responses in contexts that call for indirect interpretation, and direct responses in direct contexts (Weylman, Brownell, Roman, & Gardner, 1989).

b. Generally, given the kinds of tasks used to assess indirect requests in context, it is not clear whether the RHD patient's difficulty lies in interpreting the requests themselves, interpreting the contexts, or relating the two at some level (Joanette et al., 1990). Stemmer, Giroux, and Joanette (1994), who studied production and evaluation of request sequences rather than comprehension, suggest that the last possibility may be the case in some conditions. They examined RHD patients' production and metalinguistic judgments of requests that varied from quite direct requests (e.g., "turn down the radio") to quite indirect "hints" (e.g, "I'm having trouble concentrating"), using stimulus contexts designed to elicit relatively direct or indirect request sequences (by varying social power, familiarity, degree of obligation to comply, and degree of right to make the request). "Hints," or nonconventionally indirect requests, have specific meanings only in particular social situations, and are less direct ways of requesting than the conventionally indirect requests mentioned above (e.g., Can you/Could you) that by convention link specific forms with specific pragmatic functions. Stemmer and colleagues also examined subjects' use of elements that vary or modify the degree of imposition entailed by the request (e.g., "could you" and "possibly" to soften requests, providing reasons to establish the need for the requested behavior, or altering the focus of the request from speaker- to listener-oriented).

c. For most of Stemmer and colleagues' (1994) measures, the RHD patients were as adept as control subjects. Their problems centered primarily around the application of nonconventionally indirect requests, or "hints." In comparison to control subjects, the RHD adults produced similar numbers of hints and request modifiers, and they used a variety of request types (ranging from most to least direct) that were appropriate to the stimulus condition. They showed clear context sensitivity by virtue of the fact that they never produced strong direct commands in situations designed to elicit indirect requests, but produced strong direct commands frequently in direct request contexts. However, the RHD subjects did not take the stimulus context into account in their production of hints. For the evaluation task, direct responses to both types of stimulus contexts were judged (in terms of directness, politeness, and likelihood of occurrence) similarly by RHD and control subjects, suggesting again the RHD subjects' sensitivity to contextual factors. But the RHD adults evaluated hints as more like direct or conventionally indirect requests than did control subjects. That is, the most indirect response type was often used and evaluated more like a direct request. The combined results suggest that RHD patients can build mental representations of direct and indirect stimulus contexts and request forms. The authors suggested that RHD patients' problems might arise from difficulties applying, integrating, or revising the mental representations constructed for the various elements of the task when some of those representations are in conflict. For nonconventional indirect requests, the mental representation of the stimulus context is not necessarily compatible with that derived for the request itself (whose interpretation is not linked by any strong convention to a particular pragmatic form or function). If subjects entertain (mentally) several representations for these nonconventional forms, including possibly a conventional one, some selection or integration must eventually occur to mesh these varied representations with those that reflect the subjects' interpretation of other relevant sources of information (e.g., the stimulus context). It is under these types of conditions that RHD adults demonstrate difficulty.

d. The reader will note that most evaluations of RHD adults' indirect request comprehension have used metalinguistic association and judgment tasks. Recently, Lemieux, Goulet, and Joanette (1993) reported that RHD adults had no difficulty interpreting indirect speech acts in more natural communicative situations, such as being asked in a therapy setting: "Can you, within 30 seconds, tell me as many words as you can starting with the letter F?" Evidence from other studies of nonliteral processing has raised similar cautions against overgeneralizing from poor performance on metacognitive tasks after RHD (e.g., Tompkins, 1990; Tompkins et al., 1992).

4. **Figurative and other implied meanings.** Some RHD patients may also take idiomatic, metaphoric, connotative, or sarcastic expressions more literally than they are intended. But performance with pictured assessment materials may be confounded by problems of visuospatial and visuoperceptual analysis, or by difficulty in assessing the relative plausibility of the foils. For example, few reference situations are possible to depict the literal meaning of an idiom such as "spill the beans," with the result that these literal meanings are often portrayed in prototypical ways. By contrast, the figurative meanings of the same expressions can be depicted in a variety of ways, so more reference situations must be evaluated against the one presented in the task, potentially making it more difficult for patients to select the figurative foil (Huber, 1990).

   a. Some work that has minimized or eliminated visual demands in assessing figurative meanings raises questions about the characterization of RHD subjects as overly literal (Tompkins et al., 1992; Weylman et al., 1989). Errors often reflect a nonliteral interpretation that is related to the expected figurative meaning, rather than a literal response. For example, when defining the phrase "pull some strings," a patient may say "know some important people."

   b. Nonliteral interpretation problems often emerge when the assessment method requires metacognitive abilities such as comparing literal and metaphoric word attributes to judge similarity of meaning; associating intact appreciation of figurative expressions such as "a loud tie" with specific, task-imposed contexts; or explaining nonliteral forms such as proverbs. For instance, a dissociation has been observed between RHD patients' access to idiomatic expressions presented in sentence contexts, and their relative difficulty defining and explaining the same forms (Tompkins et al., 1992). In addition, RHD adults may comprehend nonliteral expressions that they have produced in conversation better than other common figurative expressions (Apel, Van Dyke, & Fedorak, 1992).

5. **Sensitivity to listener needs and situation.** Presupposition, and theory of mind, are two concepts associated with sensitivity to listener needs. Presupposition involves the process of forming assumptions about what a listener believes and knows and, as such, requires taking the perspective of one's communication partner. Someone's "theory of mind" reflects his or her presuppositions. These related concepts are important at a variety of levels, affecting choices rang-

ing from referential and lexical markers to conversational management devices, as speakers attempt to make their contributions appropriate to their partners.

a. Clinical observation suggests that some RHD patients have difficulty in this area. They may delve into a topic without informing the listener, they may use inexplicit referential devices, and they may attempt few conversational repairs. Some research has also suggested problems with presupposition and theory of mind for RHD adults. One study (Kaplan, Brownell, Jacobs, & Gardner, 1990) involved conversational irony. An actor's poor performance in some situation, such as a golf game, was followed by a positive comment from another character (the speaker) about how well the actor was doing. RHD subjects were provided with information about the nature of the relationship between the speaker and the actor (e.g., friends) to help guide their interpretation of these remarks. RHD subjects were less likely than control subjects to use the relationship information to decide whether the speaker was telling the truth, joking, sarcastic, mistaken, or lying on purpose. Further, the RHD group felt that actors hearing the positive comments would believe that the speaker was telling the truth. The authors interpreted this finding as a difficulty in attributing knowledge of speaker intentions to the actor. Of course, this task has a metacognitive component that may make it hard for RHD patients to perform.

b. An impaired sensitivity to listener needs and situation may be manifest more generally in social disinhibition and other social/interactional problems. Klonoff, Sheperd, O'Brien, Chiapello, and Hodak (1990) also observed that their RHD subjects had difficulty taking the listener's perspective about what was central in everyday interactions. Social awareness should receive more attention and exploration in the future, given its likely influence on a patient's everyday functioning.

6. **Humor.** Deficits in appreciating humor after RHD are potentially multifaceted. They can be linked to impairments in interpreting situational, facial, and prosodic cues that signal the emotional content of a message, and/or to difficulty integrating content across parts of a narrative. Some of the prosodic and situational cues have been considered previously. With regard to content integration, some patients appear to detect, but to have difficulty resolving, the incongruity or contradiction that is frequently necessary for a story to be perceived as humorous, although they do recognize surprise as an essential element of humor (e.g., Bihrle, Brownell, & Gardner, 1988). This is

demonstrated by a tendency to select humorous nonsequitur endings for jokes over either straightforward endings or humorous endings that cohere with the rest of the context and are preferred as punchlines by adults without brain damage. These deficits, like those with figurative language forms more generally, have been ascribed to a difficulty using context to interpret intentions, particularly when task demands are high.

Humor production has not been carefully documented for RHD patients, but clinical observations indicate that in some cases, their humor may be crude or otherwise disinhibited, and inappropriate to the situation. For example, male patients may relate lewd jokes or make suggestive comments in the presence of female clinicians. When patients behave this way, it can create great consternation for family and others around them; although we know one patient whose family members laugh heartily at his suggestive comments and are relieved that he has retained his "sense of humor."

7. **Inferences.** Inferencing, or gleaning information that is not explicitly provided, has received a great deal of attention in relation to RHD. To the extent that inference processes are a means for dealing with those occasions when speakers say something other than what they mean, inferencing may be involved in interpreting intended meanings in many of the areas covered thus far. A proposal that inference deficits are at the heart of RHD communication disorders is considered near the end of this chapter, and some normal theory and evidence regarding communicative inferencing processes is presented in Chapter 4 (section III-C-3-f). First, though, some specific aspects of inferencing performance are discussed below.

Some work shows that, although RHD subjects make few errors sorting pictures of objects, they may have more difficulty sorting pictures according to an implicit theme or gist, particularly when the pictures contain multiple contextual cues that lead to thematic interpretations (Myers, Linebaugh, & Mackisack-Morin, 1985). Similarly, some patients are poor at inferring motives and morals from story contexts (Wapner, Hamby, & Gardner, 1981). Some types of inferences may be more difficult than others as well. For example, some RHD adults may do better answering inference questions that rely on general world knowledge than those that require integration of information provided in a text; some may have more difficulty drawing inferences about spatial relationships than about nonspatial descriptions. RHD adults tend to be fairly good at drawing initial inferences from linguistic material, but may have more difficulty revising them if a reinterpretation becomes necessary (Brownell, Potter, Bihrle, & Gardner,

1986; Tompkins & Mateer, 1985). And, as reported by Kaplan et al. (1990), inferences about affectively consistent information (e.g., a person in a pleasant situation hears a positive comment and interprets it as "telling the truth") may be less impaired than those about affectively inconsistent or discrepant situations (e.g., someone in a negative situation hears the same positive comment, which may be intended ironically, or as an attempt to make someone feel better). In general, RHD patients appear to have more difficulties with inferencing when the context supports or suggests alternative interpretations.

B. Text-level Abilities: Discourse and Conversation

1. **Impairments beyond the sentence level.** Many of the pragmatic deficits reviewed above are observed beyond the single-sentence level. In addition, text-level processes, themselves, may be impaired after RHD. The material below provides a detailed discussion of discourse and conversational concepts, focused on identifying and evaluating component impairments that may lead to text-level performance deficits in RHD adults. Though this material is lengthy in places and complicated at times, it forms a necessary foundation for assessment and treatment information that is presented later in this book. Discourse and conversation deficits observed in RHD adults are also reviewed briefly.

2. **An emerging interest in discourse analyses.** Discourse analyses, concerned with production and comprehension of text units longer than single sentences, have gained popularity in speech-language pathology assessment because discourse processing calls on complex interactions of knowledge and mental operations that are presumed to underlie daily life interactions. Discourse analyses are pertinent for RHD adults because many of their communicative difficulties are manifest beyond the sentence level. The validity with which monologic discourse performance reflects conversational performance has not been established; both kinds of analyses are discussed in the sections that follow.

3. **Discourse processing: Concepts and models.**

   a. Producing and comprehending discourse require multifaceted, interactive processing skills. Any discourse unit is a reflection of the speaker/writer's knowledge and beliefs, purposes and goals, and the variety of supporting cognitive operations needed to plan content and form, organize and integrate information across sentences, realize linguistic markers and continuity of expression, and maintain situational and topical appropriateness. Similarly, interpreting discourse depends on the knowledge, goals, and linguistic and other cognitive abilities of the comprehender, which include assumptions of the speaker's or writer's knowledge, goals, and purposes.

b. Discourse takes a number of forms that differ in structure, content, and function. Among the most commonly identified and studied discourse genres are narrative, procedural, and conversational. Narrative discourse, or storytelling, is oriented around characters and events; procedural discourse informs by conveying sequences of actions associated with achieving a goal. Features of conversation specific to that genre, including dyadic skills such as turn-taking and topic maintenance, will be considered separately below.

c. Table 2–2 describes some general properties characterizing successful discourse (see Patry & Nespoulous, 1990). These, and several others, will be considered briefly below in the context of two models of discourse processing. First, however, a note is warranted on the lack of terminological unity in the discourse literature. Discourse analysis is complex, partly because its constituent processes and representations are not well understood. But another source of complexity is terminological. For example, the term "coherence" is used by some authors to refer to both the surface and intermediate levels of continuity noted in Table 2–2, while "cohesion" is used by others to refer to the same two levels. "Macrostructure" and "superstructure," terms to be introduced below, are sometimes used interchangeably and other times to refer to separable theoretical and analytic concerns. Readers of the discourse literature may be frustrated by the tendency for the same terms to be used in different ways, sometimes without explicit definition.

d. Much work in discourse analysis stems from one influential model of discourse comprehension (e.g., Kintsch & van Dijk, 1978; van Dijk & Kintsch, 1983). Mross (1990) provides a readable description of this position and summarizes some supporting evidence. The model highlights different mental representations that contribute to discourse comprehension; identifies some processes presumed to operate on those representations; and emphasizes the top-down, strategic nature of interpretation. In this model, discourse is mentally represented at three levels: a surface level, where surface structure and lexical information are retained briefly in verbatim form; a text base where units of meaning are represented; and a situation level where information from the text base is combined with expectations and world knowledge to construct an integrated interpretation.

Table 2–2. Fundamental properties of discourse and their relationship to surface structure.

Remote From Surface Structure

Unity	Discourse is perceived as a whole, not as a simple concatenation of sentences
Appropriateness	Formality, content, expression take into account the situation and the addressee's knowledge
Intentionality	Message, or purpose, is clear
Topicality	Topic is also clear
Informativeness	A reasonable amount of information is included.

Surface Structure Elements

Cohesion	Reflects continuity established through word-level semantic relations. Cohesion occurs when the interpretation of a word or phrase in a discourse unit depends on that of another in the same discourse unit. Cohesive devices are explicit linking elements like pronouns, determiners, and other lexical or syntactic forms that coreference information across phrases and sentences (see also Armstrong, 1991).

Intermediate with Respect to Surface Structure

Coherence	Reflects continuity over an entire discourse unit. Coherence is concerned with semantic relations (e.g., those involved in logical sequences and cause/effect relations) and pragmatic factors (e.g., new information should not contradict already given information, and should be relevant to what has come before). It can be overt (established directly from propositions in the text) or covert (linkages via inference and world knowledge); and local (reflecting relationships among individual propositions) or global (reflecting propositions' relation to an organizing principle or discourse theme).

Source: After Patry and Nespoulous (1990).

(1) At the level of the text base, comprehension proceeds through analysis of propositions. A proposition is a predicate (i.e., a verb, modifier, or sentential connecter) that represents the links or conceptual relations between its associated arguments (e.g., the agent, goal, and/or object of

a verb). As a discourse unit is analyzed, each proposition is maintained temporarily in the text base in a limited-capacity workspace, or memory buffer, and checked for argument overlap with other propositions. Important propositions are held in the buffer, while others are replaced and gradually cycled into a longer-term representation of the discourse (e.g., the situation model, discussed below). Among the candidates for "important propositions" are those that are thematically relevant to the interpretation being built, including those that reflect foregrounded information, which is defined as information that becomes the focus of processing because it is likely to be connected with other text elements (e.g., terms that serve as sentence topic or to which pronominal reference is made). Other propositions likely to be retained in the buffer include those that are emphasized in some way, or those that have been processed too recently to discount as unimportant without further interpretation. When interpretation depends on information that has been displaced from the buffer, a comprehender must either draw an inference from available information, or institute a search of the intermediate discourse representation. The allocation of buffer capacity depends on a number of factors, including the structure and purpose of the discourse, and the comprehender's goals and topic knowledge.

(2) Propositional representations in the text base are organized hierarchically, with the initial proposition(s) in the discourse unit taking a superordinate position. A second level is formed by propositional representations that overlap with those at the superordinate level, while propositions that share arguments with the second level but not the first form a third layer, and so on. The text base represents propositional meaning at local (microstructure) and global (macrostructure) levels, and also contains superstructure information that is retrieved from long-term memory.

(a) Microstructure corresponds primarily to the surface level in Table 2–2. Microprocessing deals with the relationships between individual propositions, conveyed by syntactic and stylistic forms like changes in word order, paraphrase, and other cohesive devices (see Huber, 1990).

(b) The macrostructure representation contains the main ideas, themes, or "gist" of the discourse. Kintsch and van Dijk (1978) suggested that macrostructure was based on microstructure, but more recently others proposed and they appear to concur (van Dijk &Kintsch, 1983) that "top-down" processes are crucial in determining macrostructure representations. Top-down processes are driven by the comprehender's goals and relevant prior knowledge, including knowledge of discourse superstructures.

(c) Discourse superstructures are abstract cognitive representations that code knowledge of conventional elements of different discourse genres, including news stories, fables, overlearned procedures, or even scientific manuscripts for those sufficiently familiar with research reporting (see Table 2–3). Presumably, superstructures are constructed and stored in the brain as a result of exposure and experience with such conventionalized forms. They are not consciously available to the comprehender: Most people cannot identify the elements involved in producing a good story and do not "decide" to consult a narrative superstructure when they are presented with a story. Even so, reliance on superstructures can be inferred from a variety of data, including some that show comprehension and memory performance to suffer when stories are presented in unconventional formats. Superstructures are thought to

Table 2–3. Elements of discourse superstructure

Narrative Discourse (Storytelling)

Essential elements are a setting, development or complicating action, and resolution; an *episode* is a segment that contains each of these elements. Complex narratives have multiple episodes. Optional elements include a summary or abstract, evaluation, and coda (end signal).

Procedural Discourse

Procedural discourse is less often studied and less well understood than that of narratives, but it may be guided in part by scripts. A simple procedure may be described as a routine series of steps that ends in the prespecified goal (target step). More complex procedures may require description of other elements, such as the conditions for performing the procedure, or any particular items required. Procedural discourse also has optional and essential steps, which may be possible to uncover empirically.

(See Cannito, Hayashi, & Ulatowska, 1988; Ulatowska, Allard, & Chapman,1990).

conserve processing resources by providing a comprehender with the outlines and expectations for interpreting a discourse unit once the genre has been identified.
Other notable discourse superstructure organizations
include scripts that represent culturally routine
sequences of events or procedures, like placing an
order in a restaurant, shopping for an article of cloth-
ing, or making a cup of coffee.

(3) At the level of the situation model, the comprehender constructs a representation of the situation described in the discourse unit. General world knowledge, beliefs, and other
sociocultural factors influence the formation and application of situation models. A situation model can be coded
spatially as well as propositionally. The influence of this
level of representation is often inferred by manipulating
factors such as a comprehender's study goals (e.g., to summarize, or to learn and apply information from the discourse unit) or the extent to which a text biases a
comprehender toward spatial processing, and then examining the effects of these manipulations on discourse comprehension and memory (see Mross, 1990).

e. Frederiksen, Bracewell, Breuleux, and Renaud (1990) recently
described a stratified model of discourse processing that focuses
on representations and operations involved in many independent
and interdependent layers. The model incorporates multiple levels of representation and processing of language and semantic
information, from linguistic elements to propositions to interconnected conceptual units. The authors' notion of conceptual
frames, or abstract structures that contain high-level knowledge
or rules, would subsume the various superstructures mentioned
above, but their frames are more general than discourse superstructures, including such structures as scripts and schemas.

(1) In the stratified model, discourse comprehension typically
proceeds largely from the top-down. Frame-level knowledge
and rules assist interpretation processes as the comprehender
activates previously stored hypotheses and expectations, or
tries to construct them when they are not available.

(2) Frederiksen and colleagues also model the processing and
control involved in discourse production. Table 2–4 summarizes hypothesized discourse production processes,
organized according to the type of structure they operate

Table 2–4. Processes operating at different levels of discourse production.

Conceptual Network Level

Generating or retrieving conceptual frames or organizing principles

Elaborating frames with semantic descriptive information (e.g., internal structures of events in the narrative superstructure)

Integrating these elaborated frames with other semantic networks (which can lead to further modification and elaboration)

Selecting and prioritizing from the fully specified conceptual structure the information that should be conveyed, and the order in which to convey it. These processes are directed by knowledge and inferences about characteristics of the comprehender, the situation, and the message genre

Propositional Level

Generating propositions sequentially to reflect selection and topicalization from the conceptual network

Generating propositions to foster coherent interpretation, whether explicitly based or inferential, on the basis of assumptions about the comprehender's likely inferences and interpretations

Generating and evaluating logical and macrostructure inferences for stretches of the text (e.g., topic sentences; summarization)

Chunking propositions for optimal linguistic encoding (e.g., number of propositions in a single clause, and "distance" between related propositions)

Language Level

Encoding clauses to reflect chunking and topicalization decisions

Specifying lexical information in clauses, including anaphora

Source: After Frederiksen et al. (1990).

on: conceptual, propositional, and linguistic. The conceptual level of Frederiksen and colleagues has also been called the message level, or the conceptualizer (see, e.g., Davis, 1993). The intention to inform activates the processes outlined in Table 2–4 (Davis, 1993). Discourse production involves a great deal of top-down processing control to retrieve stored information, rules, situational interpretations, and organizing principles. Concurrent bottom-up or text-driven control of discourse production is reflected in the monitoring and editing processes that take place during ongoing speech and writing. Frederiksen and colleagues analyze discourse production more generally as a form of problem-solving, with "planning" proposed as a fundamental strategy for transforming intent into realization.

4. Discourse production and RHD.

a. Interest in discourse production is growing rapidly, but the evidence is hard to interpret because no two investigators have used similar discourse models, sampling contexts, and dependent measures. In addition, most studies have involved few subjects, making it difficult to frame general statements about discourse production after RHD. Table 2–5 presents some of the contrasts among those that have been observed in the spoken discourse samples of RHD adults. The reader is referred to Joanette and Brownell (1990) for discussion of the complexities of sampling and evaluating discourse production. Some other specific studies are summarized below.

b. Joanette and Goulet (1990) report a comprehensive analysis of narrative discourse produced by 36 RHD and 20 normal adults, elicited with a novel picture sequence called the "Cowboy Story." In the beginning of this story, a tired cowboy arrives in a town and soon falls asleep on a bench while holding on to the reins of his horse. In the middle portion, a boy sees the sleeping cowboy and cuts the horse's reins, letting the horse run free, and replacing it with a toy horse. In the final picture, the cowboy has awakened and is puzzled about the miniature horse that is attached to the reins. The initial, middle, and final portions of this story correspond to a single episode that contains basic elements of a narrative superstructure: a setting, a complication, and a resolution.

Joanette and Goulet analyzed formal (lexical, syntactic) aspects of the sample, content (story structure and informativeness), and elements of cohesion and coherence contributing to both form and content. Their measures and results are summarized in Table 2–6 (and an appendix to their chapter contains a list of core propositions identified for the Cowboy Story). Informativeness analyses indicated that neither group was homogenous, so all subjects' data were combined for further analyses of propositional usage. Two groups emerged from these analyses. Speakers in Group 1 (75% of the control subjects and 44% of the RHD group) used more total propositions and more complex propositions than those in Group 2, and more propositions describing the story complication. However, Group 2 subjects did produce the

Table 2–5. Some contrasting findings in discourse production after RHD

Diminished informational content (propositions, t-units, episodes) versus propositional content and accuracy similar to comparable non-brain-damaged adult speakers

Fewer words than normal (paucity) versus same number of words versus more words or more words per turn (verbosity)

Wandering from the point versus topic maintenance skills similar to those of control speakers

Poor error monitoring in discourse versus as many successful repairs as control speakers

Productions based on scripts, which are common scenarios like ordering a meal in a restaurant, that include tangential associations versus those that terminate prematurely

Difficulty telling an integrated story versus producing a fully integrated story that is unrelated to the stimulus situation

Impaired organization on story recall versus impaired memory for story schema

Loss of connecting line (coherence errors) in narrative productions versus comparable proportions of propositions that are central to, supportive of, or distracting from the main story line

Higher proportions of literal concepts reflecting a tendency to itemize, rather than interpret, in picture descriptions versus no differences from age peers in proportions of literal and inferential concepts produced

Excessive detail and overpersonalization versus "unnecessary" detail and personal comments similar in extent to those produced by normally aging speakers.

Sources: Entries compiled from Baggs & Swindell (1993); Bloom, Ferrand, & Paternosto (1993); Cherney & Canter (1993); Hillis Trupe & Hillis (1985); Joanette & Goulet (1990); Kennedy et al. (1994); Mackisack, Myers, & Duffy (1987); Myers (1979); Roman et al. (1987); Schneiderman et al. (1992); Tompkins et al. (1993); Wapner et al. (1981).

most important core proposition of the complication, reflecting the gist of the story, that the boy played a trick. Joanette and Goulet noted that it would be important in future analyses to consider non-core propositions as well, to assess information that might reflect tangential and irrelevant tendencies in RHD patients.

c. Another recent multilevel analysis of discourse processing for a single, elderly patient (Frederiksen & Stemmer, 1993) revealed a particular difficulty constructing new conceptual representations of texts that contained information leading to a forced re-evaluation or reinterpretation. This intriguing finding, though in line with some other suggestions in the literature, will require replication to determine its generality. The patient's advanced age (79 years) in combination with minimal formal education (5

Table 2–6. Narrative discourse measures and results for RHD and normal control subjects (using the "Cowboy Story")

Formal Aspects

Total words

Percent nouns, verbs, adjectives,[a] adverbs

Verb/noun, adjective/noun ratios[a]

Pronoun/concept ratios, one each reflecting the number of pronouns used to refer to the cowboy and the boy

Lexicalization measures, reflecting the different lexical items used to express key concepts (cowboy, horse, boy, wooden horse, bridle/reins)

Gross syntactic indices, for example, percent subordinate clauses

Cohesion and Coherence [b]

Cohesive errors, or errors in semantic relations between segments of narratives (e.g., undetermined pronouns, inadequate lexical reiteration)

Nonprogression errors: Segments do not contribute new information

Contradiction errors: New information contradicts something previously given

Relation errors: New information is used without being related to that specified or implied previously

Story Schema, and Informativeness

Presence of complete or partial information representing elements of the narrative superstructure (setting, complication, resolution)

Total number of propositions in the referential portion of the narrative[a] (excluding modalized comments that reflect subjects' comments about the task and their performance)

Total simple propositions (propositions having no argument overlap with other propositions) and complex propositions[a] (those with arguments overlapping with another proposition)

Total propositions related to information in left half of stimulus

Total core propositions[a] (relatively invariant propositions given by at least 20% of either group)

Frequency of occurrence of core propositions, and co-occurrence patterns[c] of core propositions

Source: Joanette & Goulet (1990).

[a] RHD samples had fewer

[b] RHD samples more likely contain errors in two or more of these areas combined (attributable to about half of the RHD subjects)

[c] Subgroup differences in clustering

years) raise questions about her premorbid ability to mobilize and apply the kinds of reconstruction processes necessitated by the stimulus materials.

d. Again, one probable key to these diverse accounts of discourse production ability is the considerable variability we expect in RHD patients. Joanette et al. (1990) observed that only half of their RHD subjects made coherence errors that detracted from the main story line in a narrative production task. Many other RHD subjects overlap with normally aging speakers on various discourse parameters. Differences in stimulus conditions may also contribute to the conflicting findings, as different discourse genres have different cognitive and linguistic demands, as well as different communicative functions (Ulatowska, Allard, & Chapman, 1990).

5. Discourse comprehension and RHD.

a. Brownell (1988) notes that RHD adults appear to understand less in discourse than one might predict on the basis of their intact sentence-level linguistic comprehension. Indeed, the right hemisphere appears to contribute more to discourse comprehension than to single word processing. For example, brain metabolism increases mainly in the right hemisphere when people are asked to remember stories for later recall (e.g., Phelps, Mazziotta, & Huang, 1982).

b. As suggested earlier, the discourse comprehension problems that some RHD patients exhibit appear to reflect a difficulty in synthesizing their knowledge with a specific discourse context. For example, they may have trouble selecting a punchline that coheres with the rest of a joke, even though their choice appropriately captures an element of surprise. Or they may have problems choosing pictured representations for metaphors that they can define. RHD patients may also have difficulty answering questions about the more abstract or inferential aspects of narrative passages, such as those about relationships among events or characters. The extent of difficulty has been associated with education level, extent of premorbid brain atrophy, and neglect (Benowitz, Moya, & Levine, 1990).

c. Other discourse comprehension problems have been attributed to a deficit in altering initial assumptions: RHD patients even have difficulty at the single sentence level with tasks that require a shift in their initial assignment of syntactic roles for lexical items (Schneiderman & Saddy, 1988). As noted above, RHD subjects appear to have particular difficulty in discrepant situations when portions of the context point to competing interpretations. One example includes situations involving literally false statements where several possible meanings must be reconciled with other contextual cues. It has been suggested (Kaplan et al., 1990) that RHD patients as a group show less ability to use context effectively (e.g., knowledge of characters' relationship) to predict what a speaker intends (e.g., was the statement meant as a lie, a teasing comment, or a hurtful remark?) And a recent theoretically driven discourse analysis for one RHD patient (Frederiksen & Stemmer, 1993) points to a particular problem with reconceptualizing original interpretations to reconcile seeming discrepancies (e.g., original story events suggest that a woman is traveling in a plane and experiencing a terrible storm and a subsequent crash; but later events describe her being awakened from a dream by her husband, while they are camping out during a storm). Such problems may be related to difficulty linking the disparate mental models that patients construct while representing such texts (see also section II-A-3-c, above, regarding nonconventional indirect requests). Frederiksen and Stemmer also suggest that an abundance of inferences linked to explicit propositions, and an overuse of narrative frame structure, may contribute to perceptions of tangentiality in RHD patients. Unfortunately, it is difficult to attribute all of these problems to their patient's brain damage, given her advanced age and minimal education. (The control subject was similar in age, but had a high school education.)

d. The concepts of linking disparate mental models and shifting interpretations are nicely captured in another recent perspective on normal comprehension, that will be considered briefly here. Gernsbacher and her colleagues (Gernsbacher, & Faust, 1991; Gernsbacher, Varner, & Faust, 1990) articulated a structure building framework of comprehension, a theoretical orientation supported by extensive empirical work, that can complement existing analyses of comprehension deficits in RHD. According to the structure building framework, "the goal of comprehension is to build a cohesive mental representation or 'structure'" (Gernsbacher et al., 1990, p. 431). First a comprehender lays a foundation from incoming information: Perceptual processes that encode initial sentences (or propositions) create mental activation patterns that initiate the foundation for this structure. Then, the comprehender elaborates the structure by mapping onto it related information, encoded from the text and activated from world knowledge. When information is encountered that is not easily related to the initial structure, the comprehender shifts to begin a new substructure. Once portions of memory are activated, two modulatory mechanisms are essential to the processes that culminate in comprehension. An enhancement mechanism heightens the activation of information associated with a contextually relevant interpretation, and a suppression mechanism dampens activation of information that is less appropriate or relevant to the situation or discourse context. Given that RHD patients' comprehension problems tend to surface in incongruent conditions, with materials that require revision for successful comprehension, or in which multiple sources of information must be considered and reconciled, the structure building framework suggests that it may be useful to investigate the efficiency of RHD adults' suppression and enhancement mechanisms (Tompkins, 1993).

e. Despite their deficits, RHD patients do exhibit some strengths in discourse comprehension. Similar to non-brain-damaged persons, they understand main ideas in narrative paragraphs better than details (Brookshire & Nicholas, 1984); they comprehend explicit information, especially when it is salient or important, better than implied information (Brookshire & Nicholas, 1984); and they benefit when provided with thematic information at the beginning of a narrative paragraph (Hough, 1990). They also demonstrate knowledge of the essential elements of common scripts (Roman, Brownell, Potter, Seibold, & Gardner, 1987), and of metaphoric and idiomatic meanings (Tompkins, et al., 1992). Frederiksen and Stemmer's (1993) patient drew microproposition inferences, in fact paraphrasing more of the literal content than the control subject; showed evidence of using narrative frame structure in inferred propositions that indicated temporal, causal, and conditional links (but staying closer to the text than the control subject, who generated more summarization); and demonstrated some use of a goal structure to interpret story events. The patient also generated plausible inferences that could reconcile the two sets of events in the story, as well (e.g., that the woman was having a nightmare, at a later time, about being in an airplane crash), but did not tie them to the reconceptualization suggested in the story.

f. Finally, RHD adults are sometimes able to infer from, and profit from, contextual information (e.g., semantic or emotional contexts, explicit themes, internal discourse consistency or redundancy), particularly in conditions that limit demands on attentional or working memory resources. And, they can draw some inference revisions when attentional demands are reduced. Performance in these situations appears to vary with the "difficulty" of the conclusion or the inference task and the processing load that it places on mental resources (e.g., reconstructing or integrating mental representations that are not obviously connected, will demand processing resources), together with the availability of attentional or working memory reserves (Tompkins, 1990, 1991a, 1991b; Tompkins et al., 1992; Tompkins et al., 1994).

6. **Conversation: General principles and properties.**

   a. The structure and process of conversation differ importantly from the monologic discourse forms discussed above, in that partners must interact to negotiate topics, turns, and breakdowns in the exchange of intentions and information, in a variety of social roles and situations. Readable summaries of various conversational issues, principles, and properties may be found in Ashcraft (1989), Brinton and Fujiki (1989), and Murphy (1990).

   b. Conversational participation hinges in part on an evaluation of mutual knowledge and beliefs. For instance, a listener's inferences about communicative intent and speaker meaning, and subsequent responses to a speaker, require knowledge of the world, of the speaker, and of pragmatic conventions. Similarly, a speaker plans conversational contributions based on assumptions about the listener's perspective and knowledge. Conversational participants also develop theories about each others' presuppositions, and about what knowledge they have in common. Communicators draw inferences about the nature of shared knowledge based on several factors. These include group membership, which may be based on various kinds of relationships (e.g., professional, familial, cultural, geographic); shared access to physical objects; and shared knowledge of linguistic and pragmatic markers that occurred previously in a conversation.

   c. Conversation appears to be guided further by a number of knowledge structures or conventions. At a general level, some of these create an unspoken contract between participants, each of whom is presumed to cooperate by contributing appropriately. Speaker contributions are assumed to follow four postulates (Grice, 1975): try to be relevant, informative (e.g., convey new information), truthful, and appropriate in manner (e.g., clear, brief, and orderly). Some of these postulates may be violated intentionally for pragmatic purposes, as when a speaker uses irony or wishes to soften the truth. When one of these assumptions appears to have been violated, a listener operating under them will infer an unstated interpretation (e.g., an obvious untruth was probably told to spare someone's feelings; a request was phrased indirectly to make it more polite).

7. Specific elements of conversational exchanges.

a. Many specific aspects of conversational interactions, such as how to begin and end conversations, exchange turns, manipulate topics, and repair conversational breakdowns, also appear to be governed by conventions and rules. These rules and the cooperative signals used to mark them tend to differ across languages and cultures, and their use is highly influenced by contextual factors (including elements of external situations and internal knowledge, emotions, and beliefs). This lack of uniformity may make for difficult or confusing interactions between people of different cultures or linguistic communities, and certainly complicates research and clinical evaluation of conversation.

b. Memory Organization Packet (MOP) theory provides one theoretical framework for studying conventions that govern the organization and content of conversation (for middle-class members of mainstream American culture). Schank (1982) proposed MOPs as part of a revision of script theory, when simple scripts were found to be too rigid for governing goal-directed behavior. A MOP is a generalized cluster of events, called scenes, which are collections of high-level script components (e.g., a set of "entering" scenes for different contexts). MOPs organize, coordinate, and combine sets of scenes as indicated by specific intentions or goals. Conversational MOP theory identifies scenes that can occur and the phases (opening, maintenance, closing) in which they occur, the consistency of organization, and their progression and timing in conversations (e.g., Kellermann, 1991; see application by Kennedy, Strand, Burton, & Peterson, 1994). Some examples of scenes in first-encounter conversations include introductions; queries about occupation, interests, or people known in common; and leave-taking signals.

c. The mechanics and models of other specific conversational dimensions, such as topic control, turn-taking, and repair skills, are covered thoroughly by Brinton and Fujiki (1989). Some of the key information from their writings on these areas will be elaborated below, and considered further in Chapter 4 (III-C-4).

8. Conversational behavior and RHD.

a. Descriptions of conversational abilities after RHD are mostly anecdotal. The study of conversation is particularly challenging given the enormous normal variability in conversational parameters such as numbers of turns, durations of turns, and the like. It is also difficult to tease out the source of observed conversational difficulties, as conversation involves so many cognitive processes: developing and elaborating a context for interpreting what is said, holding in memory that which is likely to be important, resolving references and ambiguities by attempting to determine speaker intent, planning an appropriate response, exhibiting sensitivity to listener knowledge and memory load, abiding by the structure and rhythm of the exchange, responding to conversational signals, and adopting appropriate social roles, to name a few.

b. One preliminary effort examining spontaneous conversations with familiar partners (Prutting & Kirchner, 1987) found the majority of the 30 pragmatic skills investigated to be appropriately used by a group of 10 RHD adults. With conservative scoring, where any single occurrence of an inappropriate behavior in one dimension resulted in rating the entire dimension as inappropriate, about half of the RHD patients were judged inappropriate in eye gaze, prosodic pattern and variation, turn-taking contingency, turn-taking adjacency, and quantity/conciseness. Parameters such as topic selection, topic introduction, topic change, other turn-taking variables, and cohesion were noted to be deficient for 2 or fewer of the 10 subjects. One complication for interpreting these data is that all patients were receiving treatment at the time of the study, and it is not clear whether the treatment focused on these or other pragmatic parameters.

c. In first-encounter conversational dyads consisting of RHD adults and speech-language pathologists, Kennedy and colleagues (Kennedy & Perez, 1993; Kennedy et al., 1994) also noted poor eye contact for RHD patients. RHD speakers took more turns and used more words per turn in their conversations than did control subjects. But a variety of topic skill parameters, including introductions, maintenance, expansions, shades, reintroductions, and terminations did not distinguish the two groups. Those in the patient group, on average, were more likely to talk about themselves than to ask questions of their clinician partners. This may be due, in part, to their assuming a "patient role" with the clinicians, inferring that they, and their problems, should be the focus of the interaction. In addition, there were many more males in the RHD subject group than in the control group, and sociolinguistic investigations suggest that males as a whole may be more egocentric in their conversations. In their interactions with the RHD group, clinicians initiated more conversational "scenes" typical of first meetings, such as questions about where the other person lives or works, or about people known in common, than they did when conversing with non-brain-damaged partners. It is possible too that these clinicians brought unconscious biases to the situation, automatically assuming a facilitating role when a partner was observed to have some impairment. A final interesting note is that some RHD speakers initiated conversational topics after clinicians had made termination moves, suggesting that the patients were not aware that the conversation should be ending.

d. In another investigation of conversation, RHD subjects were observed to use fewer figurative expressions than non-brain-damaged speakers. However, the relative frequency of various types of figurative terms did not distinguish the groups (Apel et al., 1992). And a recent analysis of speech acts in conversations showed no differences between RHD and orthopedic control patients in percent of turns containing requests for information, responses to questions, arguments, interruptions, self-initiated comments, direct quotations, narrative comments, elaborations, self-elaborations, or taboo words (Blonder et al., 1993).

C. Auditory Language Comprehension

1. In addition to the discourse comprehension impairments noted earlier, and along with their difficulties with pragmatic aspects of language, RHD patients may have some problems with the auditory processing of literal materials. Though they studied very small groups, Adamovich and Brooks (1981) reported that RHD patients performed less well than control subjects on most of the auditory comprehension subtests of the Boston Diagnostic Aphasia Examination (Goodglass & Kaplan, 1983), and on portions of the Revised Token Test (RTT) (McNeil & Prescott, 1978). The RTT is a standardized and systematic test of auditory processing for nonredundant, single commands. It uses a 15-point multidimensional scoring system to capture more information than a typical plus/minus scoring system. The authors provide preliminary norms for 30 RHD males, about 75% of whom were more impaired than control subjects on overall scores and on a subtest involving two-part conjoined commands with six critical elements (e.g., "Touch the big green square and the little black circle").

2. Because RTT stimuli and items within each subtest are homogenous in difficulty, subtests can be inspected for evidence of patterns of processing difficulty (e.g., difficulty tuning in, reflected in lower performance on the first few items; fading or attentional fatigue, reflected in poorer performance on the last few items). McNeil, Odell, and Campbell (1982) exploited this feature in exploring item-to-item performance fluctuations in RHD and aphasic adults. They observed fewer score fluctuations for RHD subjects, but those that occurred were similar to aphasic subjects' fluctuations in the extent of change from one score to the next (e.g., from 15 to 9), suggesting some similarities between groups in the nature of moment-to-moment changes in auditory processing.

D. Word Retrieval Difficulties

1. RHD adults often have word retrieval problems: Hough, DeMarco, Bedsole, Fox, and Pabst (1993) report that 60% of their RHD subjects exhibited word-finding difficulties on the Test of Adolescent/ Adult Word Finding (German, 1990). Even so, their difficulties are typically fewer in number and less obvious than those of aphasic adults. The majority of errors can be coded as semantic confusions, and, as is the case for non-brain-damaged people, most of these are coordinate errors (e.g., naming "cat" for "dog," rather than "pet" or "animal" for "dog").

2. RHD patients also tend to make more visually based errors than aphasic patients (e.g., "extension cord" for "snake"). Some visual-semantic errors can be attributed to problems of scale in the correct semantic field (e.g., "big top" for a camping tent). It has been suggested that RHD patients with temporo-parietal damage are most likely to have visual misnaming errors due to perceptual impairments of object recognition.

3. RHD patients have been found to have particular difficulty naming categories, or collective nouns (Myers & Brookshire, in press). They may identify the individual elements in a composite picture (e.g., one depicting a hammer, screwdriver, and pliers), rather than assigning the category name ("tools"). They may also have more difficulty naming objects associated with their illness (e.g., "wheelchair"), especially when they have hemispatial neglect or anosognosia.

E. Reading and Writing Deficits

1. **Reading difficulties** after RHD have usually been ascribed to impairments of various mechanisms that cooperate in encoding and processing visuospatial information, such as premotor programming of ocular scanning, spatial distribution of attention, and construction of abstract visuospatial representations. "Lower level" deficits may include difficulties scanning across a line; tracking back to the left to find the beginning of each line; or coordinating the process of looking from the top of the page to the bottom for an answer choice, and then back up again.

   a. One of the most frequently investigated types of RHD reading impairments associated with attentional or representational mechanisms is neglect dyslexia (see Friedman, Ween, & Albert, 1993, for a review). Neglect dyslexia, a heterogenous group of reading disorders, often occurs with hemispatial neglect; left neglect dyslexia is observed in some patients with right parietal lesions. In some patients with neglect dyslexia, single word reading is impaired while the reading of text is intact; other patients show deficits in both areas. Some symptoms at the text level include neglecting the left half of a page or omitting whole words on the left. At the single word level, the beginnings of words may be omitted or changed, producing characteristic substitution errors. This latter symptom is sensitive to orientation of the word in space, so the effect diminishes when words are written vertically. The most common errors are letter substitutions that preserve overall word length (such as "pillow" for "yellow"), but some deletion errors occur ("age" for "cage"). These kinds of substitutions can occur without other features of neglect.

   b. In part, the problem in neglect dyslexia is probably related to attentional processes in the portion of the reading system responsible for coding information about letter identity and position. However, symptoms may result from disrupted scanning strategies that prevent proper input to a letter representation system, a disrupted representational system that receives adequate input, disordered attention with otherwise intact input and representational systems, or some combination of these.

   c. As the preceding paragraphs indicate, most of our knowledge about reading comes from studies of oral reading, rather than reading comprehension. But, there are some indications that RHD patients may have difficulty comprehending abstract meanings or complex written material. These problems may be linguistically based, but they are more likely secondary to other problems. For example, many of the nonlinguistic deficits considered in Chapter 1 and below could contribute to an incoherent or incomplete text interpretation that is insufficient to support abstraction or inference. Or, complex materials that require integration and retention may tax cognitive resource allocation (see section V-E, below).

2. **Writing difficulties.** Benson (1979) notes that when RHD adults have writing deficits, they are most commonly spatial agraphias, due primarily to impairments in the perceptual and executive subsystems supporting writing. In a recent study of spatial agraphias, Ardila and Rosselli (1993) found that motor deficits predominated in RHD adults with frontal damage (e.g., iterations of features and letters), and spatial deficits were most apparent in RHD patients with posterior damage (e.g., inappropriate distribution in space, such as superimposition of words or elements, and misgroupings of elements within and between words). Patients with concomitant neglect may also exhibit a tendency to leave larger margins on the left side of the page, which increase as succeeding lines are written, or to crowd their output onto the right side of the space provided. Benson observes that a commonly held assumption about spatial agraphias remains unproven: namely, that they are characterized by an excessive number of separations between letters or groups of letters.

   a. Other impairments may also contribute to writing deficits. For example, if attention wanders, patients may have a problem returning to the place where their writing left off. Difficulty organizing thoughts or formulating propositions may be reflected in ambiguous or run-on sentences.

   b. There is little evidence to estimate the prevalence, or the uniqueness, of writing difficulties following RHD in adults. On diverse writing tasks, symptoms of spatial agraphia were evident in 40–73% of RHD patients with retro-Rolandic lesions, up to 50% of frontally damaged patients, and up to 20% of control subjects (Ardila & Rosselli, 1993). In another report (Horner, Lathrop, Fish, & Dawson, 1987), the presence, severity, and pattern of agraphia in narrative writing samples did not reliably differentiate RHD from either aphasic patients or those with mild dementing conditions when rated on multicomponent scales reflecting the dimensions of organization, vocabulary completeness, grammatical completeness, spelling, or mechanics. However, as the authors cautioned, interrater reliability for assigning these ratings was low. The authors speculated that the poor reliability may have been due, in part, to the diversity of features making up each rating scale (e.g., "organization" included organization, relevance, flow of ideas, repetition of ideas, intrusions, tangentiality, and inappropriate or self-referential statements; "mechanics" included spatial-constructional form, accuracy and agility of writing, and overall readability). Assigning single ratings to such diverse composites also may have masked actual differences between groups.

F. Dysarthria

Impaired speech motor control associated with dysarthria may contribute to the perception of restricted intonational variability in some RHD adults. Kent and Rosenbek's (1982) acoustic analysis of RHD patients' ($N = 3$) speech patterns indicated essentially normal word and phrase durations with a flattened prosodic contour, and the authors noted many similarities between the RHD subjects and a larger group of patients with Parkinson disease and hypokinetic dysarthria. Both groups showed a general pattern of reduced acoustic contrast, including limited fundamental frequency and intensity variation, continuous voicing, weakly formed consonants, and reduced acoustic energy in the mid-to-high frequency range.

III. SELECTED COGNITIVE AND PERCEPTUAL DEFICIT AREAS

A. Anosognosia

As noted earlier, "anosognosia" refers to lack of knowledge of disease (Chapter 1, III-E-1-e). Generally speaking, anosognosia is worse and more persistent after larger strokes. Also, generally, the worse the hemiplegia the greater the denial (Hier, Mondlock, & Caplan, 1983a, 1983b). But, even RHD patients who do acknowledge discrete impairments may tend to underestimate their severity and to minimize their influence on daily functioning. These patients may overestimate their capacity for independent living and resist supervision or intervention.

B. Orientation

RHD patients, particularly in the acute post-onset phase, may be disoriented for time and place, perhaps related to perceptual deficits (see Chapter 1, and below). Some may be disoriented to the passage of time as well. Finally, RHD can affect orientation to other people, causing difficulty recognizing even familiar faces and voices.

C. Visual and Auditory Perception and Related Functions

1. Sensation involves receiving environmental stimuli and encoding them into the nervous system, and perception is the process of interpreting and assigning meaning to that which has been encoded. Perception is influenced in part from the "bottom-up," by stimulus-driven feature detection and analysis. But, an enormous active contribution is also made by the perceiver, who brings prior knowledge and context ("top-down" information) to the interpretive task.

2. Even without significant sensory loss, RHD patients may experience a variety of impaired visual functions, including visuoperceptual, visuospatial, and visuomotor deficits. These are identified in Table 2–7. It is not clear how any one of these disorders might contribute to the others, though, logically, there would seem to be a connection between some of them, such as oculomotor scanning and visuoperceptual impairment.

Table 2–7. Disorders of visual function[a]

Visuoperceptual

Poor discrimination of complex stimuli that differ in subtle ways

Poor recognition of objects or other stimuli, such as faces

Impaired color recognition

Impaired separation of figure and ground

Poor integration of stimulus constituents, and of relationships among objects or pictured elements

Visuospatial

Difficulty localizing points in space with fixed forward gaze

Difficulties judging direction, distance, length, depth

Topographical disorientation (see Chapter 1)

Visuomotor: Deficits in movements directed by visual stimuli

Impaired scanning

Constructional impairment (see Chapter 1)

Visual-attentional

Visual neglect

[a] See, e.g., Kolb & Whishaw (1990)

3. "Visual agnosia" refers generally to a problem combining visual impressions of known stimuli into patterns, despite adequately seeing the stimuli. Two classes of agnosias have been described: apperceptive and associative. Apperceptive agnosias, or deficits affecting the analysis of perceptual properties and dimensions of known objects, are most commonly associated with RHD. Associative agnosias are disorders in deriving meaning for objects that can be seen and perceived. The majority of patients with associative agnosias have bilateral brain damage, but unilateral left occipital-temporal lesions are sufficient to cause associative agnosias (McCarthy & Warrington, 1990).

4. Visual agnosias may result in difficulty recognizing, drawing, or copying objects or pictures. The term "agnosia" has sometimes been misused to encompass most of the deficits in Table 2–7. Since the term is often used in the literature, readers should be familiar with the varieties described in Table 2–8. Readers must also be aware that in many reports of agnosia, other possible explanations for performance deficits, such as sensory or perceptual problems, have not been convincingly excluded.

Table 2–8. Varieties of visual agnosias [a]

Object Agnosia:	Inability to name, or demonstrate use of objects. Rare, often associated with bilateral damage.
Agnosia for Drawings:	Inability to recognize drawings, including realistic representations, complex scenes, schematic drawings, geometric figures, incomplete figures.
Prosopagnosia:	Originally defined as inability to recognize familiar faces with preserved recognition of objects, forms and colors; recently observed that the deficit may encompass other familiar, nonfacial, stimuli such as buildings or makes of cars. Patients may compensate by recognizing voices or some other salient characteristic such as clothing. Rare; rarely persists; nearly always due to bilateral damage.
Color Agnosia:	Difficulty associating objects with their prototypical colors.
Visuospatial Agnosias:	Impaired stereoscopic vision; topographical disorientation; and in some literature, visual neglect.

[a] See, e.g., Kolb & Whishaw (1990); McCarthy & Warrington (1990).

5. Visual neglect, an attention-arousal disturbance discussed extensively in Chapter 1, is another common sequel of RHD in adults. It
is included in Table 2–7 as an attentional deficit, rather than a perceptual impairment. As noted in Chapter 1, the directional bias in
neglect can be modulated in various ways, through cues and body-
positioning. Some of these are identified in Table 2–9. Many of
these manipulations are thought to assist patients in allocating attention (overt or covert) into the neglected hemifield, perhaps by
increasing right hemispheric activation and arousal, or influencing
the extent or direction of visual orienting (see attention section,
below). Others (e.g., trunk orientation) appear to influence the frame
of reference for perceiving space in relation to one's body position.
These manipulations and cues suggest potentially useful techniques
for the assessment and management of neglect.

Table 2–9. Cues that may modulate manifestations of neglect.

Meaning Cues

Neglect is attenuated with meaningful materials (e.g., lexical stimuli as compared to
pseudowords and nonwords), for a variety of tasks (e.g., Brunn & Farah, 1991).

Deficits may diminish when visual stimuli are interactive and meaningfully
integrated (e.g., two women having a conversation as opposed to two objects), even
when the elements in the interactive stimuli are spatially separated (Kartsounis &
Warrington, 1989).

Contralateral processing is enhanced by the meaningfulness of information presented in
ipsilateral space. Seron, Coyette, and Bruyer (1989) asked RHD left-neglecting patients to
identify concrete objects or scenes from sequences of stimulus segments that varied in the
informativeness of the information included in the early (right-sided) segments. When
early segments resembled part of an object but did not provide sufficient information to
identify the object (e.g., an axe handle), subjects used information from the left side of the
stimulus in later segments, to identify these stimuli as accurately as stimuli that provided
early, unambiguous identity clues (e.g., a rhinoceros' horn). But when early segments
were not perceived as object-like, patients had considerably more difficulty using left-
sided information and performed more poorly.

Spatial and Motor Cues

Response times for orienting attention are improved when visual cues are provided to
alert patients to an upcoming attentional shift (e.g., Posner et al., 1984; 1987).

Neglect symptoms diminish when "jumping" stimuli are presented on the left side of a
task, perhaps by tapping a relatively preserved collicular visual system that appears to be
involved in detecting movement and generating orienting (Butter, Kirsch, & Reeves, 1990).

(continued)

Table 2–9. *Continued*

Neglect is attenuated when the left hand is used for tasks such as pointing to laterally-displayed lights (Joanette, Brouchon, Gauthier, & Samson, 1986) or cancellation and line bisection (Halligan & Marshall, 1989a).

Neglect symptoms diminish on a computerized line bisection task when the cursor used to transect the lines is placed at the leftmost end of the line before each trial, and a beep signals trial initiation (Halligan & Marshall, 1989b).

Neglect symptoms on line bisection are lessened when patients observe the experimenter move a pen along a line from left-to-right before responding (Reuter-Lorenz & Posner, 1990).

Neglect symptoms diminish when various other anchors (letters, red lines, symbols) are placed at the left end of a line to be bisected or a stimulus to be read, particularly when the patient is instructed to attend to the cue (e.g., Riddoch & Humphreys, 1983).

Neglect symptoms are exacerbated when elements within visual arrays are spatially separated. Similarly, neglect diminishes when stimuli are continuous (e.g., shapes as opposed to scattered lines or dot arrays; Kartsounis & Warrington, 1989).

Neglect patients can allocate attention further into the affected hemifield when stimuli straddle both right and left hemifields, than when they are fully contained in either (Farah, Brunn, Wallace, & Madigan, 1989).

Neglect symptoms have been compensated for by turning patients' trunks to the left, so that both left visual field and right visual field stimuli were projected to the right side of trunk space (Karnath, Schenkel, & Fischer, 1991).

6. Patients may also experience various auditory disorders in the absence of significant sensory loss. These are outlined in Table 2–10. Auditory agnosias, or impaired capacity to recognize the nature of nonverbal acoustic stimuli, are less well understood than visual agnosias, but those that have been associated with RHD are also indicated in Table 2–10.

7. The reader who wishes more information can consult Ashcraft (1989) and Kolb and Whishaw (1990) for clear discussions of a number of the constructs and functions considered in this section.

D. Attention

1. Visual and auditory events impinge on our eyes and ears regardless of our interest in them. In a similar way, internal thoughts and asso-

Table 2–10. Disorders of auditory function[a]

Audioperceptual

Impaired perception of music (e.g. loudness, harmonic structure, tonal memory)

Impaired discrimination of affective and linguistic prosody

Audiospatial

Impaired sound localization, shifting auditory signals towards the right side

Auditory neglect: Rare in comparison with visual neglect; controversy about its nature and existence. An analogue to visual neglect, where patients ignore auditory stimuli from the side contralateral to the lesion, has not been unequivocally reported (Beaton & McCarthy, 1993). This may be partly due to the anatomy of the auditory system: Both hemispheres receive input from both ears.

Auditory Agnosias

Amusias: Inability to discriminate tones in a scale; impaired melody recall or recognition; disorders of rhythm and tempo. Rare; usually associated with right temporal lesion.

Agnosia for sounds: Inability to identify the meaning of nonverbal sounds, such as a bird singing. Often associated with amusia and word deafness. Probably due to bilateral temporal damage.

[a] See, e.g., Kolb & Whishaw (1990).

ciations regularly arise without our intent, even if we are not actively aware of them. Attention is a collection of operations that forms an important mental resource allowing us to manage this information barrage, and to process and act on that which is relevant to our goals. The many facets of attention will be considered in the sections that follow, after a brief discussion of the characterization of mental resources.

2. Mental resources are parts of the cognitive apparatus that are available in limited quantities and that can be drawn upon when needed to accomplish perceptual, cognitive, or motor processing. The most common usage of the term "resource" refers metaphorically to the "fuel" or "effort" needed to execute mental operations. However, resources can also include such things as the skills involved in processing and the communication channels used (input modalities, response modes, etc.) (cf., Hirst & Kalmar, 1987). Results of dual-task studies have been used to infer that processing resources are limited in

capacity. When subjects carry out certain kinds of tasks simultaneously (e.g., tasks with similar input or output characteristics), each may be done more poorly than when it is performed singly. From this kind of interference, we infer that the demands for performing the tasks concurrently exceeded the limited quantity of a necessary, shared or overlapping, resource. The reasoning behind this inference is that subjects should be able to perform the tasks equally well in single and dual task conditions if different resources were being used, or if the quantity of a shared resource was unlimited.

3. Attention has many functions. For example, it is assumed to be responsible for selecting and prioritizing relevant aspects of the information that continuously flows into our brains, whether that information originates from the external/sensory or internal/cognitive world. It works to improve the speed or efficiency of perceptual and cognitive operations. It also facilitates the registration of prioritized information into a working memory system where it can be processed further and integrated with the products of other mental activity in service of comprehension, problem solving, and other goal-directed behavior. Moreover, attention is assumed to provide the fuel for carrying out cognitive activities.

4. There are a variety of theories of attention. Most posit that attentional processes are fixed, or limited, in capacity. Mental operations generally require attentional fuel (with the possible exception of automatic or mandatory processes, section 6 below), so the total attentional capacity available to a person usually determines how many tasks or operations can be carried out simultaneously, and the nature of complex and time-dependent processing that can occur sequentially (but see Allport, 1989, for a competing view). In addition, most theories of attention include a mechanism for controlling and allocating its limited resources to accomplish various goal-directed activities.

5. Attention often operates in a controlled and purposeful fashion. We are especially aware of this controlled mode when we concentrate on novel or unfamiliar activities, deviate from our usual routines, and/or juggle several tasks at one time. However, attentional control is also exercised when we are unaware of it. In its "controlled" or "conscious" mode, the attentional system selectively focuses on relevant internal and external stimulus representations, which are the internal records or abstract codes that are constructed as information processing proceeds. The system then allocates resources to accomplish necessary processing operations. This "effortful" expenditure of attention consumes some of the available resource capacity.

6. By contrast, some cognitive processing can operate relatively auto-matically, without requiring significant amounts of total capacity. Automatic processes call up (or "activate") stored knowledge that helps to direct routinized actions, without our intention. For example, we do not have to attend to every aspect of our usual route from home to work, or to search effortfully for familiar word meanings in our mental lexicons. But, when we drive to work from somewhere other than home or encounter less familiar meanings or usages of words, we probably engage more conscious attentional mechanisms.

   a. Automaticity results from practice and overlearning, and it is important in reducing the "load" when we interact with the world. Automatic processes run without interfering greatly with simultaneous activities or significantly reducing the attentional fuel available for other mental work. Thus, we can perform more complicated tasks, or more tasks concurrently, as we develop automaticity for relevant parts of those tasks. Automatic processing appears to be more resistant to brain dam-age than the effortful allocation of mental resources.

   b. Experimentation has also indicated that many automatic processes, such as lexical access in normal adults, should be considered obligatory or mandatory. In the case of lexical access, it has been demonstrated that when we encounter words, we cannot stop lexical access processes from operating (although they may not run successfully when lexical entries are not easily available).

   c. The nature of the interaction between automatic/mandatory processes and controlled attentional operation is important for understanding some attentional impairments that can occur after brain damage. Let us return to the domain of lexical processing to set up an example. There is ample evidence that whenever we encounter a word like "bat" that has two (or more) relatively equally dominant meanings (a balanced lexical ambiguity), we access both meanings automatically and mandatorily. This occurs even if there is a strong contextual bias toward one of the meanings (e.g., Swinney, 1979). A controlled attentional opera-tion is needed to select (albeit extremely rapidly) the sense that is most appropriate in the current context. In many instances the products of mandatory processing (e.g., activation of the unwanted meaning of "bat") are not immediately relevant to our current goals. If these competing possibilities equal or exceed the target information in strength (e.g., are more familiar, or have more environmental immediacy, personal relevance or other salient features), they may intrude into processes of perception, comprehension, and formulation. To avoid this kind of disruption, contextually inappropriate products of mandatory processing that might compete with relevant information are dampened or discarded by controlled attentional processes. Non-brain-damaged individuals routinely inhibit competing possibilities, although they may pursue "tangents" more readily in informal social contexts (and normal aging may impair the ability to discount associations that are irrelevant to specific task-imposed goals). But some brain-damaged patients, especially those with frontal lobe damage, may appear to be distractible or to have difficulty inhibiting familiar or routine actions and thoughts, perhaps because of a failure of attentional control to avoid interference from unwanted products of relatively spared mandatory or automatic processing (e.g., Shallice & Burgess, 1991a).

7. A distinction between parallel and serial processing is somewhat related to the notion of attentional control. Some mental processes occur simultaneously, or in parallel, while others operate in sequence, or serially. Examples of parallel processes include low-level visual operations that recover properties of the environment (e.g., detecting edges, color, motion), or some of the component skills of reading comprehension (e.g., letter and word identification, eye movements, and activation of stored knowledge that will influence interpretation). The mandatory access of multiple lexical meanings of balanced ambiguities, described above, also occurs in parallel. Seriality may emerge with increased need to coordinate individual cognitive operations or their products, particularly when there are precise time constraints for one process to be completed in order to serve as input to another process. Thus the lexical selection operation that follows multiple lexical access is an example of a serial process. Some authors have likened parallel with automatic processes and serial with effortful processes, in the sense that multiple operations can be carried out in parallel without consuming significant amounts of resource capacity, while each serial process places increasing (additive?) demands on cognitive resources. Although this is often the case, the situation is more complex than this, and there is no one-to-one correspondence between parallel and automatic processes, or serial and effortful processes.

8. Psychologists have distinguished a number of components of the attentional system, but there is no consensus about the number and nature of these subcomponents or the ways in which they are related to each other. Following Whyte's (1992) clear presentation, this discussion will focus on arousal, selective attention, and strategic control of attention.

a. *Arousal* can be likened to an energy source. It is mediated by the reticular activating system in the brainstem, which is reciprocally connected to cortical association areas. The right hemisphere appears to be particularly important for tonic arousal (Posner, Inhoff, & Friedrich, 1987), a relatively stable, baseline state of wakefulness that fluctuates slowly throughout the day. Arousal levels can be heightened by increasing task complexity or performance incentive, providing alerting signals, or generating compensatory effort. Moderate increases in arousal tend to speed task performance, perhaps by facilitating the effortful access to attended information. Arousal levels are diminished by factors including intoxication and fatigue, and lesions that induce neglect may produce an asymmetrical reduction of arousal in the right hemisphere of the brain. In conditions of hypoarousal, the attentional resources that are mobilized to do perceptual and cognitive work may be inadequate to meet task demands.

b. *Selective attention,* defined in Chapter 1, section III-E-1-b, determines how and where attentional resources are allocated. Filter theories of attention suggest that selective attention helps to screen out many irrelevant stimuli and thoughts that invade our minds, to focus on information that is relevant to our goals and expectations. Resource theories of selective attention hold that our finite supply of resources can be allocated flexibly to focus as needed on particular stimuli, thoughts, or actions. Thus, selection occurs for events from the external environment and from our mental world of activated knowledge and memories.

(1) Although there are many models of selective attention, this discussion will highlight one influential example that has been linked empirically to hemispatial neglect. Posner and colleagues (e.g., Posner & Petersen, 1990) described a model of selective attention in which modality specific resource pools for visual and auditory selection function under the control of a more general resource pool. At least three component operations are specified that subserve the function of orienting and shifting attention in space: disengage, move, and engage (Posner & Driver, 1992; Posner et al., 1984, 1987). These operations are inferred from changes in response times to stimuli presented in different parts of space and cues specifying where to attend. For example, before a target detection trial, subjects are provided with a cue about where in the array the target is most likely to appear. The cue is valid when the target occurs in the expected location, and invalid when the target occurs in a different location (in the same or the opposite hemifield).

When a stimulus is presented at a location other than the one specified (invalid cue condition), the disengage operation releases attention from the expected position, and the move component supports the shift to the new location. The engage component allows subjects to allocate attention to a predicted location when presented with a pre-target cue, or to the target itself after an attentional shift. These operations are attributed primarily to the covert orienting of attention, as the expected changes in response times can be observed even when eye position is fixed. When the proportion of valid cue trials is high, response times are faster on valid cue trials, presumably because the predictive cue facilitates attentional engagement. Response times are slower for invalid cue trials, and especially so when the invalid target appears in the hemifield contralateral to the brain lesion.

(2) A variety of evidence suggests that the right parietal lobe is involved in attentional shifts for both visual fields. Based on various experimental findings and arguments, Posner and colleagues (1984, 1987) characterize parietal neglect as a difficulty in releasing attentional focus when attention is engaged, especially in the intact hemifield. However, as indicated in Chapter 1, there is controversy about this position. Posner's group (1984) also observed a disruption of attentional engagement at the (unexpected) target location after an attentional shift, but this was less consistent and less severe than the disengagement deficit. Other work has linked the move component to the superior colliculus and surrounding midbrain structures and the engage function to the thalamus, particularly the pulvinar nucleus (Posner & Petersen, 1990).

c. Performance in many daily activities requires a balance between allocating attention in goal-directed ways, attending to important but unexpected events, and overriding routine (mandatory) programs when confronted with novel or technically difficult problems. *Strategic control of attention*, defined as "the goal-directed operation of attention to facilitate chosen tasks" (Whyte, 1992, p. 941), allows this balance to occur. Determining task priorities and modulating the activity of mandatory processes, differentiating relevant from irrelevant information, resisting distraction, sustaining attentional focus, dividing or switching attention, and generating compensatory mental effort are all functions that fall under the province of higher attentional control. It has been suggested that strategic control of attention is mediated largely by fronto-limbic regions of the brain (e.g., Shallice & Burgess, 1991a).

(1) Attentional control was mentioned earlier in relation to overriding mandatory and automatic processes. Shallice (1988; Shallice & Burgess, 1991a) describes a supervisory attentional system (SAS) that helps accomplish this goal (though see Kimberg & Farah, 1993, and section III-E-2-d below for an alternative view of the necessary cognitive architecture). In many cases, such as walking along a familiar route, routine actions or thought operations are sufficient to perform a task. These programs operate automatically when there is an appropriate internal or external trigger, and often more than one of these programs is working at one time. But when routine programs are insufficient to realize a goal, or when several programs are likely to compete with each other, the SAS becomes important. The SAS directs information processing according to long-term goals and task requirements by biasing and selecting among routine responses, or by interrupting them and initiating novel ones. The SAS also helps to maintain intentions in the face of competing mandatory processes and thus contributes to conflict resolution. This aspect of the SAS captures nicely the experiences that we have all had with slips of action, such as when we go into the kitchen to get a pen, but wind up organizing the desk drawer or washing the dishes. When the SAS is preoccupied so that it does not control automatic response tendencies, some aspect(s) of the immediate context, either internal or external, can trigger routine programs that are inconsistent with original goals.

(2) A related dimension of higher attentional control involves interrupting an ongoing task to attend to unexpected stimuli. When this subcomponent is hyperactive (as in failure of the SAS), patients will have difficulty resisting distraction. But if it is underactive, they could remain unaware of information that might be critical for performance. Fronto-limbic and hippocampal structures seem to be involved in detecting novel signals or events and in facilitating habituation to those deemed irrelevant.

(3) The integrity of the right hemisphere is considered particularly critical for developing and maintaining an alert state over time (Posner & Petersen, 1990; Whitehead, 1991), also referred to as sustained attention. As noted in Chapter 1, this vigilance function is important for processing high priority stimuli. It appears to depend in part on a cluster of right frontal and parietal regions (Pardo, Fox, & Reichle, 1991). Patients with RHD in those areas have evidenced reduced galvanic skin response and heart rate response to warning signals (e.g., Heilman et al., 1985; Yokoyama, Jennings, Ackles, Hood, & Boller, 1987). Also, frontal lesions (in either hemisphere) interfere with sustained performance of monotonous tasks (e.g., Wilkins, Shallice, & McCarthy, 1987), unless the subject can purposefully compensate with a higher level of autonomic activity, as described below. Sustained attention deficits may be manifest in difficulties with extended listening, maintaining eye contact, and staying on topic or task. Some research has also linked depression, in part, to a disruption of right hemisphere arousal and vigilance mechanisms (cf., Liotti & Tucker, 1992).

(4) A related aspect of the strategic control of attention is the goal-directed generation of arousal, or compensatory effort. Compensatory effort may involve "trying" to stay alert for certain simple, but very important, tasks such as driving straight on a highway. RHD patients can often generate compensatory effort to improve their performance in the short term, but no one, brain-damaged or not, can sustain compensatory effort for extended periods of time.

(5) Strategic control extends to divided attention as well. It is common in daily life to perform two or more tasks concurrently and to alternate or divide attention between them. This causes a problem for many patients, especially those with prefrontal lesions in either hemisphere. The ability to divide attention is also relevant for performing "high load" single tasks, such as comprehending discourse units that are grammatically complex, or that require backtracking and re-evaluation. In fact, comprehending most any text makes us juggle many simultaneous acts of processing and storage. To name a few, the comprehender must execute syntactic, semantic, and lexical processes to represent initial propositions; hold those propositions temporarily while others are encoded and interpreted; relate them to information retrieved from context and world knowledge; inhibit information that was automatically activated, but is not relevant to the unfolding interpretation; resolve ambiguities

such as those entailed by polysemous words, inexplicit reference, nonliteral expressions, syntactic garden paths, erroneous assumptions, or other inconsistencies; and draw inferences or other conclusions about the integrated textual interpretation. Indeed, RHD patients often complain about keeping track of lengthy conversations, complicated movies, or novels with many characters and complex plots.

9. To summarize briefly, the more attentional resources and the greater attentional control required for a particular activity, the more poorly RHD subjects (or indeed anyone) will perform. But, becoming familiar and practiced with new tasks or mental operations allows people to attend to fewer aspects of them, freeing up some of their limited capacity. This point has implications for clinical management, that will be considered later. Readers who want more overview material about attention and performance are referred to Ashcraft (1989) or Eysenck and Keane (1990).

E. Memory

1. **The multidimensionality of memory.** Like attention, memory is a multifaceted construct. The multitude of memory processes and systems is too complex to consider in this book, but Table 2–11 provides a brief summary of selected memory phenomena and terminology. For more information, consult the very readable writings of Ashcraft (1989) and Squire (1987), or the more specialized Solomon, Goethals, Kelley, and Stephens (1989). Chapter 1 (section III-E) has already recounted a number of visual and nonverbal memory deficits that can be associated with RHD. The working memory (WM) system is another important aspect of memory for RHD patients.

Table 2–11. Memory concepts and terminology

Memory Systems: Fractionation of memory systems has received much attention in the study of memory.

Sensory memory (SM) stores receive information from the external world, which decays extremely rapidly (less than 1 second) unless it is attended. The separate registers for auditory, visual and tactile information are called echoic, iconic, and haptic memory, respectively.

Short-term memory (STM) is also known as immediate memory, and is roughly similar to primary memory and portions of working memory, defined below. In traditional models, STM is a temporary storage space for information from the internal world (sensory memory stores, and long-term memory) that requires further processing. Sensory information that is attended is transferred there, together with stored

Continued

Table 2–11. *Continued*

permanent knowledge that is useful for interpreting the sensory information. Information in STM decays rapidly (on the order of 30 seconds or so) unless it is refreshed through control processes like rehearsal, elaboration, organization, or decision. The traditional view is that short-term memory has a structural capacity of 7 ± 2 units of information, with the size of a "unit" depending on strategies adopted by the perceiver. For example, chunking and recoding processes, such as remembering 4 digits of a phone number as a single date or clustering related words together, allow people to reduce the effective load on STM and increase the sheer number of items that they can retain temporarily. Traditional immediate memory measures include digit and word spans, and recency effects in list-learning experiments.

Primary memory is a reconceptualization of STM that de-emphasizes structure and time of storage, and emphasizes processing. A key distinction is that information in primary memory can be lost whenever someone is required to perform another task, regardless of the amount of time that has passed since the initial material was presented (e.g., 5 seconds or 5 minutes). But if subjects keep the target information in mind without being distracted, information in primary memory can remain longer than usual.

Working memory (WM) is another reconceptualization of STM. It extends the concept of STM by focusing on the active information processing functions of an immediate memory system, rather than on passive stores. Some elements of WM are assumed to be responsible for performance on traditional immediate memory tasks, but WM is also involved with activities like reasoning and comprehension. WM limitations are not due to time per se, or to the number of"slots" available in the system. Rather, limitations are due to the amount and nature of processing that can be carried out at one time, and thus to an individual's total processing capacity and processing skill. WM is discussed more extensively in the text.

Long-term memory (LTM) is the system responsible for storing information on a more permanent basis, in the form of knowledge that can be retrieved to guide behavior. Many divisions of the LTM system have been proposed, such as declarative (knowledge of facts and details of events that one can recount) and procedural knowledge of skills or ways of doing things, and that cannot be described), episodic (knowledge of contextually specific and personally experienced events) and semantic memory (stored general knowledge about the world including facts, word meanings, scripts or culturally routine sequences of events in particular situations, story schema, and knowledge of the skills involved in goal-directed actions). Information is encoded into LTM through comprehension and learning, by way of which currently processed information is related in some way to knowledge that is already stored in LTM. As new information is incorporated into LTM, new associations are formed so that its structure is continually reorganized. LTM is essentially limitless in size.

Secondary memory is a rough synonym for LTM. It is generally contrasted with primary memory, and so focuses on a system that retains information after a period of distraction.

Table 2–11. *Continued*

Other Types of Memory: Relatively newer concerns in the study of memory include implicit memory, metamemory, and prospective memory (or more broadly, everyday memory).

Implicit memory can be contrasted with explicit memory, which is the traditional focus of memory tests. Explicit memory involves the conscious recollection of facts, names, or events when needed. By contrast, implicit memory can only be inferred, and is revealed when some stimulus or event influences subsequent processing and performance, without the perceiver's conscious recollection of that stimulus. Implicit memory is typically less affected than explicit memory by aging or brain damage.

Metamemory involves one's awareness and monitoring of one's own memory capabilities, and beliefs about their effectiveness. Metacognitive awareness in general prompts us to initiate strategies (e.g., to rehearse or write down information that we want to remember), and provides a mechanism by which we anticipate, assess, and recognize failures, and attempt to improve our performance accordingly. Metamemory is frequently impaired after frontal lobe damage. Normal aging may also be accompanied by changes in metamemory.

Prospective memory is memory for performing future actions. The mechanisms of prospective memory, and the ways in which they can be impaired, have received little attention, but prospective memory is a crucial skill for navigating in the world. It is part of a recent concern with *everyday memory.*

Memory Processes: Fundamental processes for establishing long-term memories include encoding, storage and retrieval. These fundamental processes can be carried out along the continuum of predominant automaticity/effort that is described in the text, and they interact crucially. For instance, retrieval will suffer if encoding or storage processes are ineffective.

Encoding involves inputting information into various memory systems. Encoding activities are the processes that convert sensory information into forms that can be maintained temporarily in sensory or STM, or related to pre-existing knowledge in LTM. They constitute the initial portion of the act of remembering, and are required for learning and acquisition. Encoding can vary along "levels" of stimulus properties, such as physical appearance or semantic characteristics, or in amount or nature of elaboration and detail.

Storage processes are those that lead to formation of long-term memories, involving some kind of integration with previously-stored information. *Consolidation* is one storage process that is based on the idea that the storage of memory traces does not occur instantly. During the consolidation process, new information is gradually incorporated into LTM. If processing is interrupted during the consolidation period (e.g., by an anoxic episode or some other brain injury), the information will not be mapped into long-term stores.

Retrieval processes are those that contact stored information and mediate its recovery from memory. Retrieval is tapped by recall or recognition tasks. Recall

(Continued)

Table 2–11. *Continued*

tasks require subjects to search memory and reproduce stored knowledge, and take two forms: free recall tasks involve only a general request to recall, while cued recall tasks provide some hint to support recall (such as a category name for lexical search). Recognition tasks are considered less demanding because they involve discriminating a correct response rather than reproducing it. Recognition involves both an experience of familiarity, and a context-dependent search or retrieval process that identifies what the familiar target is.

The *encoding specificity* effect is an experimentally robust finding about the interaction between encoding and recall. That is, remembering depends on the compatibility between encoding activity and the retrieval task or situation. Learned information is more accessible for recognition and recall tasks when the purpose and conditions of retrieval match the nature and context of encoding.

Memory Disorders: Memory disorders take various forms, most of which are related to the systems, types, and/or processes summarized above. That is, different patients might have deficits of immediate memory, declarative memory, metamemory, encoding processes, or memory retrieval. Two other types of memory disorders are worthy of note.

Material-specific memory disorders were alluded to in Chapter 1, with a focus on nonverbal or spatial memory deficits for RHD patients. Dissociations observed after brain damage support the notion that memory can be laid down in very specific ways (e.g., verbal vs. nonverbal; faces vs. routes).

Anterograde memory deficits are difficulties in recognizing or recalling material or events encountered since the onset of a memory disorder, and can be contrasted with *retrograde* memory deficits, or difficulties with material and events encoded or learned before the onset of the memory disorder. Retrograde memory deficits have been associated with disruption of memory consolidation. Anterograde and retrograde deficits usually co-occur in memory-impaired patients.

Modulators of Memory: Memory processes are modulated by more factors than can be recounted here, but some include: alertness and attention, prior knowledge and expertise, meaningfulness of encoded material, depth and nature of encoding (e.g., processing for meaning), association strategies, affective states, goals for remembering, and social context. The influence of hormones and neurotransmitters on memory is also under study (see, e.g., Squire, 1987).

2. **Working memory.** Working memory is a recent reconceptualization of the passive short-term memory store. The adjective "working" emphasizes the system's active role in concurrent information processing and storage activities that pervade daily life. The reader may recall, as an example of simultaneous processing and storage, the previous discussion of processes involved in comprehending a text. For a more concrete example, try solving the following math problem in your head:

$[(6 \times 8)/3] \times [(13 - 7)/3]$.

As you work out the solution, you are probably aware of retrieving some facts while holding onto others, and while carrying out arithmetical operations or processes.

a. One influential model (Baddeley, 1986) describes multiple components of a working memory system, each of which has a limited capacity. A "Central Executive" is responsible for controlling attention, cognition, and action. Two subsidiary "slave" systems or buffers provide temporary storage for information that is being actively processed: the articulatory loop for facilitating and retaining speech-based coding, and the visuospatial sketchpad (or scratchpad) for generating and manipulating visuo-spatially coded images. These buffers are similar to modality-specific short-term stores, but when overloaded, they can draw resources from the central executive. Many who perform the mental arithmetic problem above rely on both slave systems, using speech-based codes to derive basic products (e.g., "$6 \times 8 = 48$" or "$13 - 7 = 6$, and that divided by 3 = 2"), and visual coding to imagine the process of dividing the larger product (48) by 3. As another example that would call on both buffers, imagine being asked how many windows there are in your house. To answer, you would probably try to visualize each room, and then count as you moved mentally through the house.

b. Much of the evidence leading to this multicomponent model of working memory was derived from dual task data (see Baddeley, 1986). Although the central executive component was ill-defined (Baddeley himself called it an "area of residual ignorance"), it was hypothesized to control decisions about the ways in which available resources need to be allocated to meet ongoing processing and storage requirements, which includes selecting the most beneficial strategies for relating information in the service of activities such as learning, reasoning, decision making, and comprehension. It also provides the "workspace" for active mental effort and integration.

c. Working memory limitations are attributed to the amount of processing capacity available at any time. As an analogy, consider a hospital's surgical capacity, which depends on the number of operating rooms, numbers and types of surgeries or procedures taking place, number and skill of surgeons, and so forth. Only a limited number of operations, whether surgical or cognitive, can occur accurately, efficiently, and simultaneously. But when less difficult procedures are scheduled, and/or when more skilled surgeons (processing routines) are at work, more capacity will quickly become available for other operations.

d. On the basis of the preceding discussion, the reader may have begun to wonder how working memory and attentional functions are related. The answer is, they appear to be closely related.

(1) Attentional selectivity helps to manage the load that is input to working memory; the working memory system provides for temporary storage of information, which allows attention to be allocated elsewhere. And the central executive has much in common with certain aspects of strategic attentional control. For example, the central executive sets priorities for allocating attention and other mental resources to accomplish mental activity. In fact, Baddeley (1986) invokes the Shallice model of the Supervisory Attentional System as a promising theoretical framework for specifying the functions of the central executive.

(2) It should be mentioned here that there are important alternatives to the idea of a WM central executive system, or a Supervisory Attentional System. For example, Kimberg and Farah (1993) question the need to invoke a central executive that coordinates the activities of multiple aspects of cognition. In computer simulations, they reproduced performance patterns that mimic "dysexecutive" deficits by weakening the association strengths among WM representations of environmental stimuli, behavioral goals, and stored knowledge. Thus, they argue that such deficits may be a consequence of impaired connections between various representations that generate competing activations. When these connections are weakened, behavior may be determined by potentially incomplete or less relevant sources of information and mental activation.

e. Just and Carpenter have also investigated working memory extensively, as a constraining factor in language comprehension and other cognitive activities. Their work focuses on the aspects of working memory that are akin to Baddeley's central executive component. In their model, working memory capacity can be flexibly allocated to information processing and storage functions (Just & Carpenter, 1992). These functions compete for limited working memory capacity, such that more resources are consumed when more demanding mental operations are carried out and/or when a greater number of partial comprehension products must be maintained on the way to a final interpretation. The more capacity used in working memory at any time, the less remains for carrying out further computations or for storing additional products of comprehension. Individual variations in "functional" or available working memory capacity may result from differences in the size of the resource pool as well as the accuracy, efficiency, and demands of mental operations that are executed.

f. Just and Carpenter's data demonstrate that working memory capacity constrains numerous normal language comprehension phenomena. Young adults with high and low working memory spans, reflecting differential ability to process and store information concurrently, exhibit systematic differences in a variety of processing operations, across linguistic systems. Differences between high and low span subjects emerge at critical junctures when comprehension processes are most demanding, indicating that capacity limitations affect performance as resource demands approach and exceed the available supply.

g. In a recent investigation, 25 RHD adults were found to be more limited than control subjects on a measure of working memory capacity (adapted from Just and Carpenter's work) that requires simultaneous processing and storage of spoken information (Tompkins et al., 1994). Additionally, capacity, as indexed by this task, was related to individual RHD patients' abilities to resolve textual inconsistencies and to revise initial inferences in other tasks with relatively high information processing load. And further, as predicted by Just and Carpenter's capacity theory, there was no meaningful association between capacity and performance in "light load" tasks that were not expected to overburden available resources. Working memory limitations of this sort may also be at the root of some of our patients' complaints of difficulty keeping up with fast-moving conversations and complicated story plots. As working memory capacity may modulate performance on a variety of cognitively-demanding tasks, it is discussed further in Section V with other potential accounts of RHD symptomatology.

3. **Prospective memory.** Prospective memory, or remembering to do things in the future, has not been linked specifically to RHD. However, because of its relevance to daily functioning, we would do well to assess prospective memory in RHD patients.

F. Integration

1. Integration deficits were included in the list of visuoperceptual disorders in Table 2–7. But, there have been broader characterizations of difficulties with integrating, or synthesizing, information into a whole.

2. Generally, RHD patients may have trouble evaluating individual parts in the context of an organizational framework or appreciating the relationship of discrete elements to an overall structure. Integration deficits have been described in the linguistic domain as well as the visuoperceptual domain. For example, Molloy, Brownell, and Gardner (1990) conclude that the fundamental discourse comprehension impairment after RHD is a difficulty combining old and new information. Further, Myers (1986) suggests that RHD patients may have trouble with any task that requires them to detect key elements, see relationships among them, combine them into an overall structure, and draw relevant conclusions. RHD patients' integration deficits typically have been ascribed to problems taking in and using contextual cues, but perceptual integration requires attention to features of the stimuli themselves as well as contextual information (cf., Treisman & Gelade, 1980).

3. Klonoff et al. (1990) have described integration deficits in daily living under the rubric of "seeing the big picture." Families of three RHD patients reported that the patients fastened onto small details of a discussion, without appreciating a wider perspective or another point of view. The same patients were impaired in safety judgments, including decisions to drive or to shoot guns. The patients could recite the reasons for restrictions on their activities, or for using certain compensatory strategies, but a discrepancy remained between knowing and doing. It should be remarked that these patients were enrolled in comprehensive, long-term rehabilitation, and, as such, may have been more severely impaired than other subsets of RHD patients.

G. Planning, Organization, Reasoning, and Problem Solving

1. Planning, organization, reasoning, and problem solving are multifaceted and interactive cognitive skills that contribute to executing goal-directed behavior. The extent to which these skill areas overlap and cooperate in everyday cognition makes it somewhat difficult to write about one without referring to the others, but each area is discussed briefly below. For more information, the reader is referred to Ashcraft (1989), Lezak (1983), McCarthy and Warrington (1990), and Ylvisaker and Szekeres (1994).

2. Planning is associated with formulating a framework, often a sequence of steps, for directing behavior. It involves generating alternative approaches, and selecting one based on anticipation of its feasibility, utility, and appropriateness. To develop a viable plan in unfamiliar circumstances, it is necessary to gather information

about unalterable or constraining aspects of the situation and other potential obstacles, as well as the tools and resources that are available, necessary, and helpful for carrying out any potential plan. (This kind of information-seeking activity is an important aspect of problem-solving behavior as well.) As a plan is implemented, it must be evaluated to determine how well it is serving its purpose, and to identify when some change in approach might be warranted. Generally speaking, planning is integral to, and depends on, organizational, reasoning, and problem-solving processes considered further below.

3. Ylvisaker and Szekeres note that the term "organization" has a number of senses. It can refer to a characteristic of our knowledge stores (e.g., connections among related entries in a mental lexicon) or to a product of mental activity (e.g., generating a relationship of some sort among elements in a set). In addition, organization has a process function that is directed by specific problems or goals (e.g., encoding and retrieval goals). According to Ylvisaker and Szekeres, organizing processes include noting similarities and differences, detecting relevancies, specifying temporal sequence, and combining information in superordinate units such as themes or higher-level categories. Organizing schemes can also include overlearned, implicit knowledge structures such as scripts, discourse superstructures, or conversational rules. All of these kinds of activities and schemas help to focus attention, to create plans, and to learn, remember, reason, and infer.

4. The domain of reasoning is also multidimensional. Reasoning involves drawing conclusions or inferences, or generating hypotheses and alternatives, from evidence and from experience. The term "reasoning" implies rationality and the domain of reasoning includes formal logic, but research indicates that everyday reasoning is often not very logical or rational (Ashcraft, 1989). Rather, everyday reasoning frequently reflects heuristic processes or "rules of thumb" that may or may not generate "accurate" solutions to problems that are encountered. Ashcraft recounts extensive examples of widespread biasing influences on everyday reasoning that probably result from a person's (often incomplete or inaccurate) stored knowledge and experience. Common biases include those based on representativeness (which can lead to stereotyping) and availability heuristics. For example, we tend to consider certain conclusions to be more likely if they seem representative to us or if we can easily remember examples and instances of them. These kinds of biases operate in college students (and even in their professors!) who presumably function reasonably well cognitively, raising cautions about what to

expect in terms of "accurate" reasoning performance from adults with brain damage.

5. Problem solving is a multicomponent process involved in achieving purposeful and novel goals (i.e., automatically retrieving a word from memory does not involve problem solving, but a consciously organized search through the lexicon for a less familiar term reflects a problem-solving process). According to Ashcraft, much of our nonautomatic cognitive activity represents instances of problem solving. Problem solving involves deliberately analyzing a situation, devising a plan of action, and executing and evaluating the plan. It requires focusing attention to direct action toward the problem, abstracting necessary information from its elements, analyzing the properties of the single example or situation, and identifying similarities with or differences from other examples stored in memory. In addition, planning is required to generate a framework to direct activity by identifying subgoals and alternative approaches, forming and selecting strategies, and anticipating outcomes of each step. Finally, strategy execution, shifting, and evaluation are necessary (see, e.g., McCarthy &Warrington, 1990).

Again, everyday problem solving typically involves heuristic processes and educated guesses, rather than completely rational or optimal decisions. Some research reports that expert medical diagnosticians rely primarily on a forward reasoning method, first generating and then ruling out alternative hypotheses based on an analysis of symptoms, whereas novices reason backwards, trying to confirm one specific diagnostic hypothesis (Patel & Groen, 1986). More generally, effective problem solvers focus on what Ylvisaker and Szekeres call the "front-end" aspects of problem-solving processes before attempting to solve a problem: clarifying the problem, searching for analogies, generating a variety of possible solutions, and formulating a plan to explore those solutions (Dodd & White, 1980).

6. Earlier sections of this chapter described RHD adults' potential difficulties with some component processes of planning, organizing, reasoning, and problem solving, such as appreciating and generating alternatives; perceiving relevant properties and characteristics; focusing and sustaining attention; and various aspects of integrating information and inferencing. The "abstract thoughts" element of problem solving is often tested by asking patients to define proverbs, such as "a bird in the hand is worth two in the bush," and other figurative expressions. Concrete responses on such tasks characterize some RHD patients, and many other patients with brain damage more generally. Other tasks that are commonly used to assess problem solving and reasoning skills involve classification activities, or defining similarities.

(It should be noted here that performance on many such tasks varies with premorbid education and intellectual abilities.) Impairments in these kinds of planning, organization, reasoning, and problem-solving tasks are often associated with lesions in prefrontal regions of the brain, though subcortical damage can create difficulties as well.

7. At present, one important deficiency in our knowledge base is the lack of good information about RHD adults' ability to plan, organize, reason, and problem solve in tasks that bear a closer relationship to daily life situations and demands. Some clinical observations have been proffered: Daily planning and organization tasks that may prove difficult for RHD patients include record keeping activities; following sequential procedures; keeping checklists; organizing datebooks, schedules, and notebooks; and keeping track of personal belongings (Klonoff et al., 1990). Klonoff and colleagues' patients had severe problems with time management as well, often arriving late to their rehabilitation appointments. One former professor had particular difficulty keeping his lectures within set time limits, especially when he needed to adapt them for different time constraints. Another major gap in our knowledge about RHD patients' reasoning and problem-solving skills concerns the lack of information on their application of "normal" reasoning and problem-solving heuristics and strategies.

IV. OTHER BEHAVIORAL PROBLEMS

Several other behavioral deficits of RHD that can have important consequences are summarized in Table 2–12. Some of these kinds of problems have been described

Table 2–12. Other behavioral deficits that may follow RHD in adults

Impulsivity and disinhibition

Distractibility

Response delay

Poor error recognition

Slower rate of learning

Difficulty switching sets

Apparent lack of motivation

Depression

General discrepancy between "knowing" and "doing" (often associated with poor judgment)

as personality disturbances (e.g., lack of motivation, impulsivity, distractibility) but many probably reflect cognitive disturbances of awareness and attentional control. In any case, these deficits may affect performance on specific cognitive or rehabilitative tasks and activities, causing errors to occur. They may also influence daily functions such as eating, spending or budgeting, work performance, and sexual behavior. Overall, the cognitive and behavioral problems exhibited by RHD adults can interfere with judgment and social skills, family relationships, functional living activities, and the potential to return to productive work (Klonoff et al., 1990).

V. POTENTIAL ACCOUNTS OF SYMPTOMS

A. Domain-related Factors

Some clinicians and researchers have suggested that domain-related factors may account for various symptoms of cognitive and communicative disorders after RHD. For example, Myers (1981) surmised that RHD patients rely too heavily on their linguistic systems, generating abundant and inefficient discourse, to cope with inadequate perceptions. Brownell and colleagues (Brownell, Carroll, Rehak, & Wingfield, 1992) invoked the domain level to explain RHD patients' successful integration of discourse components in a task using explicit pronouns. The authors suggest that patients were successful because linguistic information is easy for them to encode. RHD patients' difficulties processing particular components of incoming messages (visuoperceptual, emotional, nonliteral, prosodic) may also translate into problems interpreting texts containing these elements. However, domain-specific encoding deficits do not tell the entire story (see section E, below).

B. "Inference Failure"

1. Myers (1991) coined the term "inference failure" as a hypothesis about the nature of deficits in RHD patients. "Inference failure" refers to faulty inferencing, rather than absence of inferencing, and Myers proposes that it can occur at all levels of cognitive and perceptual processing.

    a. Myers indicates that inferencing involves recognizing relationships between key elements of meaning and other contextual cues. She recounts a variety of communicative symptoms and argues that each is interpretable as a manifestation of inference failure. Among these are difficulty interpreting nonliteral expressions, resolving incongruous information, and recognizing intentions and emotions signalled by prosodic and facial features. In addition, impulsivity, tangential and inefficient discourse production, labeling pictured elements without weaving together the key points, and anosognosia are described as potential failures of inference.

b. Myers (1991) further specifies some visuoperceptual problems that tend to follow RHD, particularly difficulties with ambiguous stimuli or those in degraded or atypical views. She considers these problems as instances of impaired inferencing as well, in that (1) ambiguous stimuli require context to disambiguate them; and (2) degraded visual stimuli are resolved by assigning depth cues, which requires visual inference. Myers concludes "in all levels of processing, [inference] appears dependent upon an ability to identify available cues, integrate them with one another and with other sensory input, and form relationships that specify meaning beyond the sensory data" (p.178).

2. The proposal is underspecified at present, as there are many ways in which this chain of events and operations could break down. Moreover, other impairments may masquerade as inference failures. Consider a task involving inference revision, or nonliteral interpretation, or any sentence-to-picture matching task, that requires patients to process several interpretations. RHD patients may have difficulty evaluating the relative plausibility of these multiple interpretations (Joanette et al., 1990). If so, they may make the "wrong" choice for reasons other than inference failure. One interpretation may win out simply because it is more strongly activated (e.g., more typical, familiar, or personally relevant) or because it involves less mental work (e.g., compared to nonliteral foils, literal depictions of figurative meanings can be represented in relatively prototypical ways, so there are fewer reference situations to evaluate against the one presented in the task). An additional drawback of this proposal is that it does not provide a basis for predicting when patients can be expected to exhibit inference failures.

3. Much recent research has shown that RHD adults can generate a variety of inferences. They can, and do, use contextual cues to draw inferences in prosodic, emotional, nonliteral, and linguistic domains, especially when other cognitive demands are minimized. These kinds of findings can be accommodated by cognitive resource theories such as those discussed in the Attention and Memory sections above (see also V-E, below). Findings like these suggest that it might not be inference per se that is at risk after RHD. Rather, patients may have difficulty with "higher level" or "more demanding" computations that, as is often the case with inferences, are derived from an actively constructed representation of sensory, perceptual, linguistic, and other contextual input.

These computations might suffer because the cognitive resources that remain after building the mental representation are insufficient to carry out additional interpretive operations, and/or because they are allocated elsewhere. In addition, sensory and perceptual encoding that are slow or inaccurate could deprive higher mental computations of "good data" to act on and may disrupt the timing of the meaning-construction process. For example, "inference failure" could result if the mental representations that form the basis for inference are incomplete or inaccurate at the time when (relatively intact) inference processes are ready to be executed (e.g., Tompkins et al., 1994).

Myers (1991) alludes to the problem of mental effort, suggesting that patients' effort to perceive may use up resources that would be needed for ascertaining relationships. However, she does not pursue this possibility further. Another clue about the relationship between "inference failure" and mental effort is found in the fact that depth perception is primarily problematic for RHD adults when stimuli are degraded. From a resource perspective, a faulty representation, whether derived from a degraded external stimulus or an internal computation,will require more resources to "make sense" of it. Whenever resources are diverted or depleted, or limited information is available for them to work with, an end-product interpretation may suffer. If cognitively demanding conditions lead to inference failures, then it is not clear how inference failure per se could be a central explanation of RHD communicative deficits.

C. Semantic Activation Failure

1. Beeman (1993) provided recent evidence, and a new account, for inference deficits in RHD adults.

   a. Subjects were presented with spoken stimulus stories and were given several goals to execute concurrently: to remember the texts so that they could answer questions about them when each was over, or so that they could retell some of them; and to make lexical decisions about letter strings that were presented visually at various points in each text, as they listened to the text. The letter strings were either word or nonword probes, and subjects had to decide if each was a real word or not. The word probes were either related to inferences in the stories, or unrelated. Beeman argued that if subjects were generating inferences as they processed the texts, inference-related information should have been salient and accessible when the probe stimuli were presented; thus, responses to inference-related probe words should be faster than responses to unrelated probes. This was indeed the case for the normally aging control subjects in the study.

b. In comparison with these control subjects, RHD patients answered fewer inference questions about the stimulus stories, and included fewer inferred events in recalling the stories. In addition, their lexical decisions were slower to inference-related probe words than to unrelated probe words. This response pattern suggested to Beeman that the RHD patients had failed to activate the lexical/semantic information needed to draw inferences during comprehension. He attributed their generally reduced performance with inference questions and inference judgments in his study to this presumed failure.

2. Beeman's interpretation again runs into the questions raised in the preceding section about resource demands and the timing of conceptual activation and representation.

a. First, the subjects were asked to coordinate a variety of cognitively demanding activities. The task clearly required a multiway division of mental resources: The stories for recall were interspersed with the stories for comprehension questioning, so subjects had to be prepared to respond flexibly on different occasions, and they had to divide their attention between building representations of the stories and making lexical decisions. Further, Beeman alludes to subjects having left-sided neglect and indicates that they were either trained or reminded to look to the left for visual stimulus strings. This element of intentional compensation would add another source of demand on the overall resource pool. In addition, the stimuli were long and the sentence structure more complicated than is typical for materials used with brain-damaged adults. We do not know how RHD subjects prioritized each of these demands, but it appears that they allocated resources so that they could give some response to each part of Beeman's task. They answered factual questions about the stories accurately, and they made accurate lexical decision judgments for the most part. It has already been suggested that higher-level computations and processes like those involved in generating inferences may suffer as task demands exceed the available supply; this seems likely for Beeman's task.

b. Beeman's conclusion that RHD patients fail to activate information to generate inferences also appears to be premature, because activation processes could simply be protracted in time.

If semantic activation and/or inference generation proceed more slowly after RHD, the relevant conceptual information may not have been sufficiently activated ("available") to contribute to lexical decision judgments when the probe stimuli were presented. This is particularly likely given the other demands for attentional and working memory resources in this study. If the activation failure hypothesis were tested in a more straightforward task, it might be less attractive. Other work using less demanding tasks indicates that RHD patients do show evidence of activating metaphoric facets of word meaning, and emotional inferences (Tompkins, 1990, 1991a), although they do so more slowly than normally aging control subjects. Beeman's ideas offer food for thought, but the multiple task demands obscure clear interpretation.

D. Integration Deficits

1. Difficulties with integration, associated with problems evaluating and formulating gestalts, were discussed in section III-F, above. Molloy et al. (1990) categorized common RHD discourse problems into two classes, involving difficulties in using context either (a) to deduce meaning from ambiguous (especially nonliteral) utterances or (b) to alter original inferences when new information necessitates a change in interpretation. As indicated above, the authors attributed these discourse comprehension impairments to a primary problem of integrating textual and contextual information. Similarly, Kaplan et al. (1990) concluded that difficulties integrating information of different types, perhaps exacerbated by problems imputing mental states to characters, are likely candidates to explain RHD patients' deficits in conversational exchanges. Stemmer et al. (1994) hypothesized as well that integrating conflicting mental representations of request contexts and forms created problems for RHD adults. And, in some early work, Myers (1979) reported evidence that certain verbal expressive deficits may reflect an extension of RHD patients' difficulties integrating distinct elements into a perceptual whole. Finding that visual integration deficits went along with a paucity of interpretive remarks in picture description, Myers concluded that RHD adults have trouble integrating information on perceptual and more formal levels.

2. Although these descriptions and those recounted above suggest its appeal, the term "integration deficits" has been used rather globally. As is the case with the "inference failure" hypothesis, ascribing a symptom to an integration deficit may not be very helpful in determining how and why performance breaks down. Brownell and his colleagues

(1992) have become more specific in recent work, examining problems with integrating multiple or disparate aspects of a discourse context, such as cues to speaker mood or motives, and plausibility.

3. Another difficulty with a global appeal to integration deficits is that it is possible that they may be traced to other sources. For example, many of the tasks and situations linked to integration deficits can be argued to place relatively heavy demands on mental resources. Thus, a patient who seemingly cannot integrate information at some level might be able to if attentional/working memory demands are reduced, and/or if cues and structure are provided regarding the key elements, or the overall framework, for the situation. In fact, Brownell and colleagues (1992) reported that RHD patients integrated discourse components successfully in a task using explicit pronouns. Rehak, Kaplan, and Gardner (1992) similarly reported successful integration in tasks requiring patients to choose a continuation for short conversational scenarios, when the stimuli conformed to expectations of cooperative interactions.

4. Finally, some writings are not clear about how to distinguish between integration and inference deficits. Integration is a component of perception and inference, as the terms have been used in work described above; and perception and inference certainly contribute to integration, particularly at the discourse level. Specifying clear operational distinctions and expected performance differences would aid the search for underlying causes.

E. Resource Factors

1. Limitations on the availability or allocation of mental resources have been emphasized throughout this chapter as potential reasons that RHD patients exhibit many characteristic deficits and behaviors. This position has developed primarily from a line of research (all Tompkins references) indicating that:

   a. RHD patients' difficulties in domains typically considered problematic (nonliteral, emotional, prosodic, inferential) vary with information processing demands placed on cognitive resources;

   b. RHD patients can use context to predict, infer, and integrate when resource demands are limited; and

   c. RHD patients' ability to perform in conditions of higher processing load covaries with their functional working memory capacity, operationalized as the ability to process and store information concurrently. Furthermore, problems identified by other researchers are often observed in the context of tasks that can be argued to place high demands on patients' mental resources: when ambiguities or inconsistencies are built in, when revision is necessary for successful comprehension, when multiple sources or representations of information must be considered and integrated to form a final interpretation (particularly when there is some incongruity or conflict among them), or when divided attention demands come into play.

2. In addition to its intuitive appeal to account for high-level processing deficits, a resource perspective could accommodate the impact of domain-specific encoding deficits on comprehension impairment. Slow or otherwise faulty component processes could deprive subsequent comprehension operations of sound representations to act on and of resources to act with. Thus, difficulties in encoding individual aspects of a signal could generate effective differences in resource capacity and in comprehension skill, particularly as the limits of capacity are approached. And, a resource perspective can account for the partially correct performance that is often observed. For example, the finding that RHD patients can detect, but not resolve, incongruity in appreciating jokes is predictable from a resource perspective; resolving incongruity, a later stage process, would require more resources than merely detecting and representing incongruity. For further arguments about this perspective, and more discussion of its implications, the reader is referred to the primary references.

3. One major risk of a resource perspective is that it can be too seductive. Invoked after the fact, it can be made to fit almost any outcome and, as such, runs the risk of explaining nothing. It is critical to formulate and test specific predictions in pursuing this explanatory focus. It will also be important to explore the interaction between resource limitations and impaired sensory, perceptual, or higher cognitive component processes. For example, in our work, we are currently pursuing the possibility that RHD patients do not suppress irrelevant or incompatible information efficiently once it is activated (Tompkins, 1993). Ineffective suppression could underlie a variety of performance observations, could allow "bad data" to influence various processing operations, and/or could divert cognitive resources needed for other mental work.

4. The potential power of resource explanations justifies more rigorous work along these and other lines. But the performance variations that can be achieved by manipulating processing demands have immediate relevance for clinical management.

5. Decreased arousal, or capacity for cognitive activation, has also been suggested as a general factor that may underlie some deficits after RHD. The evidence for this position is mixed. But hypoarousal, often associated with neglect (Coslett, Bowers, & Heilman, 1987; Heilman, et al., 1985), may influence the allocation of mental resources for processing. In all of Tompkins' work, patients with more severe or long-lasting neglect have routinely done more poorly than patients with minimal or no neglect, in the conditions of higher processing load. This is consistent with the suggestion that neglect influences the availability or allocation of mental resources.

F. Processing Complexity

1. Joanette and Goulet (1994) have recently noted that, although it is not a very intriguing hypothesis, many of the symptoms that we observe after RHD might reflect a complexity effect. That is, RHD patients tend to be most impaired on task elements and processes that can be considered to be most difficult (e.g., those requiring the most attentional effort, those involving less plausible or less frequent representations, those demanding rapid serial responding, and so forth). It is possible that the more complex a task is, the more we need both hemispheres to carry it out. This position can be related broadly to the resource perspective described above, but the resource perspective also allows for impaired low-level (e.g., sensory and perceptual) processes to influence (relatively intact) higher level operations.

2. The notion of task complexity may seem intuitively clear, but explanations based on processing complexity turn out to be difficult to test (see, e.g., Salthouse, 1988). Presumed task complexity is usually manipulated along qualitative dimensions, by varying, for example, the syntactic structure of sentences, or the discriminability of perceptual elements, or the number of postulated different operations involved in the tasks to be compared. Salthouse notes that in cases like these, poorer performance that is attributed to increased complexity may actually be due to impairments of the new and different processing operations or strategies entailed by the "more complex" tasks. He advocates manipulating complexity along quantitative dimensions by varying the number of repetitions with which a single processing operation must be carried out to complete a task. Accordingly, he has studied complexity effects with tasks that vary, for example, the number of line segments to be integrated into a pattern for visual discrimination. This approach to complexity focuses on how much processing is required, rather than what kind of processing is required. Even with this kind of quantitative approach, it remains difficult to compare complexity across different tasks or

domains, because the effects of increasing the number of process repetitions may be different for some operation A than for another operation B. Increasing time pressure for responding might also be expected to increase task complexity, but when time is limited subjects may adopt atypical, and less successful, strategies such as responding on the basis of partial information; again, presumed complexity may be confounded with variations in the accuracy or efficiency of processing operations that differ from those in the "less complex" task. Differential task sensitivity is also an important issue. We can try to equate dependent measures for sensitivity, by matching them on reliability, item difficulty, and shapes of distributions of item difficulty (e.g., Chapman & Chapman, 1973, 1978). Those who wish to pursue a complexity explanation for the communicative and cognitive deficits observed after RHD will have to grapple with complicated issues like these.

G. Pragmatic Attitude

1. Joanette and colleagues (1990) have also raised the possibility that RHD patients fail on many (artificial) communicative tasks, because they do not assume the pragmatic attitude required of a "good subject" when faced with violations of pragmatic principles and conversational practice. Our assessment and treatment tasks often fail to respect these principles. For example, to ascertain how RHD patients deal with inconsistent or misleading information, we use tasks that violate the expectation that speakers generally strive to be unambiguous when interacting with others. According to Joanette and colleagues, RHD subjects may justify or accept incongruous elements, in part, to try to make them fit with this expectation. Other tasks do not allow an informative exchange, violating the principle that speakers attempt to convey only that which is relevant, and unknown, to the listener. When a patient's appreciation of jokes is assessed with a task like selecting punchlines, the examiner already knows the correct choice, so the patient does not have the opportunity to convey new information. Role playing activities that are popular in treatment, and that are included in pragmatic assessments such as the CADL test, also require a metapragmatic attitude. For example, stating or acting out how one would interact with another person he or she has just met, require different abilities from those involved in striking up an actual conversation.

2. Joanette et al. (1990) recommend more attention to this global, pragmatic component through more natural communicative tasks. Unfortunately, such tasks are difficult to develop and to administer in

controlled ways. But giving patients plenty of demonstration, examples, and practice may help to reduce some of the metapragmatic demand involved in figuring out what exactly is expected of them.

H. Conclusion

None of these proposals in their current forms provide adequate accounts of RHD communicative difficulties. All potential accounts must be more rigorously specified, to make predictions that can be tested. Furthermore, it would be surprising if any single explanation could account for RHD communicative symptoms; an integrated framework will have to be developed. In the meantime, though, the proposals reviewed above can provide some guidance to clinicians attempting to document patients' deficits and to focus treatments as effectively as possible.

CHAPTER

3

Appraisal, Evaluation, and Diagnosis: Objectives and Orientations

I. CLINICAL CHALLENGES

A. Infrequent Referral

Referral for communication evaluation after RHD may be rare in some settings. Clinicians may have to educate referring agents and potential consumers on the points listed below.

1. In casual conversation, patients with right brain lesions often "talk" perfectly well; as a result, speech-language referral may not be considered. Some physicians may not be attuned to the fact that more specific and subtle communicative deficits can occur after RHD or that these impairments may be quite socially handicapping.

2. In addition, physicians, other hospital staff, and family members may not be aware that speech-language pathologists can provide beneficial clinical diagnostic and/or management services.

3. RHD patients who are unaware of their deficits will not refer themselves and will be unlikely to accept someone else's request to seek assistance.

B. Premorbid Factors and Heterogeneity of Outcome

By now, heterogeneity is a familiar theme. Communicative and cognitive outcomes of RHD are heterogenous, partly due to the nature of the brain injury, but also partly because of each patient's unique history. Along with specific stroke-related deficits, each patient's premorbid abilities, skills, and concerns should influence diagnostic decisions, prognostic estimates, and the focus of treatment.

C. Measurement Concerns

As mentioned earlier, there are few norms or standardized instruments to help us attribute abnormality, determine severity, or measure what we think we are accomplishing in treatment with RHD adults. In addition, as outlined in Chapter 1, the tests and rating scales that do exist may be of questionable psychometric value. Some guidelines for evaluating our assessments are discussed in section V below.

II. OBJECTIVES AND PRINCIPLES OF INITIAL ASSESSMENTS

There is no mystery in determining initial assessment objectives for RHD patients. Regardless of the etiology of a communication disorder, our initial assessments will include a structured set of observations for a variety of purposes, as outlined below. Specific tools to help accomplish these assessment objectives are discussed in the next chapter. In general, initial assessment data should help us to document premorbid function, specify tentative diagnoses, formulate prognoses, determine candidacy for treatment, and plan initial directions when treatment is indicated.

A. Establish a Behavioral Profile

The first and most familiar assessment objective for many clinicians is identifying a patient's abilities and deficits, or behavioral strengths and weaknesses. The behavioral profile will document both cognitive and practical skills, such as those addressed in Chapter 2. Much of this information will come from formal, standardized measures, but non-standardized assessments and observations also have an important place in clinical activities, when used judiciously and interpreted responsibly (see section V-C below). Behavioral data gathered in the initial assessment may also contribute to establishing pre-intervention baselines, for monitoring the effects of treatment.

B. Render a Diagnosis

As Wertz (1986) reminds us, tests do not diagnose; well-informed clinicians do. Aligning the behavioral data with relevant medical and biographical information (see Chapter 4, section II, and Table 4–1), we are positioned to make a tentative, general diagnosis about the nature of observed symptoms. For patients with RHD, we must make our best guess, often in the absence of appropriate normative information, about whether the observed behavioral profile differs from what we would expect of non-brain-damaged adults with similar sociodemographic characteristics and medical histories. In addition, we need to weigh the evidence to postulate whether communicative performance is consistent with relatively focal damage to the right hemisphere or with multiple or diffuse brain lesions more commonly associated with language of confusion or language of generalized intellectual impairment (see Wertz, 1985). These distinctions will affect our decisions about offering treatment, as well as prognoses and treatment focus.

C. Estimate Severity and Determine Candidacy for Treatment

An assessment should help us to estimate the relative severity of impairments in various communicative areas. Severity estimates will be useful particularly for articulating prognoses, determining candidacy for treatment, and planning treatment procedures and directions.

D. Identify Functions Hypothesized to Underlie Overt Symptoms

1. Another critical purpose of assessment is to generate and test hypotheses about the reasons for patients' successes and failures. Comprehensive tests, as well as isolated tasks, are only means to an end. They provide a context for observing impaired and spared functions, for ascertaining common threads in performance, and for detecting factors that facilitate or impede cognitive processing and communicative behavior.

2. Experienced clinicians know that poor performance on any assessment measure can reflect a variety of deficits. Even the single tasks included in comprehensive measures typically require many component processes, at the levels of perception, interpretation, and/or response, that may contribute to the overall error score. Consider a subtest of confrontation naming. A RHD patient's performance may be deficient because of problems including diminished arousal and task orientation, fluctuating attention, visuoperceptual deficits (including some associated with normal aging) that degrade input to the lexicon, impairment of the conceptual knowledge base or of knowledge retrieval operations, lexical-semantic confusions, impulsiveness, articulatory impairments, or some combination of these.

3. As diagnosticians, we must guard against what Davis (1983) has called "pure task blindness": a tendency to describe the tasks that are difficult for patients (e.g., naming; repetition; discourse production) when asked to specify diagnoses and treatment goals. Rather, it is important to analyze the measures that we select and to postulate which of their features or requirements may cause difficulty for our patients. It is also important to look at our patients' performances across the various measures that we administer, to try to identify symptom patterns and component processing deficits that might account for such patterns. Both item comparisons and task comparisons can provide insights about the nature of observed impairments (see Davis, 1993).

4. Generally we will also need to apply specialized tests or specially designed probe measures to follow up on our initial hunches about the nature of performance deficits, probing areas such as attentional /resource factors, or "inference failure" (see Chapter 2, section V). Informed judgments about why patients succeed and fail are important for developing reasoned treatment approaches, and, logically, would seem to contribute to crafting effective treatments for many areas of difficulty (see also section IV-C, below). This problem-solving aspect of the assessment process is one of the most critical, and, generally, will continue after treatment is initiated.

E. Determine Effects of Deficits on Daily Functioning

If treatment is indicated, priority should be given to ameliorating symptoms (e.g., socially inappropriate or unsafe behavior) and/or underlying processes (e.g., ineffective allocation of mental resources) that are hypothesized to cause important disruptions in daily activities and interactions. At the same time, it may be possible and desirable to defer or forego treatment for deficits with minimal functional impact (e.g., some word-finding difficulties, or mild dysarthric symptoms). Of course, the severity of impairments in processes deemed critical for daily functioning will also influence prognostic statements.

F. Identify Patients' and Families' Concerns and Goals

As much as possible, a rehabilitation program should respect the wishes of the patients and families involved. It is always important to mesh our concern about objectively identified problems and functional deficits with the patients' and families' agendas. A mismatch in goals and expectations may occur if we judge some deficits to be trivial in their effect on daily living (e.g., mild spelling impairments or dysarthrias), but they cause considerable concern for patients or family members. If these deficits make appropriate targets for direct intervention, then they can be given priority. But even if they are not appropriate as direct treatment targets at a particular point in time, they will most likely need to be addressed through counseling before we will be able to convince the patients or their families to focus on other treatment goals. There is clinical value in listening to patients and their families for other reasons, as well. For example, they may be able to provide insight into problems that we cannot observe with our structured assessments or in the rehabilitation environment.

G. Formulate Initial Prognoses and Treatment Focus

As indicated in the preceding sections, the determinations made in accordance with our assessment objectives will influence prognostic estimates and treatment focus. Prognosis is always inexact, but especially so for RHD patients, because there is so little information to guide our predictions. In any case, the nature of the behavioral profile, the most probable diagnosis, the severity of impairments, their apparent modifiability, and their fundamental importance in daily life environments and interactions will provide useful clues for relative prognostic statements about the form that we think a patient's progress will take, and about eventual performance levels in various situations. When we have determined that our patient is a candidate for treatment, our data about these factors, our hypotheses about functions underlying impaired performance, and our knowledge of patients' and families' concerns, will guide our decisions about short-term and long-term intervention goals. Initial treatment targets can be selected to address:

1. Deficits that are most detrimental for communicative activities (e.g., impairments in fundamental processes and abilities, or in necessary prerequisites for communicative behavior);

2. Impairments that are most problematic in daily life, or most distressing to the patient and those around him or her;

3. Bad habits and unproductive strategies; and

4. Behaviors that we expect to be able to modify quickly.

III. OBJECTIVES OF REPEATED ASSESSMENTS

A. Purposes of Repeated Assessment

The *purposes of assessment* change as time passes. For example, repeated assessments begin with pre-treatment baseline measures and then are given periodically to monitor the effects of treatments that were developed as a result of our initial assessments. Initial treatment decisions may be validated by the changes documented in periodic assessments. Conversely, a lack of progress, or minimal generalization accompanying treatment, should suggest a re-evaluation of treatment procedures or goals. Repeated assessments may also spur us to revise our prognostic statements, as we learn more about our patients' abilities, expectations, and resilience, and the demands of their placements or roles in society.

B. Focus of Assessment

The relative *emphases of assessments* may vary over time, too, along with the focus of treatment. In the early post-onset stages, we are typically most concerned with identifying abilities and deficits, and the functions or processes underlying them, so that we can try to remediate particular processes and skills in treatment. As time passes, neurological recovery wanes, and performance stabilizes, we may focus more on functional abilities, daily life impact, and future plans. Many months post-onset, it will become more important to identify ways to cope with, and compensate for, residual impairments.

C. Other Influences on Assessment

We should remember to monitor *patients' and families' goals* periodically, as well. As they confront changing obstacles and reach ultimate levels of acceptance their priorities and concerns may shift, and our assessments should reflect this.

IV. COMPLEMENTARY ASSESSMENT PROCEDURES

To develop a performance picture consistent with our multiple assessment objectives, both neuropsychologically oriented and behavioral assessments are important, as are task analysis and nonstandardized probe procedures.

A. Neuropsychologically Oriented Assessments

Formal, neuropsychologically oriented assessments revolve around standardized tests (see section V below, and Chapter 4). The best of these measures provide contexts for observing processing skills and strategies that are relatively impaired or spared, supply general indicators of severity and type of disorders, assist in determining levels of functioning vis-à-vis normative expectations, and render information relevant to prognosis. These kinds of assessments typically lack information about where and why performance breaks down, what kinds of everyday communicative difficulties are likely, and what kind of management is most relevant. As such, their relationship to treatment planning is often indirect.

B. Behavioral Assessments

Behavioral assessments include structured observations, interviews, checklists, and questionnaires. They can yield information about the likelihood of everyday communicative and cognitive failures, and how severe and distressing they are, and as such, can help to guide treatment decisions. Behavioral assessments focus on identifying a problem by operationalizing it (e.g., "concentration" = working for 10 minutes on a specific treatment task or social activity, or number of head turns away from a task) and by gathering information from various observers about its frequency, consistency, and disruptiveness in a variety of situations.

C. Task Analysis and Other Nonstandard Probe Procedures

Task analysis and other nonstandard probe procedures help clinicians to unravel the nature of performance breakdown and to identify cues and contexts that may facilitate performance, both of which will assist in focusing treatment.

1. Task analysis involves a number of steps:

   a. describing the components of a selected activity or skill, by referring to current theory, empirical evidence, and logical analysis to hypothesize its constituent and prerequisite elements (see Chapter 6, section II-E-2 for further guidelines);

     b. developing probe tasks to evaluate which of these component steps
or processes the patient does well, and which create difficulty;

     c. analyzing which of the potential sources of difficulty appear to inter-
fere most with performance, might be fundamental to other activities or components of activities, are most bothersome, and/or can be
remediated relatively quickly. These can become intermediate or
prerequisite treatment goals, to be achieved on the way to a longer-
range goal of performing the targeted activity.

  2. Other nonstandard probes are designed to identify performance
facilitating factors, by manipulating parameters expected to affect
task familiarity, difficulty, and/or demands on mental resources.
These kinds of manipulations are discussed liberally in later chapters (see Chapter 4; Chapter 6, section III-A; and Chapter 7).

V. ASSESSING THE ASSESSMENTS

A. Conceptual Foundations

Because clinical practice cannot wait for exhaustive theory development, and because the development of adequate assessment instruments
requires years of intensive effort, our neuropsychologically oriented
assessment measures are usually only peripherally related to contemporary theories of cognition. This problem is particularly acute for RHD
patients, because hypotheses about the nature of their communicative
deficits have only recently been proposed. None of the existing positions has been articulated sufficiently to achieve the status of a theory
or a model, and none has been tested to determine its potential utility.
Consequently, the standardized instruments that are available are, for
the most part, independent of current views about cognitive-communicative function in RHD.

B. Psychometric Principles and Test Interpretation

How confident can we be that our assessments measure what we expect?
How consistently do they allow us to measure functions of interest? The
answers to these questions depend in large part on the validity and reliability of the assessments.

  1. *Validity* refers to the "truth" of measurement. Perhaps the definition
of validity is best illustrated with the following question: Are we
measuring what we think we are measuring? Test manuals should

document the extent to which the test items measure the construct or domain of interest and should provide evidence that the construct of interest is indeed being tapped by the measure. For instance, if we want to assess attention, we do not want to use a purported test of attention that measures problem solving, or general intellectual ability, instead.

Many of us assume that, once documented, validity is an inherent and invariant property of tests and measurements. But, the term applies better to the inferences that we derive from these measurements: the conclusions we wish to draw, the nature of the individuals we tested, and the procedures we followed all influence claims of validity. The validity of a measure will also depend, in part, on the fit between the developer's and the user's definitions and assumptions. If, for example, a measure is designed to provide an overall index of attention, but the tester embraces a cognitive theory that fractionates attentional capacities and processes, the measure will not be a valid assessment from the tester's point of view.

2. *Reliability* refers to the stability, consistency, or repeatability of measurement. Chapter 1 referred to tester or observer reliability (interjudge and intrajudge) in discussing the difficulty of quantifying subjective phenomena like aprosodia and flat affect. Interjudge reliability helps to guard against idiosyncratic scoring or unintended bias; intrajudge reliability is critical to ensure that changes in a rater's criteria or judgments (sometimes known as "observer drift") are not interpreted as changes effected in treatment. Test-retest, or parallel forms, reliability is also crucial for the same reason: We want changes in scores to reflect the patient, not the instability of the test. If the measure itself is not stable, we cannot be confident in the data that it generates: item or subtest scores, severity estimates, behavioral or classification profiles. Standardized procedures, operationalized scoring criteria, and carefully selected items help to maximize measurement reliability.

3. Several important aspects of *interpreting reliability data* are covered briefly below.

   a. Correlation coefficients are often used as evidence of reliability. But two sets of scores can be highly correlated without being consistent: A high correlation simply means that the relative ordering of individual scores from high to low is consistent across testers, test forms, or occasions. Point-to-point agreement is a better measure of tester (or observer) reliability. Each observation or score is compared with the observation or score for the same item, which has been generated independently by the other observer, or at a later date by the same observer. Then agreement ratios are computed. For each summary score that is to be interpreted, the number of scoring agreements is divided by the number of agreements plus disagreements. Tester reliability is usually considered acceptable if point-to-point agreement exceeds .80 for each interpreted score.

Though point-to-point agreement data are rarely used to assess test reliability, it would be possible to do so. When correlational data are provided for reliability assessment, significance tests for differences between mean scores provide important supplemental data for determining whether correlated scores are statistically "equivalent" or consistent (at the level of subtests or overall means).

b. Another valuable concept in the interpretation of reliability is standard error. Standard error reflects the precision of specific statistics (means, medians, correlations, proportions, differences between means, etc.) by estimating the random fluctuations that would be obtained if they were derived on repeated occasions. Relatedly, a statistic called the standard error of measurement estimates the consistency with which particular tests would measure performance on repeated administrations. The larger the standard error relative to the magnitude of the obtained scores, the more difficult it is to tell whether any one score is truly different from some other score (e.g.,whether there is a change after treatment). When assessing whether a change is clinically meaningful, we must remember first to account for the variability that can be attributed to unreliability.

c. Finally, reliability is necessary for, but does not guarantee, validity. By way of example, a scale that is consistently off by one-half pound is a stable measure, but it is not a valid one.

C. Standardized Versus Nonstandardized Measures

1. Most formal, standardized measures provide some evidence of validity and reliability and describe established procedures that enhance our confidence in the results when we administer them. But generally, standardized instruments are not developed to provide opportunities to test potential strategies for facilitating performance, do not allow detailed probing into functions presumed to underlie impaired performance, do not reveal daily life problems and concerns, and are not sufficiently sensitive to detect changes in behaviors or processes targeted in treatment. In addition, most standardized tests are lengthy to administer. Accordingly, clinicians often modify standardized instruments or supplement them with special-purpose nonstandard observations and probes.

2. There are pitfalls to modifying standardized instruments: most importantly, the reliability, validity, and normative data will not apply. When the intent of assessment is to gather baseline data or to document progress, clinicians should probably complete a test as designed. When we do use modified instruments or informal measures, we should aim to maximize their reliability and validity.

3. We can maximize the reliability of nonstandard measures by:

    a. generating, and adhering to, administration and scoring procedures that are well-specified, clearly operationalized, and consistent;

    b. including as many items as feasible to tap the content domain of interest;

    c. administering the measure at least two times prior to implementing treatment, to estimate test-retest stability; and

    d. examining the consistency of administration and scoring, with assessments of intrajudge (same observer) and interjudge (different observers, working independently) agreement.

4. We can provide preliminary evidence for content and construct validity by computing an index of internal consistency (such as Cronbach's alpha; see Nunnally, 1978) that indicates the extent to which the items "hold together" to form a coherent indicator of a single construct (.80 is usually considered acceptable), and by generating rational arguments about the nature of the construct that the probe is measuring. If we establish and follow well-specified procedures like these, we will be better able to compare performance across patients, and within patients over time.

CHAPTER

4

Appraisal/Evaluation: Procedures and Data

I. GENERAL CLINICAL CHALLENGES

A. Limitations of Tests and Measures

It has been noted that few measures are targeted for assessing cognitive-communicative performance in RHD adults. Those that are available tend to have only a tangential relationship to current theories about cognition and right hemisphere function, are generally psychometrically weak, and are usually standardized on very small patient samples (section III-A, below). In large part, clinicians are left to their own devices to develop behavioral probes and improvised measures of RHD functioning. When developing such tools, we should bear in mind the recommendations in the last chapter for maximizing reliability and validity of nonstandard measures (Chapter 3, V-C).

B. Questions of Professional Expertise and Test Application

1. Other, more specialized tests that are appropriate for assessing RHD adults tap domains such as attention and perceptual function, areas that transcend the traditional "communication" or "language" realm of speech-language pathology expertise. Many of these areas have been claimed as the province of neuropsychologists, neurophysiologists, and/or occupational therapists (see Chapter 8, section II-A, for a discussion of these and other members of the rehabilitation team). Speech-language clinicians need to walk a fine line in deciding what tests and measures they should administer in their assessments of RHD adults. But the answer to the dilemma of which tests to give is not to be found in something as simple as "professional boundaries." Some speech-language pathologists have particular training and expertise in nonlanguage cognition, while some neuropsychologists are especially well versed in language theory and evaluation.

2. One answer to the question about who can give what tests is that it depends on a mix of factors, including expertise, training, and working environment. In terms of working environment, when a speech-language clinician enjoys a position in a hospital or rehabilitation center staffed by expert members of other disciplines, that clinician has the luxury of consulting with other professionals to determine how best to cooperate and collaborate in evaluating any patient. For instance, a neurophysiologist could assess sustained attention with evoked potentials, a neuropsychologist could administer a standard test of sustained attention, and a speech-language pathologist could assess sustained attention for communicative tasks behaviorally or could gather data from an experimental paradigm (e.g., Rizzo & Robin, 1990, discussed below). In this kind of environment, both interest and special expertise will determine who carries out these sorts of overlapping assessments. In any case, cross-disciplinary cooperation and communication in the work setting are crucial so that each patient receives the most appropriate care and so that no one steps on any other professional's toes. The situation is more complicated when speech-language clinicians are not in a position to refer patients to other professionals. In such cases, when the patient's profile warrants it, speech-language clinicians will need to take on nontraditional evaluation tasks, within the limits of their training and expertise.

3. In most cases it is quite simple to pick up a manual and administer a test. But skilled test analysis and interpretation require a working familiarity with pertinent theories and constructs, expert observational abilities, and attention to behavioral nuances that can supply critical clues suggesting to the astute diagnostician how to follow up with other probes and measures. Plainly, the more formal training and clinical experience one has administering and interpreting specific tests or related assessments, the better. Ethics should restrain those in any discipline from dabbling in areas for which they do not have appropriate training and expertise.

4. Regarding who should administer and interpret specific tests, it is possible to conceptualize published instruments along a continuum with respect to the need for specialized training and expertise. By virtue of explicit requirements for training, tests such as the Porch Index of Communicative Ability (PICA) (Porch, 1981) specify who should administer and interpret them. General neuropsychological batteries like the Wechsler Adult Intelligence Scale-Revised (Wechsler, 1981) and the Illinois Test of Psycholinguistic Abilities (Kirk, McCarthy, & Kirk, 1968) fall toward the "high" end of the continuum in terms of amount and type of training and experience required for valid administration and interpretation. Other tests, such as the Behavioural Inattention Test (Wilson et al., 1987), are designed to be easy to administer, score, and interpret, regardless of discipline and without specialized training; and demographic estimates of premorbid intelligence can be generated by anyone who has access to the data. Somewhere in the middle are tests like the Wechsler Memory Scale-Revised (Wechsler, 1987), that speech-language pathologists should not try to interpret without receiving training from appropriate experts, either during their academic work, or in continuing education. Clinicians should consult test manuals for information about tester qualifications and then abide by the stated requirements. When such information is not provided, clinicians must consult their own consciences to decide if they are sufficiently knowledgeable to administer and interpret a particular test or procedure.

C. Potential Confounds and the Unfolding Assessment

In any cognitive-communicative assessment, we must keep in mind that effective task performance can depend in large part on the accuracy and efficiency of the primary skills, or basic building blocks, associated with its completion. To take an obvious example, we would not say that a blind man was aphasic (or visually agnosic) simply because he failed items on an aphasia test. Similarly, even when a test is designated as a measure of some form of attention, patients may fail that test for reasons other than attentional ones. For instance, normal changes in sensation, perception, and speed of processing that are associated with advancing age can deprive higher-level cognitive operations of accurate and timely input and of processing resources. Such normative changes can interact with and exacerbate those due to a stroke. Premorbid factors such as poor literacy or reasoning skills will also confound certain kinds of assessments. Lower-level stroke-related deficits, such as problems with sustained attention or spatial perception, can impair performance on higher-level abstraction and inferencing tasks; and time pressure together with demands to coordinate many simultaneous processes may strain higher-level cognitive skills such as abstraction and inferencing. To isolate the nature of a patient's difficulty on any evaluation task, clinicians should try to identify component steps, skills, and processes by referring to published literature and rigorous logical analysis (for more information on this process, see Chapter 6, section II-E-2). Then as necessary when the evaluation unfolds, clinicians can assess the accuracy and efficiency of those component operations to pinpoint sources of difficulty and to identify strengths and weaknesses that will contribute to the process of focusing treatment. The well-prepared diagnostician keeps task components in mind while administering a test or procedure and can follow up shortly thereafter with focused probes or supplemental tests to evaluate hypotheses about where and why a patient is having trouble.

D. Attributions of Abnormality

For many of the cognitive-communicative abilities that appear to be compromised by RHD, the range of normal performance is unspecified, and potentially vast. Pragmatic skills, interpretation and production of discourse, conversational content and style; all of these are shaped by numerous sociocultural and individual experiences and expectations. Some pragmatic and discourse functions appear to change with the normal aging process as well. Thus, clinicians should exercise caution in designating individual communication signals or behaviors as abnormal or inappropriate. Identifying the existence and severity of a "problem" in these areas may require thorough exploration and discussion with the patients and those close to them, to determine which behaviors are new or atypical since the stroke, and which appear to create social, cognitive, and communicative barriers.

II. THE APPRAISAL PROCESS

Appraisal involves collecting medical, biographical, and communicative/perceptual/cognitive performance data that will lead to diagnosis, prognosis, and treatment planning (as noted in Chapters 3, 5, and 6; see Table 4–1 for some relevant medical and biographical factors). In an inpatient setting, appraisal is usually initiated after receiving a consult, or a request to evaluate a patient, from the responsible physician; clinicians can often request consults from physicians as well. In an outpatient setting, appraisal may be initiated at the request of patients, their friends, their families, or other professionals. A brief overview of appraisal steps and procedures is provided below.

Table 4–1. Medical and biographical appraisal data

Medical Data

Present cause, complete diagnosis, previous episodes, coexisting neurologic and major medical problems, lesion size and location

Vision (acuity, fields, perception, neglect), hearing (acuity and discrimination), mental status, neurologist's estimate of severity and type of language and cognitive impairment (e.g., neglect, anosognosia)

Reflexes, limb involvement, sensory deficits, gait impairment, signs of brainstem or cerebellar involvement

Laboratory findings, medications (type, dosage, duration, effects)

Rehabilitation assessments or treatments, planned or received

Biographical Data

Name, address, contact person, birthdate, education, marital status, gender, ethnicity

Age at onset, date of onset, institution(s) with prior records

Premorbid and present status for: handedness, occupation, living environment, general health, special skills and interests, language usage, motivation, awareness, cooperation, other personality characteristics

Familial left-handedness for first-order relatives

Premorbid communicativeness, intelligence, languages used

Pre-existing speech, language, cognitive, or learning deficits

Social support, cooperation of persons in living environment

Source: Adapted from Wertz (1985).

A. The Record Review

Whenever possible, the clinician's first step should be to obtain and consult available records, to collect pertinent medical and biographical information. This information provides a framework of expectations about the nature of a patient's cognitive/communicative deficits and premorbid abilities, and knowledge against which to check the patient's self-awareness and response accuracy.

B. Initial Contacts and Impressions

1. If the patient is hospitalized, a bedside screening visit allows opportunities for patient and clinician to get acquainted and for the clinician to make informal observations that can guide further evaluation when it is deemed necessary. During the visit, the clinician should make mental notes about areas that may require structured or formal assessment, such as general awareness, apparent ability to sustain attention and resist distraction, impulsivity, awareness and understanding of deficits, error recognition and correction, other spontaneous or elicited strategy use, amount and appropriateness of communication and social interaction, and specific pragmatic skills outlined in Chapter 2. For an outpatient, these kinds of observations can be made while conversing with the patient (and family) about their reasons for coming to the clinic and while taking case history information. It may be informative to conduct at least part of the initial session with patient and family member together so that interactional patterns and skills can be observed.

2. Early on, it is also useful to gather other types of information through patient and family interviews, questionnaires, or inventories (see Table 4–2 for types of information to obtain). As outlined in Chapter 3, knowledge of abilities, histories, personalities, needs, complaints, and goals should bear on selection of specific evaluation contexts and tasks, attribution of deficit, determination of severity, estimates of prognosis, and focus of treatment. In addition, these same types of information can contribute to selecting generalization probe tasks for evaluating treatment outcomes (see Chapter 6, section III-A-2-b). It is important to obtain this kind of information for patients at all levels of severity, but in particular, patients who are mildly affected, and who are aware of their problems, may report

Table 4–2. Information to obtain in early patient/family contacts[a]

1. Patient's premorbid communication abilities, interests, and style; personality characteristics; learning and coping strategies: to estimate pre-stroke baselines against which to judge current and future predicted cognitive and behavioral functioning, and to select evaluation contexts, tasks, and/or methods.

2. Patient's communication needs in a variety of contexts (current and projected work skills, social/leisure activities, living environment): to identify behaviors, skills, and contexts that would have high priority in assessment and direct patient management, and to select functional outcomes. Assessment might cover, for example, typical communication partners and situations; types and complexities of messages to be processed in typical contexts; family and social roles.

3. Patient's and family members' complaints, concerns, and rehabilitation goals: to identify behaviors and skills that would have a high priority in assessment and management, and/or in counseling and family instruction.

4. Patient's activities, family context, educational and occupational background, and other life history: to identify topics with high knowledge, interest and relevance for assessment and treatment.

[a] Much of this information can be gathered in cooperation with other members of an interdisciplinary rehabilitation team (see Chapter 8, II- A).

difficulties in a structured interview situation that would go undetected in standardized testing.

C. Formal Contacts and Structured Evaluation

If further evaluation is warranted, formal contacts are scheduled. The clinician should quickly complete the process of gathering case history and interview data, and continue qualitative and behavioral observations throughout the formal evaluation period (see section IV, below). The principal goals of formal assessment are to evaluate communication strengths, weaknesses, and needs, and when impairments are identified, to probe potentially contributing communicative, perceptual, and cognitive factors. Specific tests, tools, and procedures for formal evaluation are outlined in section III, below. It is also important to assess the integrity of prerequisite skills and abilities (e.g., auditory and visual acuity and perceptual functions) that are necessary for performing the assessment tasks of interest. Along with the kinds of information from Table 4–2, an estimate of premorbid intellectual function, generated from demographic data (e.g., Barona, Reynolds, & Chastain, 1984; Wilson, Rosenbaum, & Brown, 1979) or from performance on the National Adult Reading Test (Nelson, 1982) may provide a benchmark for selecting evaluation and treatment materials that are likely to have been within the patient's capacity before the stroke.

III. TESTS, TOOLS, AND PROCEDURES

After some overall measures are described, this section considers assessment tools and procedures following the organization established in Chapter 2, the symptom review. The overall measures, and some of the pragmatic assessments (III-B) are discussed in a fair amount of detail. However, page limitations prevent in-depth discussion and analysis of many of the other measures. To gather the best available information on tasks and measures that they are considering, readers are urged to consult the original references, compendiums of assessment tools (e.g., Lezak, 1983; Spreen & Strauss, 1991), and other sources of normative data and psychometric properties.

A. Generalized Measures of RHD Function

This section describes and evaluates the few published tools that focus on cognitive-communicative deficits of RHD adults. In preview, test development and standardization are inadequate in most cases. Standardization samples are typically quite small. It is usually impossible to determine what subset(s) of RHD patients the norms would apply to, because pertinent medical, sociodemographic, and cognitive characteristics are not described or are not related to test performance. The manuals for a number of these tools claim adequate validity and reliability, but inspection of the evidence often raises questions about these claims. Clinicians need to evaluate the nature and quality of the evidence provided to support psychometric adequacy of any instrument, whether commercially available or advocated in professional seminars and publications. We must remain cautious about the conclusions we draw from poorly developed tools.

1. The *Right Hemisphere Language Battery* (RHLB) (Bryan, 1989) consists of 7 subtests: metaphor-picture matching, written metaphor choice, inferred meaning comprehension, humor appreciation, lexical semantic recognition, emphatic stress production, and discourse production (for which 11 parameters are rated on 5-point scales). Examiners are instructed to note changes in emotional sensitivity and other common problem behaviors throughout the test session.

The RHLB manual reviews some of the major consequences of RHD and some evidence for right hemisphere language processing capacities. It also describes the test and provides administration and scoring instructions along with a brief summary of background research. Some information is given on test interpretation and applications. One appendix provides the rating scales for scoring the discourse sample, and another appendix contains a table for converting individual subtest scores to T scores (normalized, standardized scores ranging from 0–100, to allow comparisons across individuals and subtests).

Standardization data (means and standard deviations) are summarized for 30 non-neurologically impaired hospitalized control subjects, 40 patients with (presumably unilateral) RHD, and 40 with LHD and aphasia. Each brain-damaged group consisted of 30 patients with vascular etiologies, and 10 with unspecified nonvascular etiologies. Subjects were described very generally as being between 20–80 years of age, without history of hearing loss, and matched across groups for social background. The manual does not provide details about these characteristics, so it is difficult to generalize the normative data. Gender distribution is identified as 18 males and 12 females in each group, leaving the sex of 10 subjects unaccounted for in each brain-damaged sample. The RHD subjects made more errors on all tests than did control subjects. No performance breakdown is provided along the lines of age, education, etiology, or gender.

Data on the psychometric properties of the RHLB are sparse. Construct, concurrent/discriminative, and predictive validity are not addressed. The author partially addresses content validity by relating subtest selection, in a general way, to a selective literature review. However, the test areas sample very narrowly from the content domains that are included. Potential problems are evident with the content that is included in many of the subtests as well. For example, the metaphoric stimuli are not equated (or analyzed) for familiarity, syntactic structure, or cues provided in the associated linguistic contexts. Cultural differences in lexical use may also influence performance (e.g., "green fingers" is used in the test for what United States speakers refer to as "a green thumb"). The inferred meaning subtest mixes various types of inferences with presumably different processing demands, provides no criteria for determining the accuracy of a response to an inference question, and makes no provision for scoring partially correct or related inferences which frequently characterize RHD patients' performance. For the subtest requiring production of emphatic stress, there is no validation or verification of the "correct" answer; more than one stress placement seems possible on a number of items. In addition, there is too little control over the discourse production task, as sampling procedures are entirely unspecified. Different types of discourse samples are likely to lead to different patterns of results. Poor control over sampling context and procedures leads to another problem as well: Some of the parameters to be rated (e.g., humor) simply may not have occurred in the sample obtained.

Reliability data are mostly lacking. There are no data provided on intrajudge scoring reliability. Interjudge reliability data were reported only for the discourse subtest, and only as a correlation coefficient (recall caveat from Chapter 3). It is doubtful that independent raters could achieve high point-to-point agreement for the discourse evaluation parameters, because the scores to be assigned are imprecisely defined (e.g., "reduction in questioning due to aphasia"; "reduction in prosody that is compatible with aphasia").

Some test-retest data are provided, for brain-damaged subjects only. The brain-damaged subjects were tested initially between 1 and 6 weeks post-onset, and 79% were retested 14–20 weeks later. (There is no indication of whether patients received treatment in the interim). Paired t-tests for the RHD group indicated significant differences from the first to the second test, only for the lexical semantic test and discourse analysis. On the basis of these data and correlation coefficients ranging from .62 to .83, Bryan claims adequate test-retest reliability for RHD subjects. Standard error data are not provided. The fact that performance was stable on most subtests between 1 month and 4 or more months post-onset leads to questions about test sensitivity: Patients should have been improving spontaneously (or as a result of treatment) during that time interval.

2. The *Mini Inventory of Right Brain Injury* (MIRBI) (Pimental & Kingsbury, 1989) is a 27-item screening tool. The authors indicate that it can be used to identify adults exhibiting deficits in areas typically compromised by RHD, determine relative severity of damage, identify specific deficit areas, catalog strengths and weaknesses that may provide the basis for treatment goals, document progress in treatment, and serve a measurement function for research.

The MIRBI consists of 10 subsections, 8 of which are measured with 3 or fewer items. The subsections are identified as (a) visual scanning; (b) integrity of gnosis; (c) integrity of body image/body schema: examiner observing patient for signs of neglect; (d) visuoverbal processing: oral reading and reading comprehension, spontaneous writing and writing to dictation; (e) visuosymbolic processing: performing "serial 7s"; (f) integrity of praxis: drawing a clock and indicating a specific time; (g) affective language: repeating a neutral sentence in a happy and then a sad voice; (h) higher level language skills: understanding and interpreting humorous statements and conversation; explaining incongruities, absurdities, figurative language, and similarities; (i) emotion and affect processing: examiner observing patient for flat affect; (j) general behavior and psychic integrity: examiner observing patient for impulsivity, distractibility, and poor eye contact.

The test manual provides a rationale and overview for the MIRBI, instructions for administering and scoring the test, a section on interpreting results, and information on test development and standardization. Performance can be recorded on summary and profile sheets. In addition to total scores, four other types of scores can be generated: a RHD versus LHD differentiation subscale score, which reflects performance on 10 individual items chosen for their ability to differentiate the brain-damaged standardization groups; a percent correct per subsection score; a percent correct for the total test; and an overall severity rating, which links category labels (profound to normal) to specified ranges of total scores.

The 27-item MIRBI was developed after analyzing the performance of 50 RHD adults on a 63-item MIRBI. The 27 items were those that were failed by 54–98% of this 50-person RHD sample. The current test was standardized on 30 subjects with RHD (presumably unilateral, and more than 25% of whom had subcortical damage), 13 LHD aphasic subjects, and 30 normal controls matched for age, sex, and education with the RHD group. Samples were characterized, by mean scores only, for age, education, and days post onset; and by frequency of gender, race, and lesion site characteristics. Mean MIRBI total scores are provided for each group (without any indication of variance), and correlations are reported between MIRBI total scores and age, education, and time post-onset. All control subjects scored between 38 and 43, and a cutoff score of 38 yields 99.97% diagnostic accuracy for classifying normal versus brain-damaged subjects.

More psychometric detail is provided for the MIRBI than for the RHLB, but the MIRBI is lacking in important respects, particularly in terms of validity. Content validity is claimed by appeal to a limited literature review. But a screening measure simply cannot sample broadly from a content domain, and any instrument with so few items in each subtest cannot be valid for a number of the purposes identified by the authors. The evaluation of construct validity is rudimentary. The underlying construct evaluated was "presence of right brain injury," a coarse anatomical designation rather than a theoretical or psychological construct. The authors argue that construct validity is partially demonstrated by the fact that MIRBI total scores are strongly related to the presence of a lesion on a CT scan, and by the finding that some items allow differentiation of LHD and RHD subjects, for whom hemisphere of lesion is verified by CT scans. Arguments for concurrent validity are also, based on the association of total scores or Right-Left Differentiation scores with either the presence or the hemisphere of lesion documented on CT scans, again a gross anatomic criterion. Predictive validity is not addressed.

Reliability for MIRBI total scores was assessed in terms of internal consistency, interrater reliability, and standard error of measurement. Internal consistency is high, indicating a strong intercorrelation among items, but the other reliability indices are problematic. Interrater reliability was reported for only 4 subjects, in the form of correlation coefficients across the 27 items (all correlations below .90). The standard error of measurement was provided for total scores only, for subjects in 10-year age bands between 20–90, and ranged from 0 to 5.5 for the RHD group. One wonders whether the "0"'s reflect some empty age bands: stratifying small samples of subjects (e.g., 30 RHD) into seven age bands must leave very few in each group, but the numbers in each age range are not provided. There is no reliability information for the other derived scores, and intrascorer and test-retest reliability are not addressed.

3. The *Rehabilitation Institute of Chicago Evaluation of Communication Problems in Right Hemisphere Dysfunction* (RICE) (Burns, Halper, & Mogil, 1985) was originally marketed in 1985 as the first comprehensive evaluation for RHD patients. Its five sections focus on general behavioral patterns, visual scanning and tracking, assessment and analysis of writing errors, assessment of pragmatic communication violations, and metaphorical language.

The original assessment was not standardized, and provided no specific administration or rating instructions, no normative information, and no reliability or validity data. For these reasons, the

RICE has been recommended as a source of ideas rather than a formal test. In a recent conference presentation, Halper and Cherney (1991) provided preliminary data on the internal consistency of the major sections of the RICE, along with minor modifications of content, instructions, and scoring for most sections. Operational definitions and procedural instructions remain underspecified. Psychometric studies of a revised RICE (RICE-2) (Halper, Burns, Cherney, & Mogil, 1991) are reportedly underway, but much more development is needed before this instrument can be used confidently to measure communicative abilities in RHD patients.

4. Available at nominal cost from the New York University (NYU) Medical Center Institute of Rehabilitation Medicine is a compendium of normative data on a variety of standardized and experimental tools (Gordon et al., 1984). Norms are provided for tests and evaluation procedures that are organized into seven sections:

   a. visual scanning deficits and visual inattention, assessed with cancellation and line bisection tasks, Raven's Coloured Progressive Matrices, and a test for subtle inattention deficits. For the last two measures, norms are provided for overall scores and for bias scores that reflect the extent to which subjects ignore one side of the page in choosing responses.

   b. basic activities of daily living, evaluated with simple arithmetic, address copying, oral word reading and scanning, and reading comprehension tasks.

   c. sensory-motor integration, assessed with tasks involving response to double simultaneous stimulation, estimate of body midline, and manual dexterity and coordination measures.

   d. perceptual (visual) integration, assessed with tests of facial recognition, figure-ground discrimination, visual memory span, and visual stimulus reproduction.

   e. higher cognitive and perceptual functions, measured by the verbal and performance subtests from the original Wechsler Adult Intelligence Scale (WAIS) (Wechsler, 1955).

   f. language and cognitive flexibility, evaluated with conceptual analogies for verbal abstract reasoning, word fluency tasks, a version of the Token Test, and immediate story retelling.

g. evaluation of affect state, assessed through affect adjective checklist, depression inventories, and tasks requiring comprehension and discrimination of emotional prosody and facial affect interpretation.

Some of the measures included in the manual are standardized, formal tests, and others are research procedures. The authors do not evaluate or describe the psychometric adequacy of the original measures; that is left up to the user. The manual does provide information on the utility of each test or procedure, a brief description of the measure and its reference citation, special administration and scoring instructions, and normative data.

A total sample of 385 RHD patients is described in the publication. They were predominantly NYU Medical Center inpatients; all had suffered unilateral right hemisphere CVA. On average, the sample was 65 years of age and had a high school education. Males and females were represented approximately equally. Initial testing was conducted on average 10 weeks after CVA onset. Different subsets of these 385 subjects provided norms for each test or procedure. Each set of norms indicates the number of subjects on which it was based, along with data about age, education, sex, visual field impairment, and time post-onset of CVA for that subsample.

Norms are stratified for age, extent of visual field deficit, and education when these factors influence performance. Correlations with age and education are typically very small and only occasionally significant, so the most relevant stratification is that for extent of visual field impairment. Norms are provided as raw scores, T scores, and percentiles. Either raw score conversion can be used to interpret individual performance, but T scores are based on a common metric, so performance expressed in T scores can be compared across test domains. Test-retest data (correlation coefficients) based on small samples are available for each procedure in the first 3 sets of measures, and for some of the perceptual and higher cognitive measures. There was typically a 2-month interval between test and retest.

This publication has several strengths, and some shortcomings as well. Generally, the norms in this document are based on much larger samples than those for the published commercial tests or procedures considered above. The norms take into account important subject characteristics like visual field deficits, when samples are large enough to do so. And a wide range of domains is covered, providing clinicians with a valuable source of information in many areas relevant to assessing cognitive and communicative functioning in RHD adults. Among the limitations is the fact that no normative data are provided for normally aging, non-brain-damaged control subjects for the nonstandardized measures. Additionally, many of the standardized measures are now available in revised forms (e.g., the WAIS and the Wechsler Memory Scale, portions of which are included here, have both been revised), and other measures do not reflect current advances in analyzing or understanding performance. Some relatively recent concerns, for example, those involving discourse or language inferencing, are barely represented and only in atheoretical tasks. Despite these limitations, the procedures that are included provide the clinician with a great deal of information about expected performance levels after RHD of varying severity.

5. The *Ross Information Processing Assessment* (RIPA) (Ross, 1986) consists of 10 subtests purported to assess memory (recent, immediate, remote), spatial orientation, orientation to environment, general information recall, problem solving/abstract reasoning, organization, and auditory retention and processing. The early portions of the manual exclusively refer to assessing information processing deficits in persons with closed head injury. However, the section on test development indicates that the RIPA was normed on adults with unilateral RHD as well as closed head injury patients, and some clinicians report using the RIPA with RHD patients. The manual neither indicates the number or characteristics of the RHD adults tested, nor separates RHD from traumatically brain-injured patients in reporting test norms or test-retest data.

Regardless of its population focus, this test is severely limited in terms of validity and reliability. The manual does not define "information processing" or provide a theoretical model of the construct(s) of interest, so it is difficult to assess construct or content validity. Content validity is limited by the fact that all RIPA subtests tap the auditory-verbal domain. There are no data on internal consistency reliability or scorer reliability (either inter- or intrajudge), despite the recommendation to describe responses qualitatively using poorly operationalized diacritical scores. Standardization data are also insufficient.

B. Pragmatics Domain

1. General measures and assessments.

a. The *Pragmatic Protocol* (Prutting & Kirchner, 1987) was introduced in Chapter 2. It was designed as a general index of pragmatic abilities, not as a complete diagnostic procedure. Thirty parameters represent three aspects of communication: verbal, paralinguistic, and nonverbal. The verbal measures include speech acts, topic skills, turn taking, lexical selection/use, and stylistic variations. Paralinguistic aspects include intelligibility and prosodics. The nonverbal dimension focuses on kinesics and proxemics. The examiner rates each parameter after observing the patient in a 15-minute, unstructured conversation.

Parameters are scored as "appropriate" (i.e., having a facilitative or neutral influence on conversation), "inappropriate" (i.e., detracting from the exchange and penalizing the individual), or "no opportunity to observe." When there is no opportunity to observe some parameters, additional samples should be gathered. Behaviors noted as inappropriate should also be examined further to assess their communicative consequences. Interscorer agreement was reported to be high for raters who received 8–10 hours of training with the Pragmatic Protocol and reached a 90% criterion during that training.

b. The *Profile of Communicative Appropriateness* (Penn, 1988), another general index of pragmatic behavior, includes 51 parameters in six areas: response to interlocutor, control of semantic content, cohesion, fluency, sociolinguistic sensitivity, and nonverbal communication. The speech sample to be scored should be 20 minutes long. Though its content is not specified, the sample generally will include conversational (topics of shared interest and reference), narrative (description of onset of communication problems) and procedural discourse components (how to change tire; make cup of tea). Scores are applied using a 5-point "appropriateness" rating scale, along with a category to indicate inability to evaluate a behavior in a particular sample. Ball, Davies, Duckworth, and Middlehurst (1991) reported that interscorer reliability was unacceptably low; this may be due to the poor operation-alization of both the parameters to be rated and the labels at-tached to points along the rating scale.

c.   The *Communicative Effectiveness Index* (Lomas et al., 1989) was designed to measure change in functional communication ability over time in aphasic adults. Significant others rate communication performance for 16 situations, determined in pretesting to be important to family members of aphasic patients. The items focus on basic needs, health threats, life skills, and social needs. Ratings are marked on visual analogue scales, ranging from "not at all able" to "as able as before the stroke." The authors argue that noncomparability among raters using this kind of scale is unimportant, since the measure documents within-patient change using each rater as his or her own control over time. The authors assessed internal reliability, test-retest stability for a chronic aphasia group, and interrater reliability. Evidence for criterion-related validity was gathered by comparison with Western Aphasia Battery and speech questionnaire data, and by analysis of sensitivity to change in performance for an acute, recovering aphasia group. Although the test was not designed or validated for RHD adults, and most of the behaviors that are rated are too low level for RHD patients (e.g., getting someone's attention), the report provides a useful procedural model for interested clinicians.

d.   Gerber and Gurland (1989) described an *Assessment Protocol of Pragmatic Linguistic Skills* to analyze breakdowns in social exchanges between familiar and unfamiliar partners, at the level of conversational turns. The profile focuses on the synergy between pragmatic and linguistic functions in several areas: nature and consequence of breakdowns, partner and speaker resolution strategies (signals for repair and revision attempts), and linguistic and pragmatic behaviors that contribute to successful turn exchanges. Again, the profile was not designed or validated for RHD adults, but it could be used as is, or adapted as necessary to capture other types of breakdowns and repairs, for individual RHD subjects.

e.   Holland's (1980) *Communicative Abilities in Daily Living* (CADL) was designed for aphasic adults, but it too can highlight pragmatic strengths and weaknesses in RHD subjects. The test consists of 68 items that assess performance in several simulated everyday activities (e.g., going to the doctor, going shopping). The items require a variety of pragmatic skills, ranging from using and interpreting speech acts and social conventions, to comprehending humor, idiom, and absurdity, to interpreting verbal and nonverbal context. A 3-point scoring system was designed to capture the adequacy with which a patient gets a message across, regardless of modality or strict linguistic accuracy. Norms are provided for non-brain-damaged and aphasic adults stratified by age, gender, and living environment (home or institution). Evidence documenting the test's validity and reliability is included in the manual.

f. Referential communication tasks, or barrier tasks, can be constructed to elicit information about many of the specific pragmatic abilities considered in Chapter 2. They can be designed as general screening tasks, or to probe further into areas of concern identified with other assessments, such as the Pragmatic Protocol.

   (1) These kinds of activities include at least one sender and receiver. Typically the sender is asked to describe or otherwise transmit a message about some stimulus (e.g., a picture sequence) that is hidden from the receiver's view. The receiver's task depends on the goal of the activity, and may include, for example, guessing what the sender has described, selecting from several choices a representation that is most like what the sender has conveyed, arranging a series of pictures and statements to reflect the description, or duplicating the sender's stimulus in a drawing. The receiver can ask the sender to clarify or elaborate as necessary, varying requests from open-ended (e.g., "What?") to maximally directive ("Say that again?"). To assess whether the sender can infer message adequacy and adapt accordingly from the most open-ended cues, the receiver might simply reveal each response to the sender, rather than request further information. Data can be recorded for a variety of aspects of cooperative performance, including, for example, the accuracy of the receiver's first and subsequent responses to a single message, the numbers and types of receiver requests for more information, the ways in which the sender modifies the message based on feedback from the receiver, and the number of turns or cues needed for the receiver to accomplish the specified task. Presupposition and sensitivity to partner can be inferred by noting factors such as lexical selection, conciseness and relevance of information, and formality, as well as contingent responses and feedback-based adaptations.

(2) The materials and instructions used in this kind of activity can be structured to tap comprehension and production of many pragmatic forms and functions. Consider the following possibilities for assessing the patient in the role of sender. The materials to be conveyed might include humor, emotion, or nonliteral meanings as key elements; could be words or phrases that are distinguished by prosody (e.g., "greenhouse" vs. "green house" or statement vs. question); or could be pitch patterns that are represented as a series of high and low notes on a scale. In each case, the receiver would be given a duplicate stimulus item and several foils, selected to represent the possible confusions that might result if the patient had difficulty conveying the feature of interest. In another modification of this type of task, the patient functioning as sender could be provided with stimulus messages auditorally through a personal headset, rather than (or as a supplement to) the more standard visual stimuli. To tap production and control of specific message types or forms, rules could be designed to limit the ways in which the patient can transmit the information. For example, for emotional material patients might be told that on the initial attempt, they would be restricted to using only vocal inflection or facial expression to convey the stimulus.

(3) To assess whether and how the sender-patient tries to modify a message, a clinician acting as receiver could simulate general or specific misunderstandings whether or not the original message was adequate. In so doing, the clinician-receiver may want to test the patient's awareness of and response to different types of cues that can be used, implicitly or explicitly, to request more information. Among these could be emphatic stress cues ("Did you say greenhouse or green house?") or implicit questions signaled by rising intonation ("You said it has a . . . ?"). Other types of indirect or implicit requests might include the most conventional (e.g., "Can you tell me something else about X?") or some hints that incorporate figurative elements ("That went right over my head"). Nonverbal signs might also be used as implicit requests (e.g., a shrug, or a nonverbal expression of confusion).

(4) With a patient in the receiver role, the clinician-sender can similarly use prosodic cues, emotional information,

nonliteral forms, or different types of speech acts (e.g., direct command to "draw a horizontal line" vs. indirect "can you draw a horizontal line" or "it has a horizontal line") to convey various message stimuli. The clinician-sender can also give vague information purposefully, to elicit requests for clarification and possibly other speech acts.

2. Focused measures and assessments.

a. The preceding paragraphs describe some of the many ways in which referential communication tasks can be structured, and performance documented, to provide some clues about patients' strengths and weaknesses in particular pragmatic areas. As always, failures should be followed up to evaluate the possible source(s) and modifiability of the problem. For example, if the patient as sender does not generate a meaningful change in the message after seeing a receiver's (inaccurate) response, then the patient's ability to adapt to more constrained requests for clarification may be evaluated.

b. Some other possibilities for assessing specific pragmatic areas are noted in Table 4–3, though most of the published measures were not developed for RHD patients or elderly adults. Several tools were mentioned above in the descriptions of RHD evaluation instruments (e.g., the affect assessment section of the NYU battery, section III- A), and some are considered in the next section (III-C) on discourse and conversation. Clinicians can also refer to the research literature (much of which is reviewed by Joanette et al., 1990, or cited in Chapter 2) to develop their own tools. Published studies may help to identify theoretically relevant component steps, skills, or processes that should be tapped in an attempt to unravel the nature of a particular deficit performance (see also Chapter 6, section II-E-c, and Table 6–3). In addition, researchers are often happy to share their stimuli, materials, and ideas with clinicians who request them.

3. As always, informal observations and interviews with family or staff about patients' daily living and social skills can provide valuable information for structuring pragmatic assessments and for designing generalization probes to evaluate the effects of treatment.

C. Discourse/Text Level

1. Discourse processing: Some general concerns.

a. When choosing discourse elicitation procedures and tasks, and when interpreting performance, clinicians need to remain aware

Table 4–3. Some assessment tools for specific pragmatic areas[a,b]

___

Prosody

Seashore Tonal Memory test (Seashore, Lewis, & Saetveit, 1960): Subjects listen to sequences of 3–5 musical tones; after each sequence, they hear another in which one tone differs, and indicate which tone has changed. Performance for 3-note sequences (a) has distinguished RHD and normal control groups, and (b) for RHD subjects, correlates with performance on tasks requiring discrimination and interpretation of speech prosody (Tompkins & Mateer, 1985; Tompkins, 1991a, 1991b). However, overlap among groups is extensive; non-brain-damaged adults who do not consider themselves "musical" also do poorly on this measure.

Tennessee Test of Rhythm and Intonation Patterns (Koike & Asp, 1981): Subjects imitate nonsense syllable stimuli that vary systematically in intonation, stress, and number of syllables. RHD adults with adequate speech motor control do more poorly than normal controls on intonation patterns, having particular difficulty with rapid midstimulus changes of pitch direction (Tucker & Hamby, 1987).

See also Emotion and Nonverbal Communication, below.

Emotion and Nonverbal Communication

Profile of Nonverbal Sensitivity (PONS) (Rosenthal, Hall, DiMatteo, Rogers & Archer, 1979): A standardized recognition test of decontextualized emotional behaviors. Includes 20 different posed affective situations varying in intensity and valence (positive and negative), expressed by one sender through 11 channels: visual (films of face, body from neck down, and entire figure); auditory (randomized spliced or content filtered speech); and all 6 possible paired combinations of visual and auditory. Subjects select responses from a choice of two. Various shortened forms of the PONS have also been developed (see Buck, 1984). One report of PONS assessment indicated that RHD adults are impaired in perceiving emotion from isolated facial, body, and speech channels (Lundgren, Moya, & Benowitz, 1984).

Communication of Affect Receiving Ability Test (CARAT) (Buck, 1976): A 32-item videotape shows 25 different senders' spontaneous reactions while viewing emotionally loaded color slides. Receivers guess from facial/gestural expressions what kind of slide was viewed (scenic, sexual, unpleasant, unusual). Internal consistency and test-retest reliability are reported to be satisfactory. Variations are possible, including adding or substituting information from the content-filtered audio track to the task (Buck, 1984).

Slide-viewing technique (Buck, 1978, 1984): Elicits spontaneous emotional reactions to slides of the types used for the CARAT test. Senders watch and discuss their reactions to these slides, while unknowingly being videotaped. Facial/gestural responses are viewed and judged by receivers who rate pleasantness, type of slide being watched, etc. Receivers' judgments are compared with the type of slide presented and sender's rating of emotional response. RHD adults exhibit less spontaneous expressiveness with this technique than do LHD and control subjects (Buck & Duffy, 1980).

Florida Affect Battery (Blonder et al., 1991): Part 1 includes face discrimination, expression labeling, and matching tasks; Part 2 requires comprehension of emotional and nonemotional prosody; Part 3 involves tasks of matching facial and vocal

(Continued)

___

117

Table 4–3. *Continued*

emotional expressions. RHD patients as a group do less well than control and LHD groups at discriminating faces, facial emotions, question and statement intonation, and emotional prosody; naming emotions conveyed prosodically; matching facial emotions and faces to voices.

Speech Acts

Sections of CADL, pragmatic rating instruments, referential communication tasks, conversational analyses (see Wambaugh, Thompson, Doyle, & Camarata [1991] for an application of McShane's [1980] speech act categories in conversational speech analysis).

Figurative Meanings

Familiar and Novel Language Comprehension protocol (Kempler & Van Lancker, 1986): A 4-choice picture pointing format is used to assess comprehension of spoken familiar phrases (e.g., idioms, proverbs) and novel sentences matched for grammatical structure, length, and word frequency. RHD subjects do better on the novel than the familiar subtest, and aphasic subjects show the reverse pattern.

Gorham Proverb Test (Gorham, 1956): Includes a section for free interpretation of proverbs, with responses scored on a 3-point scale to represent concreteness; and a multiple choice format with foils that provide inaccurate, partially correct, and concrete interpretations. Interrater reliability is reportedly poor, and clinical validity is questioned because increasing difficulty seems to be achieved by decreasing proverb familiarity (Van Lancker, 1990).

California Proverb Test (Delis, Kramer, & Kaplan, 1984): Also uses verbal explication and multiple choice formats, and expands Gorham scoring system to 10 categories for classifying responses. Has similar limitations to the Gorham test (Van Lancker, 1990).

Sensitivity to Listener and Environment

Social Comprehension and Judgment screening test (Sohlberg & Mateer, 1989a): Given open-ended questions about social situations, a patient is asked to explain reasons, actions, consequences, and social appropriateness. A 3-point scale reflects quality of response.

Adult Social Communication rating scale (Hough & Pierce, 1994): A measure of prosocial awareness or conversational style. Scale evaluates communication behaviors in conversational situations, as assessed by a variety of partners. Behaviors are rated in clusters that include skills for initiating and maintaining conversations, dealing with feelings, generating alternatives to aggression, coping with stress, and advanced social conversation and planning skills.

Humor

Linguistic Humor Comprehension measure (Spector, 1990): A research instrument developed for adolescents that describes and analyzes how humor is generated through irregularities or ambiguities in phonological, lexical, morphological, and syntactic elements. Requires metalinguistic judgments: pinpointing source of ambiguity and explaining meanings that could be derived from that ambiguity.

Table 4–3. *Continued*

Other Forms of Inference

Pragmatic rating instruments, referential communication tasks, sections of CADL examining interpretation of verbal and nonverbal context and cause-effect relationships, discourse tasks and conversational analyses (see sections III-B and III-C).

Tests of visuoperceptual and integrative function, and higher-order inferences required for problem solving and reasoning (see Tables 4–7 and 4–9).

[a]For specific tests, some comments are provided about application and interpretation for RHD subjects when this information is available.

[b]For each of these areas, clinicians can also construct, adapt, or use tasks from the research literature (see Chapter 2), being careful to maximize their reliability and validity (see Chapter 3).

of the various types of knowledge and skills that the tasks may tap, and of the ways in which any particular patient's deficits in "supporting" areas, such as attention or perceptual processing, might influence performance. As an example, perceptual deficits can influence the workings of the conceptual level of discourse processing, by providing the conceptual system with wholly or partially inaccurate information about facets of the context in which communication is occurring; information that is critical for activating knowledge and expectations that drive discourse comprehension and production.

    b. Also, as for any test or procedure, unless measures derived from discourse samples are sufficiently stable, they cannot be considered representative or used to assess change. In general, stability increases with the number of utterances and the number of occurrences of the particular behaviors to be coded and analyzed. There are no universally applicable requirements for ensuring the stability of monologic discourse or conversational samples, especially when infrequent behaviors are of interest. In addition to acquiring longer speech samples, clinicians can consider repeated baseline assessments to estimate stability and representativeness of individual samples.

2. Monologic discourse production: Methods and measures.

    a. The selection of specific discourse sampling methods will depend on the type of discourse that is of interest. Cannito et al., (1988) describe various methods for sampling, segmenting and analyzing connected discourse, that are considered briefly below.

(1) Narrative discourse can be elicited through storytelling, storyretelling, and picture or scene narration, each of which can be further subdivided. For example, to elicit discourse through storytelling, a subject can be asked to generate a story about a memorable experience (focused on a personal event, or a high profile historical incident such as the assassination of President Kennedy or the Challenger explosion), or to narrate a story or fable that is familiar from childhood (e.g., Cinderella). Picture narration can involve a single picture, a picture sequence, or an extended videotape stimulus, about which patients are asked to tell a story. Each of these methods places different demands on attention, memory, formulation, and perceptual analysis, and these demands must be kept in mind when results are interpreted.

(2) Each of these elicitation methods also has advantages and disadvantages. When tasks involve picture or scene narration, or telling well-known childhood tales, the examiner retains more knowledge and control over topic and content than when individualized experiences are reported. Story-retelling tasks allow even more control over discourse form and content, facilitating comparisons within and across individuals. They can be tailored, as well, to assess subjects' facility with various kinds of story elements (e.g., syntactic, semantic, episode components). But if the stories are novel and more than a few sentences long, a retelling task can place heavy demands on attentional and working memory resources. Individually generated samples, while difficult to control, have the benefit of tapping overlearned knowledge and interests, potentially maximizing results. Multiple narrative discourse samples, elicited with multiple methods, will help provide a complete picture of patients' abilities, especially since deficits in perceptual, attentional, or memorial domains may confound performance on any single elicitation task.

(3) Procedural discourse is elicited by asking patients to talk about how to do something. Target procedures can be relatively routine or specialized (Ulatowska et al., 1990): routine procedures (e.g., brushing teeth or making a sandwich) are learned early and performed frequently, while specialized procedures (e.g., going bowling or changing a tire) may never be learned or performed. Superstructure elements may vary for relatively simple

and complex procedures (see Table 2–3). When elicitation instructions are general (e.g., "Tell me how to make a sandwich"), clinicians can observe the inclusion and organization of essential and optional elements of the target procedure. Providing more specific instructions (e.g., "Tell me the three most important steps in making a sandwich") allows a window on patients' grasp of selected aspects of the target procedure, in this example the central aspects.

(4) Descriptive discourse is often elicited by presenting subjects with a picture or an object, and asking them to tell everything they can about it. Picture description tasks from standardized aphasia batteries sometimes elicit stories from non-brain-damaged persons, but for brain-damaged adults in particular, these picture description tasks tend to elicit a listing of elements, with little syntactic variation or meaning integration.

b. Methods for segmenting discourse samples also depend on the user's purposes. Cannito et al. (1988) report different segmentation procedures for analyzing sentential surface structure and referential clarity (T-units, or independent clauses plus their associated dependent clauses); superstructure (episodes for narratives, or steps for procedures); and information structure and content (propositions). In another example, Armstrong (1987) segmented samples into clauses for a cohesive harmony analysis, designed to index textual coherence.

c. Similarly, a variety of methods can be used to analyze discourse comprehension and production. Researchers in discourse analysis have developed some sophisticated tools, such as a computer program that is used for propositional and frame analysis (Frederiksen et al., 1990). Several clinically applicable analysis systems are considered next.

d. Analyses of discourse production after RHD.

(1) Joanette and Goulet's (1990) comprehensive narrative analysis system is outlined in Table 2–6 (and an appendix to their chapter lists core propositions identified for their stimulus story). The authors recommended analyzing non-core propositions as well, to assess information that might reflect tangential and irrelevant tendencies in RHD patients.

(2) Sherratt and Penn (1990) also took an integrated approach to discourse analysis, assessing narrative and procedural samples produced by an adult male with a right parietal lesion and a sociodemographically matched control subject. Narrative samples were elicited using single and sequence picture storytelling tasks, and an account of a memorable experience. Procedural descriptions were requested for changing a tire and buying a jacket. Each task was analyzed according to four profiles: subjective evaluation of appropriateness of discourse grammar (superstructure) components, frequency counts of syntactic measures, frequency counts of components that disrupt clarity and continuity, and subjective ratings of organizational skills (see Table 4–4). Sherratt and Penn do not provide operational definitions of the discourse elements that they evaluate, so clinicians interested in applying portions of their system will have to develop working definitions and determine coding and scoring reliability. Clinicians should also remember that even if subjective judgments of this sort can be made reliably, they do not allow us to infer much about the level of impairment or the processes that might contribute to disruption (Frederiksen et al., 1990).

(3) Webster, Godlewski, Hanley, and Sowa (1992) devised a new scoring procedure, that relies in part on retold narratives, to examine discourse comprehension in RHD adults. Because their method was designed to quantify comprehension, it is reported below in the comprehension section (III-C-3-d). However, the propositional analyses conducted on patients' retold narratives are relevant for discourse production assessment as well.

(4) Several authors have examined circumscribed aspects of discourse production, usually in the context of picture description. For example, Myers (1979) distinguished between literal and interpretive concepts produced in picture descriptions; Mackisack et al., (1987) outlined a scoring system to evaluate labeling behavior for explicit and inferred concepts; and Tompkins et al. (1993) operationalized and evaluated some commonly ascribed features of connected speech, including excessive detail, overpersonalization, and value judgment.

(5) The results of this research, considered together, underscore the behavioral heterogeneity of RHD adults.

Table 4–4. Discourse analyses of Sherratt and Penn (1990)

Narrative/Procedural Superstructure (appropriateness ratings)

Narrative: abstract, orientation/setting, complicating action, evaluation, result/resolution, coda

Procedural: introduction/orientation, sequence of steps (essential and optional), target step, coda

Syntactic Measures (frequency counts)

Number of words, T-units, and clauses
Mean words per T-unit and clause; mean clauses per T-unit
Number of ungrammatical, incomplete, and unintelligible utterances

Discourse Clarity Measures (frequency counts)

Empty phrases, indefinite terms, deictic terms
Neologisms, paraphasias, circumlocution
Repeated words, phrases, ideas
Semantic perseveration
Comments on the task, personal value judgments
Intrusive words or phrases
Incorrect reference
Incorrect use of "and"
Inappropriate use of conjunctions
Elliptical error

Organizational Skills Components (appropriateness ratings)

Temporal sequencing
Topic control
Tense use
Relevance

---

e. Analyses of discourse production in other neurologic groups.

(1) Ulatowska and her colleagues have for many years taken an integrated linguistic approach to discourse analysis (e.g., Cannito et al., 1988; Ulatowska et al., 1990), focusing on sentential surface structure, superstructure, informational structure and content, and referential structure and clarity. They have reported results for various types of subjects, including adults with aphasia and Alzheimer's disease, and those without brain damage who are healthy and active. In a useful summary, Cannito et al. describe a variety of discourse elicitation, segmentation, and analysis methods and procedures; provide a priori propositions for

several frequently used elicitation stimuli; and refer the reader to original sources of preliminary normative data on independently living, highly educated and active, elderly adults.

(2) Nicholas and Brookshire (1993a, 1993b) have described sensitive and reliable measures for quantifying discourse content in aphasia that also hold promise for RHD adults. They developed a standard set of elicitation stimuli (single and sequence pictures, procedural requests, requests for personal information) and two measures of connected speech: main concepts (1993a) and correct information units (CIUs) (1993b). A main concepts analysis indicates how accurately and completely a speaker communicates central information, like an analysis of core propositions or essential steps. A CIU analysis assesses informativeness irrespective of importance by indexing the number of words that are intelligible in context and that convey information relevant to the stimulus. Calculated measures of percent of words that are CIUs, and CIUs produced per minute of speech are generally more stable for aphasic adults than are CIU counts. In another important contribution, Brookshire and Nicholas (1994) demonstrated that test-retest stability improved greatly over that for single task samples, when samples from five connected speech tasks were combined for analysis.

f. Each of the reports reviewed above exemplifies analyses that may be useful in assessing discourse production after RHD. Syntactic deficits have not been prominent in this group, suggesting that syntactic measures may not be very informative. Joanette and Goulet's (1990) work in particular reminds us that not all RHD adults will exhibit discourse production impairments.

g. Planning and conducting discourse assessments.

(1) When a discourse processing problem is suspected, one could refer to available models, devise tasks to tap various components, and draw inferences from performance patterns about relatively spared and impaired processes. Table 4–5 provides some examples of possible tasks based on the model of Frederiksen and colleagues. For most clinical purposes, we can focus on analyzing skills that are

Table 4–5. Some tasks for assessing discourse production processes

General Principles

Assessment at any level should initially be open-ended, allowing patients to develop their own approaches and strategies. Then if patients have difficulty, feedback, task structure, or cuing can be provided (from general to specific to step-by-step) to determine their facility when performance is guided and constrained. Structure and cuing help us infer what processes patients are capable of carrying out, by providing adequate input to those processes. It is useful as well to manipulate the speaker's knowledge of the topic and discourse genre, in order to determine whether familiar topics or overlearned forms offer a spared skill base from which to build. At each level, it is also important to observe patients for self-monitoring and repair skills, initiated with and without questions or cues from the examiner.

Conceptual Network Level

1. Generating or retrieving conceptual frames or organizing principles.

   - Examine patients' manipulation of conceptual narrative knowledge using tasks that involve organizing pictures or written propositions. Stimuli can be organized into complete stories, or into smaller subsets of elements that "go together" (e.g., the introduction of the setting and the introduction of the main character).

   - Contrast performance on discourse tasks when elements are provided in conventional narrative or procedural formats, and when they are scrambled or incomplete.

   - Contrast discourse processing measures when a patient is given organized stimuli as opposed to disorganized ones; when given a starter cue (e.g., general or specific thematic information) to assist with accessing a common script or superstructure, as opposed to having to self-start; and with stimuli that are high or low in familiarity.

   - Assess completeness and organization of superstructures produced for different genres or purposes (e.g., to summarize a story, explain a process or element of a story, orient someone to a new topic); or extent to which a patient's comprehension improves when provided with explicit, complete, and organized macrostructure or superstructure information.

2. Elaborating frames with semantic descriptive information (e.g., internal structure of events in the narrative superstructure).

   - As above, plus:

   - Examine number, accuracy, and completeness of elements included in each component of the superstructure; optional or essential elements; and number and pattern of irrelevant elements.

   - Assess performance on tasks of recognizing and correcting irrelevant elements, or event and procedure sequence errors.

(Continued)

Table 4–5. *Continued*

- Assess performance on tasks of recognizing and correcting irrelevant elements, or event and procedure sequence errors.

3. Selecting and prioritizing from specified conceptual structures the information to convey explicitly, and order in which to convey it.

- After providing a patient with a fully elaborated set of story propositions (personal or nonpersonal narrative information) or procedural steps, or a nonverbal demonstration of a complete procedure, have the patient identify those elements that are essential for different listeners or communication purposes (e.g., expert vs. novice listener; familiar vs. unfamiliar communication partner; when theme or topic is familiar or not; when theme or topic is known vs. unknown; when listener's task is to summarize main points vs. repeat as many details as possible).

- Examine patients' presuppositions or beliefs about what their listeners already know, need to know, and/or consider centrally important in situations like those above, by (a) asking patients to state or select from several choices what they think the listener knows and what is essential for the listener to know; and (b) observing patients' sensitivity to these issues in role-playing, barrier task, or conversational interactions.

- After providing ambiguous or implicit forms (e.g., lexical ambiguities; conventionalized indirect requests or other nonliteral forms) in various contexts, assess patients' judgments of contextually relevant and irrelevant interpretations, knowledge of differences between surface and intended meanings, and/or attributions of communicative intention.

Propositional Level

1. Generating propositions sequentially to reflect selection and topicalization from the conceptual network.

- Provided with essential information to be conveyed from situations as given above, ask patient to describe it, arrange it in sequence, or indicate what should come next.

2. Generating propositions to foster coherent local interpretation, whether explicitly based or inferential, on the basis of assumptions about the comprehender's likely inferences and interpretations.

- Construct tasks manipulating (a) expectations of a comprehender's topic or situational knowledge (manipulated either explicitly from information provided by the comprehender or a third party, or implicitly through interactions with partners more or less likely to be familiar with or interested in the topic or situation), or (b) the situations or purposes for communication. Then assess differences in areas such as (1) amount of detail and elaboration provided; (2) use of indicators of shared knowledge; (3) judgments of listener's

Table 4–5. *Continued*

likely inferences and other possible inferences (even inaccurate ones); (4) use of cue phrases that indicate discourse structure, intention, or change of focus (e.g., "by the way;" "that reminds me;" "similarly"); (5) use of other markers of cohesion and coherence, including accuracy and specificity of reference considered against the range of possible available referents; (6) use of intonation and gesture to indicate or infer linguistic boundaries and focus of attention, or to resolve ambiguities.

3. Generating and evaluating logical and macrostructure inferences for longer stretches of the text.

   • As above for longer stretches of the text, and:

   • Examine patients' generation or identification of topic sentences, gists, main characters, central events, title, lesson or moral, and appropriate discourse summaries.

   • Assess patients' use and/or interpretation of macrostructure content to summarize prior information or episodes, to predict upcoming developments, to explain something that has been introduced, or to mark a change in focus or topic.

4. Chunking propositions for optimal linguistic encoding

   • When information is complex, or listener knowledge minimal, assess for a decrease in propositional density (number of propositions per clause).

   • Examine patients' prosodic markings of clauses and phrase structures.

   • Examine patients' alterations in density and prosodic marking when asked for clarification, either explicitly or implicitly.

Language Level

1. Encoding clauses to reflect chunking and topicalization decisions.

   • Examine, for example, the number of clauses between pronoun and referent; or the number and sequence of clauses in which the same information is maintained in topic position.

2. Specifying lexical information in clauses, including anaphora.

   • Assess many of Joanette and Goulet's (1990) formal aspects, and their "cohesive errors" (see Table 2–6).

Source: Based on Frederiksen et al. (1990) model, in Table 2–4.

most likely to contribute to or detract from RHD adults' successful communication via connected speech, such as conveying a reasonable amount of essential information that is appropriate to the situation and the listener.

(2) Brookshire and Nicholas (1993a) note that listeners routinely make sense of a lot of normal disruptions and deviations. Normal speakers digress without giving advance warning, presuppose too much or too little, use vague terms, and have slips of the tongue that result in inaccurate productions; but listeners can often fill in or make corrections without much apparent effort. Based on many previous empirical findings, Brookshire and Nicholas hypothesize that the extent of communication handicap for aphasic adults may vary in large part with the presence and accuracy of main concepts and also perhaps with the extent to which cohesive ties are realized throughout a discourse unit (presumably contributing to overall coherence).

(3) These factors together with pragmatic considerations (e.g., relevance and social appropriateness) are also likely to be important predictors of communicative success and acceptability for RHD adults. A number of elicitation stimuli and procedures have associated with them lists of main ideas, core propositions, or essential information that can be compared with patients' productions (e.g., Cannito et al., 1988; Joanette & Goulet, 1990; Nicholas & Brookshire, 1993a; Webster et al., 1992). Various types of cohesion and coherence analyses have also been described (e.g., Armstrong, 1991; Joanette & Goulet, 1990; Mentis & Prutting, 1991) that index the extent to which speakers integrate information at several levels in discourse production. Relevance can be captured in part by CIU analyses (Nicholas & Brookshire, 1993b), which are not tied to particular elicitation stimuli. It may also be useful to code non-essential or non-core information according to its contextual relevance. Other social discourse factors can be examined using one of the pragmatic tools described earlier in this chapter (section III-B).

3. Discourse comprehension and RHD.

a. Discourse comprehension is typically assessed through free recall, question answering, and/or recognition tasks. These kinds of measures are known as "off-line" or "product-oriented" measures, because they index the end-product of a comprehension task, rather than the emerging structures and component processes that contribute to a final interpretation. They contrast with "on-line" or "process-oriented" measures that are used to try to identify the nature of representations available at different points during comprehension, and the accuracy and timing of component processes that operate on those representations. Such measures include response times to probe words that are related to or included in the test stimuli, and eye fixation durations during reading comprehension. These measures can be difficult to implement and interpret for brain-damaged patients, and there is controversy about their meaning with non-brain-damaged adults; but they can suggest useful hypotheses about the timing and interaction of spared and impaired comprehension processes in brain-damaged adults. Clinicians should be alert for more literature focusing on the contributions of on-line measures to our knowledge about discourse comprehension.

b. In free recall tasks, one can assess a variety of measures of comprehension, such as the number, accuracy, and completeness of propositions recalled (explicit; inferred from text or general knowledge; those that state the key elements that are crucial for generating inferred propositions; core, essential, optional, self-generated; local [closely related to specific propositions in the text] vs. global [those that evaluate, summarize or otherwise augment the explicit text]; those representing different elements of discourse superstructures or conceptual frames; and so forth). Since recall measures often do not reveal all that has been comprehended, they should be supplemented by cued recall or choice recognition tasks, carefully constructed to avoid suggesting the answer through the questions or probes themselves. With brain-damaged patients, it is common to construct paired questions about each explicit or inferred proposition being tested, one to be answered affirmatively and the other negatively, and to give credit for comprehension only when both members of the question pair are answered correctly. If different recognition foils or probe questions are designed to contrast comprehension of various types of information (e.g., explicit vs. inferred, or literal vs. nonliteral), they should be comparable along other important dimensions, such as syntactic complexity and the range of possible reference situations (recall the discussion in Chapter 2, section II-A-4, about pictured representations of literal and nonliteral interpretations).

c. One standardized measure of discourse comprehension is available. It uses a question-answering format, and focuses on distinctions between discourse macrostructure and microstructure, and explicit and implied information.

(1) The *Discourse Comprehension Test* (Brookshire & Nicholas, 1993b) was put forward to assess comprehension and retention of spoken narrative discourse by adults with aphasia, RHD, or traumatic brain injuries. Comprehension is assessed for stimulus stories (two sets of five each) followed by yes/no questions about stated and implied main ideas and details. The test can also be administered to assess silent reading comprehension. The manual indicates clearly what the test is and is not designed to do; it is designed primarily to identify problems that may affect daily life function.

(2) The test was standardized on 40 normals adults, between 55–75 years of age (10 subjects per 5-year interval), and on 20 each with aphasia, RHD, or traumatic brain injury. The aphasic and RHD adults were at least 1 month post-onset of CVA and were matched in age and education with the normal control group. Age and education did not affect brain-damaged subjects' performance on the test. For each group of subjects, means, standard deviations, and ranges are provided for stated and implied main ideas and details, and for an overall score. Cutoff scores specify "normal" performance overall and for each type of comprehension question.

(3) Extensive evidence and arguments are provided to document the test's validity and reliability, although test-retest and standard error data were based on extremely small samples (14 aphasic and 7 RHD adults) and were provided only for overall scores. There are also two particularly noteworthy features of content validation. First, the authors report evidence of acceptable passage dependency, which reflects the extent to which the answers to comprehension questions depend on the information provided in the stimulus rather than general world knowledge. Second, they demonstrate that the content words chosen for the stimulus stories and questions are closely representative, in terms of frequency of word usage, of those found in adult-to-adult conversations. Comprehensive instructions for administration and scoring are provided.

d. As noted in the discourse production section, Webster and colleagues (1992) proposed a new scoring method to capture discourse comprehension of RHD subjects on the Logical Memory subtest of the Wechsler Memory Scale (Wechsler, 1945). For this subtest, subjects retell each of two narrative paragraphs. The original scoring system is based on verbatim recall of bits of information (the surface level of van Dijk & Kintsch, 1983; see Chapter 2, section II-B-3-d). Webster et al. focused on the text level, classifying propositions in each story as essential or nonessential to the plot. Essential propositions contained relational cues needed to establish the theme, plot, and story resolution. Nonessential, or detail propositions, were rated as unnecessary to represent those elements. The authors also scored subjects' responses for intrusions (self-generated propositions that were incompatible with a story proposition, unless explicitly identified by the subject as a tentative assumption). Interjudge agreement for classifying the propositions was adequate. A single prompt was provided to ask for any additional information after immediate retelling, and delayed recall followed 30 minutes later. After delayed recall, cued recall or multiple choice tasks were used to probe specific points.

The RHD group produced fewer detail propositions and more self-generated propositions than controls (though the absolute number of self-generated propositions was small for both groups). Cued recall performance was normal for RHD subjects, indicating that they had encoded the propositions that were omitted from their retold narratives. Two findings underscored the validity of the scoring system: control subjects recalled essential propositions more accurately than detail propositions, and essential propositions were better retained for delayed recall than were detail propositions.

e. Hypotheses about an individual patient's discourse comprehension skills and deficits can be evaluated in part by constructing assessments based on processes presented in discourse models. We can refer again to Table 4–5 for some guidelines:

   (1) In most cases where the sample tasks in that table refer to discourse production outcomes, related measures can be designed to assess the influence of the same task variables on discourse comprehension. Consider the first process at the conceptual level, generating or retrieving conceptual organizing principles. If a patient is consulting his or her knowledge of conceptual discourse frames, then conventional, well-organized, familiar stimulus formats accompanied by thematic cues should be more beneficial than stimuli without those features, for either production or comprehension tasks. Using examples from lower in the model, the influence of propositional density can be assessed on indices of interpretation as well as production, as can the interpretation of prosodic markings of phrase structure and communicative intention.

(2) Many of the discourse comprehension problems associated with RHD (see Chapter 2, II-B-2) can be addressed with tasks like those sketched in Table 4–5. For example, a number of tasks are proposed at Conceptual Level 3 and Propositional Level 2 for evaluating the patient's ability to build integrated comprehension structures by synthesizing knowledge with task context (e.g., resolving ambiguities or discrepancies, revising or suppressing inappropriate or irrelevant interpretations, etc.). Similarly, the table includes many tasks that focus on presupposition or sensitivity to listener knowledge, beliefs, or social variables. It should be noted that a number of these tasks are metalinguistically oriented. However, with some variations, question-answering or recall/recognition tasks could be constructed to assess similar variables. Clinically, we also want to examine whether RHD patients profit from manipulations designed to improve discourse comprehension, such as providing orienting tasks and instructions, introducing themes, heightening semantic redundancy, and increasing textual explicitness.

f. Inferencing is central to text comprehension, as it is often required for coherent interpretation. Because inferencing deficits have been associated with RHD, a number of issues related to the assessment of inference are considered below. This material is lengthy, but it leads logically to hypotheses about assessing and treating various inference processes.

(1) Two major areas of research interest for normal adult comprehenders include the conditions and principles that guide and constrain the encoding of inferences, and the ways in which early (automatic) inferences are used to support further cognitive processing. The first area has received the most attention. A great deal of work has

focused primarily on determining what types or categories of inferences (e.g., causal, script-based, backward looking) are routinely constructed during comprehension. One problem with interpreting much of this research stems from the use of off-line methodologies, which usually cannot distinguish those inferences that a subject generates during the comprehension process from those that are cued at the time of test by the post-task questions or probes. That is, an inference may be suggested by an examiner's question, even if it was not generated as comprehension operations took place.

(2) More recently, using on-line measures, some researchers (e.g., Swinney & Osterhout, 1990) have drawn contrasts based on processing issues rather than inference categories, between inferences that are automatically and immediately derived and those that are not. For example, McKoon and Ratcliff (1992) propose a minimalist hypothesis that delineates the limited conditions under which automatic/routine inferences are made. Unless a comprehender adopts special goals or strategies, the only inferences encoded automatically during reading (and presumably listening) comprehension are: those based on information that is easily available from explicit statements in the text or from general knowledge; and those required for local coherence of parts of the text that are processed concurrently. Local coherence is defined for propositions that are in a working memory buffer at the same time (i.e., those no farther apart than one or two sentences). It is important to understand these automatically encoded inferences, as they provide the first-pass representation of the text information from which more strategic, goal-directed (non-automatic) inferences are constructed. If they operate without appropriate modification in brain-damaged patients, they may contribute to a perception of text-boundedness such as that observed by Frederiksen and Stemmer (1993; see Chapter 2, section II-B-5-c).

(a) The first of McKoon and Ratcliff's conditions is consistent with a number of findings. General knowledge inferences (e.g., what should happen next in a story; attributes of concept meaning; category exemplars) that are not necessary for local coherence are generated during comprehension only if they are very predictable or highly typical. Inferences based on explicit textual information that are routinely drawn during comprehension are those used to establish local coherence, including connections among instances of the same concept, pronominal reference, and perhaps local causal relations.

(b) Local coherence is achieved when a set of two to three sentences can stand alone, or makes sense in combination with easily available general knowledge (e.g., inferring a relation between "the collie" and "the dog"). When neither explicit text information nor general knowledge lead to a coherent local text representation, other processes (such as strategic problem-solving inferences) are engaged to provide local coherence.

(3) Under McKoon and Ratcliff's (1992) two conditions (when information is easily available, or when used to establish local coherence), there are a number of candidates for automatically encoded minimal inferences:

- inferences linking anaphora with antecedents in nearby text
- inferences based on argument overlap and inferences about causal relations for propositions concurrently in working memory
- inferences drawn from overlearned, script-based and schema knowledge or expert knowledge
- general knowledge inferences when highly typical, as above
- perhaps inferences supported by knowledge of argument-taking properties of verbs (e.g., for a statement that lacks an argument, such as "He cleared the papers off," readers infer the missing argument when the information is easily available from prior mention).

(4) Some researchers assert, mostly on the basis of off-line tasks, that comprehenders reliably draw other backward-looking inferences during comprehension, particularly bridging inferences that connect some element from a current proposition or sentence to a representation of prior text. The minimalist prediction for the bridging inferences that do not meet McKoon and Ratcliff's conditions would be that they are constructed by relatively slower, strategic inference processes, but this prediction has not been tested.

(5) Contrasting with these rapidly and automatically generated inferences are inferences that are not required for local coherence, including those that summarize or elaborate on explicitly stated pieces of information (whether forward or backward looking in a text) and forward-looking expectation inferences. Some examples include instrumental inferences that fill in the typical instrument for a verb (e.g., a spoon for the verb "stir"), and predictive inferences about what should happen next. McKoon and Ratcliff report data supporting the minimalist hypothesis for these types of inferences: They are not reliably drawn during the comprehension process unless the two conditions above are met. Similarly, global inferences connecting goals to outcomes, which meet neither condition above, are not automatically generated.

(a) These and other strategic inferences (many types are discussed in Graesser & Bower, 1990) work on the database generated by automatic inferencing processes. Knowing what inferential information is quickly and easily available may thus help to predict to some extent the ease with which associated strategic inferences can be drawn. Strategic inferences are also critically important for language interpretation, problem solving, and learning.

(b) Britton, Van Dusen, Glynn, and Hemphill (1990) trace some of the time and cognitive resource costs that accompany strategic inference generation. Allocating processing capacity to strategic inferencing may deplete or divert resources from other critical comprehension operations. For example, computing strategic inferences may interrupt ongoing processes in a working memory buffer. While an inference is being constructed, the current status of any original process must be maintained until the inference computations are completed; then the original process(es) must be recovered and restarted. Difficulties with any of these interleaved steps might be manifest in comprehension impairments for connected discourse.

(6) Several other factors have been identified that influence the ease and strength with which inferences are encoded. These could be interpreted in McKoon and Ratcliff's perspective, but would have diverted the discussion above and so are added here:

- text internal factors such as the distance between elements needed to construct an inference, or the amount of intervening information (e.g., number of intervening first-mention nouns or propositions that require processing).
- text external factors such as a comprehender's script knowledge or domain expertise; processing perspective (e.g., given instructions to interpret a paragraph about a house and its contents from the perspective of a burglar or a home buyer, comprehenders draw inferences congruent with the assigned perspective); or congruence of the text with the comprehender's affective state (e.g., depressed people selectively process depressing information).

(7) Inferencing problems have often been attributed to RHD adults, but surprisingly little work has been done to document or characterize these presumed deficits. One consistent finding is that most adults with RHD appear to generate highly predictable inferences (e.g., Bloise & Tompkins, 1993; Brownell et al., 1986) though some more severely impaired patients have difficulty re-evaluating them when contradictory information comes along. Frederiksen and Stemmer (1993) also described a RHD patient whose primary discourse difficulties were attributed to problems with reconceptualizing an initial, obvious interpretation.

The results of some other work are consistent with McKoon and Ratcliff's hypothesis as well. For example, providing related prior context information immediately before a target judgment and heightening the semantic redundancy of that context (i.e., keeping readily available in working memory the information on which inferences are to be based) improve the speed and accuracy of inferences drawn from emotional prosody (Tompkins, 1991a, 1991b; Tompkins, Spencer, & Boada, 1994). However, few of the theoretical and empirical distinctions from the normal research literature have been used to structure assessments of inferencing after brain damage.

(8) Given other research indicating that relatively automatic processes are less impaired after brain damage than effortful processes, it is likely that automatic inferences will be easier than the strategic types for RHD adults.

Consistent with this suggestion, Frederiksen and Stemmer's (1993) patient demonstrated relatively intact local/automatic inference processes. It may be important to assess speed and accuracy of automatic inferencing, the foundation from which slower, strategic, goal-directed inferences are generated. Inefficiency in drawing automatic inferences might divert the resources that are available for generating strategic inferences, including those needed to construct an integrated reconceptualization of a text. Strategic inference abilities could be assessed somewhat independently of automatic inferences, by making local coherence links explicit in a stimulus text, reducing the need for automatic inferences. The normal research references cited above describe many possible tasks for examining relatively automatic and strategic inference processes.

(9) Some manipulations to influence the ease or difficulty of inferencing can be derived from this normal literature, including:

- to elicit relatively automatic inferences, make the inference supporting information quickly/easily available from general knowledge or from the text. This might involve providing themes prior to presenting a text; using materials that are highly predictable (e.g., based on well-known scripts) or familiar (e.g., based on a patient's specialized domain knowledge); increasing semantic redundancy to keep relevant information in focus or to increase propositional argument overlap; keeping inference supporting elements in close proximity with few intervening first-mention nouns or propositions. In addition, probes can be developed to focus on inferences that are based on this quickly/easily available knowledge, and/or that are required for local coherence. For example, queries can be related to highly predictable or typical instances or events, local causal relations, and connections between referents/anaphors or instances of same concept.
- for inferences that are typically more strategic (e.g., predictive, global causal, or consequence inferences), first minimize the need for automatic inferences as described above. A patient's performance should be enhanced by explicitly providing or representing in some fashion the key elements on which the inferences

are based. The ease or likelihood of drawing strategic inferences should also be influenced by variations in the factors associated with automatic inferencing in the preceding paragraph (e.g., predictability, typicality, subject knowledge or expertise, degree of redundancy or consistency in the text, and distance or amount of material between inference supporting elements). In addition, it would be informative to examine other factors that should induce particular inferencing strategies. Among these are changing the perspective that a patient is asked to adopt when interpreting a text, either explicitly (e.g., the burglar vs. home buyer example) or implicitly (e.g., inducing a mood through various scenarios, such as imagining oneself as a member of the team that won or lost the World Series).

4. **Conversation evaluation for RHD adults.**

   a. The available literature suggests that some RHD adults will have conversational impairments. The nature of these impairments and some assessment strategies are considered below. (For more information on conversational evaluation, consult Brinton & Fujiki, 1989.)

   b. Topic control difficulties may include problems with:

      (1) engaging a listener's attention to establish a topic.

      (2) orienting listeners to topics, introducing unshared referents, and/or identifying the global connection or relevance of a contribution. Problems in these areas may be due to difficulties taking into account what a listener knows or what has gone on before, or to grasping the "big picture" that establishes global relevance.

      (3) controlling amount and relevance of output, with resultant wandering from the point.

      (4) determining socially and situationally appropriate topics and contributions.

      (5) maintaining a balance between self- and other-oriented topics and contributions.

      (6) giving up a topic or ending a conversation when others are ready.

(7) changing/shading topics prematurely or inappropriately. Topic shading involves a subtle shift of focus from one topic to another with some elements of the new topic related to the first (see Brinton & Fujiki [1989] for criteria). If not realized carefully, topic shading may seem inept (e.g., the "shader" did not recognize the main focus or concern of the conversation) or simply rude (e.g., he or she chose to ignore the main focus). Topic shading is more common in relaxed situations with spouses and close friends, but the juncture at which it occurs and its effects on a listener are important in all contexts. Topic shading may be particularly disruptive if it occurs at a critical point in the development or exploration of the previous topic or if it is used in response to a direct question.

c. Turn-taking difficulties may include problems with:

(1) relinquishing turns and responding to signals suggesting that a conversational partner wants to take a turn.

(2) using or responding to cues that signal intent to yield or maintain speaking turns (appropriate cues include, e.g., lengthy pauses, drop in pitch or loudness, completion of a gesture, and/or establishment of eye contact as signals of intent to yield; averting gaze during pauses to maintain a turn).

(3) inhibiting disruptive interruptions of other speakers.

(4) producing back-channel behaviors that indicate interest and involvement in the exchange (e.g., nodding to signal attentiveness or agreement).

d. Conversational repair problems may include:

(1) difficulty responding to various forms of implicit or explicit requests for clarification or elaboration.

(2) difficulty adjusting according to the perception of the trouble source motivating the request (e.g., whether a requester fails to hear, to attend, or to understand the identity of a referent or the relevance of a contribution).

e. A clinician can form initial impressions of a patient's facility with parameters like those outlined above by observing the patient conversing with different partners about various topics. Interviews of family members or other significant conversational partners should also help to point up particularly disruptive behaviors and to identify those that reflect premorbid traits or interactional patterns rather than stroke-related impairments.

f. If screening and informant report suggest a problem with these or related conversational behaviors, a more detailed conversational assessment may be initiated.

(1) When a conversational sample is gathered, it should be long enough (e.g., 15–30 minutes) to maximize the likelihood that it represents a patient's typical communication patterns and skills. To increase representativeness and determine consistency of performance, the context (nature and amount of prior information provided, topics of discussion, partners, etc.) and purposes for conversing can be varied as recommended previously for discourse sampling. Structuring and specifying elicitation procedures and potential topic/question sequences before gathering the sample will maximize replicability across partners and measurement occasions.

(2) The sample should be recorded for transcription, and then segmented into speaker turns and utterances. Some guidelines for segmentation are described by Brinton and Fujiki (1989).

(3) Existing rating scales such as the Pragmatic Protocol and the Assessment Protocol of Pragmatic Linguistic Skills (see section III-B-1) help to focus the level of analysis more specifically than an informal screening observation. While applying an existing profile, clinicians can note antecedents to inappropriate behaviors, and effects of inappropriate behaviors on the conversational structure and partner behaviors. As always, clinicians should work with explicit operational definitions, to enhance coding reliability.

(4) When potential problem areas have been isolated, several steps can be taken to obtain more detail or to establish baseline data.

(a) Before characterizing areas of strength and deficit more fully, clinicians may need to develop structured probes to increase the opportunities for a patient to display a target behavior. It is difficult to draw conclusions about any conversational behavior or function with fewer than five-to-ten opportunities to observe it.

(b) Referential communication tasks (see section III-B-1-f) are one option for structuring conversational evaluation and exchange. This format provides a particularly useful window for viewing responses to requests for clarification. Various kinds of message breakdowns can be feigned if necessary, and requests can be varied in specificity. The patient's responses can be evaluated for appropriateness (e.g., appropriate to form of request, represents an adjustment to listener) and for variety of strategies used (e.g., repeating, elaborating, defining terms, providing background information; see Brinton & Fujiki, 1989). As noted earlier, barrier tasks also allow observations about presupposition, speech act use, and awareness of message adequacy independent of listener queries.

(c) Turn-taking skills could be observed in any cooperative endeavor. Referential communication tasks provide a semistructured context in which turn exchange is expected. To evaluate turn-taking skills in a less structured context, a patient and family member might, for example, be asked to plan an outing together, or patient and clinician might interact to select a set of topics for future conversations or activities (in the latter case, the clinician could evaluate the social appro-priateness aspect of topic control as well). When acting as partner, the clinician can plan to interject turn-taking signals that vary in explicitness and number, to observe the patient's response. The clinician may also be able to structure the exchange to elicit more examples of specific kinds of turn-taking problems by incorporating knowledge gained from prior observations of the contexts that lead up to them (e.g., recreating conditions that tend to precede interruptions). Dimensions of topic control can be evaluated when, for example, a patient is asked to converse about a topic that is not revealed to the communication partner(s). Again, the clinician can manipulate elements of the exchange to increase the opportunities to observe performance in areas that seem to be problematic. For more ideas about analyses of topic manipulation and turn taking, the reader is referred to Brinton and Fujiki (1989). In addition, Mentis and Prutting's (1991) system for multidimensional topic analysis might be useful when detailed information is desired about topic management and conversational coherence (see Table 7–3).

(d) Table 4–5, introduced earlier, describes a number of tasks and contexts for examining the potential bases for discourse processing difficulties. These probes can be applied to the analysis of many conversational discourse behaviors as well (e.g., conceptual and organizing principles, presupposition and understanding of listener knowledge, features of coherence and relevance).

(e) Kennedy and Perez (1993) applied the MOP perspective to analyze first-encounter conversations between speech pathologists and RHD adults or non-brain-damaged speakers (see Chapter 2, II-B-8-c). They used scene coding and analysis procedures described by Kellermann, Broetzmann, Tae-Seop, and Kitao (1989) and noted as well which partner initiated each scene. Scene inclusion and ordering were assumed to indicate knowledge of the ways to initiate, progress through, and end a conversation. Scene initiation was deemed to reflect acquaintanceship goals. If a conversational scene analysis suggests difficulty following a typical conversational format, the bases for impairment can be unravelled with probes like those described in Table 4–5. For instance, a patient can be given tasks requiring discussion, description, organization, and/or evaluation of conversational goals, scenes (or elements of conversations), and their interrelationships. Results of these kinds of tasks should be interpreted with appropriate caution, because patients' behavior may be dissociated from their performance on such meta-cognitive probes. Some patients will do better on the probe tasks than in actual conversations, while other patients will show the opposite pattern of performance.

(f) Brinton and Fujiki (1989) remind us that conversational strategies and behaviors will almost certainly vary with factors such as the nature of the topic, nature of relationship and shared history with the conversational partner, speaker mood, physical setting, discourse context, and purposes of speaking (e.g., including or excluding someone from a social group; fulfilling politeness requirements). Thus, it is important to vary some of these factors in assessing conversational behavior, to distinguish what patients cannot do in certain situations from what they do not do on a regular basis.

g. Hough and Pierce's (1994) Adult Social Communication rating scale, described in Table 4–3, adds another dimension to the assessment of conversational awareness and appropriateness, as evaluated by frequent communication partners.

D. Other Language and Speech

1. Auditory language comprehension.

Discourse comprehension measures were emphasized above and are probably most clinically relevant for RHD adults. A decontextualized measure of auditory processing ability can be obtained from the Revised *Token Test* (RTT) (McNeil & Prescott, 1978). The RTT is a standardized measure of auditory processing that uses a 15-point multidimensional scoring system to capture qualitative dimensions of responding (accuracy, need for repetitions or cues, completeness, promptness, motoric efficiency). The test consists of 10 sections with 10 commands per section. Subtests vary syntactic construction and length of commands (number of critical elements). Normative data are based on 90 non-brain-damaged adults (mostly males), 30 in each of three age bands. Performance is also described for 30 RHD (exclusively male) and 30 LHD adult subjects. The test yields a variety of scores, including a combined overall mean, subtest mean scores, and an analysis of performance for linguistic elements and command types. Test-retest reliability data are available for a small subset of brain-damaged subjects; both interscorer and intrascorer reliability are high. The manual provides evidence and arguments for construct and concurrent validity. Content validation is particularly strong, but predictive validity is not addressed. The homogeneity of item difficulty within subtests allows a tester to evaluate patterns of impairment, such as problems tuning in or fatigue. When the overall score is the only performance index desired, a shortened RTT, consisting of the first 5 items from each subtest, can be used to predict it (Arvedson, McNeil, & West, 1985).

2. Word retrieval.

a. The *Boston Naming Test* (Kaplan, Goodglass, & Weintraub, 1983) is probably the most widely used assessment of confrontation naming, despite its lack of specificity for administration and scoring, its unreported reliability, and persisting questions about the relationship of confrontation naming performance to daily life word retrieval difficulties. The test consists of 60 black-and-white line drawings for naming, which generally decrease in familiarity throughout the test. Function cues and phonemic cues are specified for each item. Norms are provided for 84 non-brain-damaged adults (ages 18–59) and 82 aphasic persons. Nicholas, Brookshire, MacLennan, Schumacher, and Porrazzo (1989) reported revised administration and scoring procedures, coding reliability data, and extended norms for non-brain-damaged adults.

b. The *Test of Adolescent and Adult Word Finding* (German, 1990) is a psychometrically sound instrument, with 107 items for naming in five types of tasks: picture naming of nouns; sentence completion naming; description naming; picture naming of verbs; and category naming. Responses are evaluated for accuracy and speed. A brief version consists of a sample of items from each section. The test was standardized on a large national sample, including 150–200 adults at each of three age bands between 20–80. Standard scores and percentile ranks are provided by age and grade level. Reliability (including standard errors) and validity are extensively addressed. The category naming task may be particularly useful for assessing word retrieval in RHD adults (see Chapter 2, II-D).

c. The *Test of Word Finding in Discourse* (German, 1991) was designed to assess children's word-finding skills in connected speech. Three stimulus pictures are used to elicit a language sample. The manual describes procedures for transcribing and segmenting the sample into T-units, fragments, and lists. Then samples are scored to generate two productivity indices (total T-units and total words), and a word-finding behaviors index (a frequency measure of substitutions, word reformulations, repetitions, empty words, time fillers, delays, and meta-cognitive comments). Raw scores can be converted to standard scores (with confidence intervals determined from the standard error of measurement) and percentile ranks. The test was standardized on children, and the manual reports extensive psychometric data.

3. Reading and writing.

a. Premorbid literacy, education level, and interest or need play a large part in deciding whether and how to evaluate reading and writing for any client. If reading or writing have played minor roles in a patient's life, evaluation may be unnecessary unless there are complaints about "vision" problems in the context of daily life reading or writing activities, or specific concerns about reading or writing themselves. When an evaluation is planned, performance expectations must be guided by available information and inferences about a patient's premorbid skill.

b. As noted in Chapter 2, RHD patients' reading difficulties are often attributable to, or at least complicated by, lower level scanning and tracking deficits, visuoperceptual impairments, and/or attentional factors, including neglect. The NYU battery (Gordon et al., 1984) described above includes a number of measures designed to tap these areas, particularly the scanning and perceptual functions. Other assessment methods and procedures in these areas are discussed below (section III-E). It may be useful to have a patient read orally at least some portion of any written stimulus materials, to gain some insight about what information is being passed on from perceptual or attentional systems to central comprehension processes. Another window on the extent to which lower level visual processes may be influencing reading can be gained by asking the patient to locate some element (e.g., word, phrase, or idea) in the stimulus context, or by probing with visual matching or discrimination tasks for various elements of written stimuli.

c. Table 4–6 lists some reading comprehension measures that might be applied fruitfully with RHD adults. When the materials do not indicate the reading grade level, a readability index (e.g., Fry, 1978) may help to determine whether they are within the client's capabilities.

d. Further reading evaluation might consist of:

(**1**) analyzing comprehension operations potentially contributing to reading difficulties that cannot be attributed to perceptual or attentional impairments. The Boning Specific Skills Series (Boning, 1976) may be useful for this purpose. It includes materials at several levels of difficulty that examine, for example, a reader's ability to follow directions, use context, extract facts and main ideas, and draw conclusions. For a more detailed assessment, any of the discourse comprehension measures listed above could

Table 4–6. Some tools for reading evaluation

Nelson Reading Skills Test (Hanna, Schell, & Schreiner, 1977): vocabulary and paragraph comprehension sections for grade levels 3–9; passage dependence is good (i.e., comprehension questions cannot be answered solely by consulting knowledge of the world).

Gates-McGinitie Reading Tests (Gates & McGinitie, 1978): vocabulary and paragraph comprehension sections for primary grade levels. Brookshire (1992) recommends adapting the task so that stimulus pictures and text are not in view at the same time.

Revised Token Test, reading format (Odell, McNeil, Collins, & Rosenbek, 1984)

Discourse Comprehension Test, reading format (Brookshire & Nicholas, 1993b)

Modified Metropolitan Achievement Test passages for reading comprehension (from NYU battery; Gordon et al., 1984): patient answers multiple choice questions about three reading passages.

Reading comprehension sections of other achievement tests, including the Peabody Individual Achievement Test (PIAT) (Dunn & Markwardt, 1970), or the Woodcock-Johnson Psychoeducational Battery (WJPEB) (Woodcock & Johnson, 1977).

be evaluated in discourse reading tasks. Of course, potential impairments of written input processing could significantly impede these kinds of analyses. It would be necessary to account for, and to minimize to the extent possible, visual signal processing decrements that might complicate such assessments. Combined auditory and visual modality presentation might assist in a comprehension evaluation, but it may overload some patients.

(2) screening for neglect dyslexia in oral reading, noting the characteristic substitutions and omissions described in Chapter 2, and the extent to which they can be modified with manipulations that tend to minimize the impact of neglect (see also neglect assessments, section III-E-3-b).

(3) determining the literacy requirements for individual social, vocational, and recreational pursuits, and assessing the patient's abilities in those areas. The Behavioural Inattention Test (Wilson, Cockburn, & Halligan, 1987), introduced below (in III-E-3-b), includes functional tasks of menu-reading and newspaper article-reading. The CADL (Holland, 1980) includes items like reading a prescription and directory assistance listings. Clinicians

can design similar informal probes for examining skills and contexts that are individually relevant for a given patient.

e. Writing can be evaluated using various achievement tests, such as those listed in Table 4-6. In addition to the standard information that they provide about writing abilities, these tasks furnish a context for examining problems of spatial orientation and detail (as outlined in Chapter 2 and described further below in section E-3). Informal assessments can also be developed to probe functional writing skills, when they are individually relevant (e.g., taking a phone message, writing a note on a birthday card, recording an appointment in a daybook). When in-depth assessment is desired, written discourse samples can be obtained and characterized using the procedures and recommendations for spoken discourse. Evaluating performance is likely to be extremely difficult without good examples of or information about prior abilities. Letters, other documents, and/or the personal judgments of individuals who know a patient well may shed some light on the extent and nature of written discourse changes.

4. Dysarthrias may be associated with RHD, as noted in Chapter 2, and may contribute to perceptions of dysprosody. For comprehensive information about the nature and assessment of dysarthrias, the reader is referred to the contributions of authors including Rosenbek and LaPointe (1985) and Yorkston, Beukelman, and Bell (1988).

E. Cognitive/Perceptual Assessment

Most procedures included in this section will receive only brief mention. Many are described in further detail by Lezak (1983), Kolb and Whishaw (1990), Sohlberg and Mateer (1989a), Spreen and Strauss (1991) or in the primary references cited with each. Lezak (1983) and Spreen and Strauss (1991) also provide valuable information about the psychometric characteristics and confounding factors for interpreting many of these measures (e.g., correlations with age or education).

1. **Anosognosia.** Anosognosia, impaired awareness of deficits or disabled body parts, is generally evaluated through observation and interview. Interview questions for the patient might include:

- Why are you here in the hospital/for evaluation/for treatment?

- How has your illness affected you?

- What things are difficult for you to do now?

- Do you make more mistakes or have more accidents now?

- Are you concerned about being able to go back to your usual activities, like driving?

- How do you think you will do (on any particular task that is about to be administered)?

- How do you think you just did (on a particular task, especially those for which a patient predicted success but exhibited difficulty)?

Family members can be asked the same kinds of questions to note discrepancies. Observational clues about anosognosia include lack of interest in going to or participating in evaluation or treatment sessions. Failure to attempt self-correction or to adapt to listener reactions may also indicate unawareness. Examiners should keep in mind that some patients or family members may engage in some motivated denial, as a psychological coping mechanism.

2. **Orientation.** Orientation to person, place, and time is frequently examined with screening questions that ask patients to provide basic biographical information; to tell where they are and why they are there; and to indicate the day, date, month, and year. The Galveston Orientation and Amnesia Test (Levin, O'Donnell, & Grossman, 1979) provides a specific set of orientation questions and scoring guidelines (see Levin, Benton, & Grossman, 1982), as does the Wechsler Memory Scale-Revised (WMS-R) (Wechsler, 1987). Benton, Hamsher, Varney, and Spreen's (1983) Temporal Orientation Test is a brief but standardized procedure that examines only for temporal disorientation, with some normative data to assist in interpretation.

Lezak (1983) describes several procedures for estimating topographical disorientation. Among them are three tasks tapping geographical knowledge and orientation, that require patients to indicate the states in which certain cities are located, describe the direction one would travel between two locations, and mark locations on a United States map (Benton, Levin, & Van Allen, 1974). Testing for topographical orientation is not easy, because patients who are clearly disoriented, even in familiar surroundings, may perform relatively well when asked to describe familiar floorplans, landmarks, or routes (Lezak, 1983).

3. Visual and auditory perceptual and related functions.

a. Some tests used to examine various visual functions are listed in Table 4–7. Assessment of neglect is considered more extensively below. Several other pertinent evaluations of auditory function were described above (III-A, B), and Lezak (1983) provides suggestions for examining impaired music perception. A formal battery for assessing several components of musical function was recommended by Benton (1977).

b. Neglect is typically tested in the visual modality. It should be evaluated in different visuoconstructive tasks and daily life activities, because many patients will not exhibit deficits in all assessment contexts.

   (1) The *Behavioural Inattention Test* (BIT) (Wilson et al., 1987) is a comprehensive, standardized measure for assessing unilateral visual neglect. It includes six conventional subtests to evaluate the presence of neglect (line crossing, letter cancellation, star cancellation, figure and shape copying, line bisection, and drawing from memory). It also has nine behavioral subtests to examine the types of everyday problems that are likely to occur (e.g., telephone dialing, menu reading, article reading, telling and setting time, navigating by map). Several subsequent articles have been published, including one evaluating a modified version of the BIT for acute stroke patients (3 days post-onset; Stone, Wilson, Wroot, & colleagues, 1991). Another study assessed performance of normal elderly persons (Stone, Halligan, Wilson, Greenwood, & Marshall, 1991), and as a result, the criteria and cut-off scores for identifying neglect were adjusted. No control subject made a right-hand start on tasks that conventionally require left-to-right scanning (the menu and newspaper tasks) or showed crowding on the figure copying tasks. Accordingly, these behavioral criteria were put forth as good indicators of abnormal performance. Stone, Patel, Greenwood, and Halligan (1992) also described a Visual Neglect Recovery Index to characterize severity of neglect on the six conventional subtests. The index expresses performance as a percentage of the maximum measurable neglect on those subtests.

   (2) The Bells Test (Gauthier, Dehaut, & Joanette, 1989; Vanier et al., 1990) was designed for the quantitative and

Table 4–7. Some measures of visual function

Visual Perception and Integration

Benton Facial Recognition test (Benton & Van Allen, 1968; Benton et al., 1983): manipulates lighting conditions and angle of view to degrade facial representations

Gollin Incomplete Figures test (Gollin, 1960): drawings of familiar objects are presented for identification, in gradations of completeness

Gottschaldt Hidden Figure test (Gottschaldt, 1928): examines figure-ground differentiation

Hooper Visual Organization test (Hooper, 1958; 1983): line drawings to be labelled are cut up and scattered in unusual orientations. Several items are associated with a frequent tendency to assign different names to separate parts of a stimulus (Lezak, 1983).

McGill Picture Anomalies (Hebb & Morton, 1943): unusual elements are included for identification in visual scenes

Mooney Visual Closure test[a] (Mooney & Ferguson, 1951): complex shadow patterns must be integrated to identify objects, often faces

Rey Complex Figure Copy Test[a] (Rey, 1941, 1964): a complex line drawing is presented for exact replication

Rivermead Perceptual Assessment Battery (Whiting et al., 1985): overall measure for subjects with brain injury, designed for professionals without advanced training in psychology, neurology, or test administration (see Braden, 1992, for review).

Visuospatial

Judgment of Line Orientation test (Benton et al., 1983): involves choosing a line from an array to match position of a single line segment

Structure of Intellect Learning Abilities Test (SOI-LA), Cognition of Figural Systems subtest (Meeker, Meeker, & Royd, 1985): requires selecting a shape to match an original as if viewed from a different perspective.

SOI-LA, Cognition of Figural Transformations subtest (Meeker et al., 1985): requires mental rotation of shapes.

Woodcock-Johnson Psychoeducational Battery Spatial Relation subtest (Woodcock & Johnson, 1977): requires spatial retention and mental rotation.

Tests of spatial discrimination, such as line bisection (e.g., see Behavioural Inattention Test (BIT); Wilson et al., 1987)

Tests of spatial search, including

- simple cancellation: Albert (1973); BIT subtest

- target detection among distractors: Bells test (Gauthier et al., 1989); BIT subtest

Table 4–7. *Continued*

- counting individual stimuli (e.g., dots) in a display

Other informal tasks: assessing spatial relations by evaluating alignment on the page for writing and copying tasks, or numbers in arithmetic problems.

Visuomotor

Block Design and Assembly subtests of WAIS-R (Wechsler, 1981).

Rey Complex Figure Copy Test[a] (Rey, 1941, 1964).

Visual Reproduction (immediate) subtest of Wechsler Memory Scale-Revised (WMS-R) (Wechsler, 1987).

Three-Dimensional Block Construction test (Benton & Fogel, 1962; Benton et al., 1983): reproducing block models at several difficulty levels.

Visual scanning: inferred from performance on reading tests or visual tests of target detection from distractors (e.g., Bells Test).

Visual Problem Solving and Conceptual Functions

Raven's Coloured Progressive Matrices (RCPM) (Raven, 1965): patient identifies the missing part of geometric patterns. Calls on processes ranging from simple completion to reasoning by analogy. Horner and Nailling (1980) present error type and problem type analyses. The CPM is sensitive to visuo-perceptual and spatial-organization abilities as well as nonverbal reasoning and abstraction. Odell, Collins, Dirkx, and Kelso (1984) describe a computerized version.

Wisconsin Card-Sorting Test[a] (Grant & Berg, 1948; and Nelson, 1976, modification): patient must induce a sorting/classification rule that is switched without warning. See also Heaton (1981).

Porteus Maze Test (Porteus, 1965): patient traces routes through mazes of increasing difficulty, without violating rules.

Visual/Spatial Memory

Benton Visual Retention Test (Benton, 1974): reproducing (or recognizing, Benton, 1950) designs after various delay intervals.

Corsi Block Span (Milner, 1971): tapping a series of blocks of increasing length, following examiner's model. Block span is generally one less than digit span (Kolb & Whishaw, 1990).

Recognition Memory Test for Faces (Warrington, 1984): selecting from a recognition set the photo from each pair that was seen before.

Rey Complex Figure Reproduction: drawing figure from memory after copy task (45 minutes after copy[a])

Figural memory, visual paired associates (immediate and delayed), visual reproduction (delayed) and visual memory span subtests of WMS-R (Wechsler, 1987).

[a]Summary of published means for neurologic patients is provided by Kolb and Whishaw (1990).

qualitative evaluation of neglect. It is patterned after a widely used line cancellation task (Albert, 1973), but it includes distractors. Subjects must circle the drawings of bells that are interspersed among drawings of other common objects. The examiner notes the order in which a subject circles each target, to infer the qualitative approach to the task. The authors report preliminary normative data, and indicate that the task is more sensitive than a traditional cancellation task without distractors.

(3) The NYU battery (Gordon et al., 1984), introduced previously, provides normative data for a variety of measures of visual scanning and inattention, including a bias score for the Raven's Coloured Progressive Matrices (RCPM) (Raven, 1965; see Table 4–7) that reflects the extent to which patients ignore the response alternatives on the side contralateral to their brain lesions. Some of Gordon and colleagues' tests of basic activities of daily living (e.g., address copying, oral reading) also provide contexts for observing errors typically associated with visual neglect.

(4) Caplan (1987) described a paragraph reading test designed to detect left-sided neglect. It consists of a printed passage from Reader's Digest, with highly variable and unpredictable left margins. Subjects read the passage aloud, and performance is scored for the first word read on each line, omissions, and time to completion.

(5) Neglect has also been associated with deficits of orienting and shifting visual attention, but patients without neglect may also exhibit attentional orienting/shifting problems. Some measures for examining attentional orienting and shifting will be discussed with other attention measures, below (section III-E-4).

(6) Several other observations may point to visual neglect in RHD adults. To attribute such impairments to neglect, visual field deficits must be minimal or absent. These impairments include tendencies to:

(a) omit left-sided detail (especially in the lower quadrant) in picture descriptions and visuoconstructive tasks;

(b) crowd graphic output to the right side of a page;

(c) omit whole words or phrases on the left side of a page when reading;

       (d) make substitution or omission errors for the left-hand portions of words (evaluate with no possible substitutions);

       (e) leave progressively larger left-hand margins on writing tasks;

       (f) ignore left-sided response alternatives; and/or

       (g) ignore obstacles in immediate environment, and personal care, on the left side of the body.

    (7) To evaluate the influence of various factors on the manifestation or severity of neglect, an examiner can manipulate the cues or features outlined in Table 2–9 and in the discussion of neglect dyslexia (Chapter 2, section II-E-1-a). To examine whether a patient is relying on visually-based compensations, the patient can be asked to perform some tests (e.g., midline estimation) with the eyes closed. Caplan (1988) also evaluated and recommended a nonstandard version of the RCPM for patients who exhibit neglect. The modification aligns the response alternatives in a single column to minimize lateral scanning requirements.

  c. Few assessments of auditory neglect are clinically available. In one informal technique, the examiner stands behind the patient and delivers, separately and simultaneously, soft sounds to each ear (e.g., rubbing together the thumb and first two fingers on each hand; Lezak, 1983). Auditory inattention is suspected when the patient shows extinction to simultaneous stimulation; that is, for the ear contralateral to the brain lesion, the patient detects the signal when presented separately, but ignores it in the simultaneous condition. A more controlled variant of this task could be developed, in which a single signal is presented monaurally or split for binaural presentation, but potential differences between ears in auditory function would make it difficult to interpret the results of such a task for any patient, in the absence of data to document that the signals were equally audible (e.g., from audiologic assessment).

4. Attention.

  a. Clinicians can make informal observations of attentional control skills during early screening and interviewing sessions and in the context of other evaluations, by noting a patient's apparent ability to sustain task focus, shift tasks or strategies, resist distraction, alternate or divide attention between several tasks or task elements, and orient to sudden or attention-demanding stimulus events often arranged with the help of a confederate (such as the ring of a telephone, or the sound of a family member's voice). When an impairment is suspected, a more in-depth assessment will be in order. Much of this assessment may be carried out collaboratively with a neuropsychologist.

b. As noted in Chapter 2, attention is a complex area. Its assessment is difficult for a number of reasons. Some attempts have been made to break attention into component skills for evaluation. However, most measures require more than one attentional process, and performance usually depends on other cognitive abilities, making it difficult to attribute poor performance to attentional mechanisms. As always, the examiner needs to remain cognizant of factors other than the ones of interest that may account for impaired performance.

c. With these caveats in mind (see further discussion in Lezak, 1983; Sohlberg & Mateer, 1989a) some typical measures of attentional components are included in Table 4–8. Some novel or less well-known tests of attentional function have been described and evaluated in a recent study with normally aging adults (Stankov, 1988).

d. Robin and his colleagues have designed a number of potentially valuable measures to assess subcomponents of attentional processing. They have applied these tasks in several clinical studies, finding them to be more sensitive for detecting attentional impairments in head injured patients than several traditional neuropsychological measures (Lodge-Miller, Robin, & Schum, 1993). Their contributions include:

(1) A "Starry Night" task, to examine sustained attention over a complex visuospatial array (Rizzo & Robin, 1990). Subjects watch a computer monitor that displays a pattern of dots, resembling a starry night. Their task is to respond to the appearance or disappearance of any "star," at unpredictable locations and intervals. Star density is manipulated, with either 50 or 1,000 dots per display.

(2) Several variations of spatial selective attention tasks, based on Posner's paradigm (see Chapter 2, section III-D-8-b), to examine orientation of attention to single targets, presented in vision, audition, or combined modalities (Robin & Rizzo,

1989). Target stimuli are preceded by cues that may or may not predict target location accurately. Visuospatial orienting can also be examined for complex spatial arrays, by pairing location cues with the Starry Night display (Rizzo & Robin, 1990).

e. Table 4–8 includes some tests believed to evaluate strategic attentional control (as defined in Chapter 2, section III-D-8-c), but there are no standard measures for some elements of this construct. Many aspects of attentional control are thought to be the province of a supervisory system that directs information processing according to task requirements (but see Kimberg & Farah, 1993; Chapter 2, section III-E-2-d). Stroop-type tasks (see Table 4–8) are often used to evaluate some parts of this system. But because the Stroop Test and its variants typically require only one type of attentional override (e.g., inhibiting a habitual reading response to produce a less preferred color-naming response), they may not be very sensitive tools. The clinician can gather additional information in informal probes by introducing tasks that require more numerous, or more frequent, changes of automatic or habitual set. At the same time, Stroop-type tasks offer good contexts for observing when patients seem to be distracted by over-learned routines that conflict with expected responses. As such, these tasks can provide indirect information about how well a patient has allocated attention for determining stimulus relevance and task priorities, or about the integrity of automatic processing systems. If trouble is suspected in these or other areas of strategic attentional control, informal probes can be designed to elicit a behavior sample sufficient to evaluate the extent and consistency of component problems.

f. The influence of arousal on performance can be estimated by manipulating some of the factors listed in Chapter 2 (section III-D-8-a), such as the importance of the task, other kinds of performance incentives, and alerting signals.

g. Sohlberg and Mateer (1989a) have published an Attention/Concentration Rating Scale to characterize broadly a patient's level of attentional functioning. Patients are rated for how well and how independently they perform a familiar recreational activity, a basic activity of daily living, a standardized test or treatment activity, an exercise program, and familiar environmental tasks. The authors recommend the scale for evaluating

Table 4–8. Some conventional measures of attention

Selective

Stroop Color Word Test (Stroop, 1935): Color adjectives (e.g., the word "red") are printed in various colored inks; word and ink colors are either congruent or conflicting (e.g., "red" printed in blue ink). Patient either names ink colors or reads words. In a color naming control condition, color adjectives are replaced with Xs, color patches, or noncolor words; in a word naming control condition, the color adjectives are printed in black ink. For naming ink colors, a conflicting color word may create significant interference. McLeod (1991) provides an integrative review of studies using this test; Stankov (1988) uses several modifications to elicit Stroop-like phenomena.

Goldman-Fristoe-Woodcock Test of Auditory Discrimination (Goldman, Fristoe, & Woodcock, 1970).

Sustained Successful performance on any attention test requires sustained attention; vigilance tasks examine duration and consistency of sustained attention itself.

Sequentially presented stimuli in lengthy and monotonous tasks, including cancellation or target detection activities (e.g., counting the number of clicks presented at a slow, regular rate; tapping when one or several targets are perceived; responding to target items only when they follow other specified items).

Trail Making Test, part A (Army Individual Test Battery, 1944; Reitan, 1958; Reitan & Wolfson, 1985): has been used as a test of sustained attention, but does not tax vigilance in the manner of the tests above. Patient connects a series of numbers on a page.

Divided Tasks involving more than one activity to be performed at once, or multiple stimuli to be processed.

Paced Auditory Serial Attention Test (PASAT) (Gronwall, 1977): String of digits is presented at different rates; patient sums each digit with the one immediately preceding. Performance predicts difficulty at work for traumatically brain-injured patients (Gronwall, 1977). Performance highly correlated with education, especially at fast presentation rates.

Attentional Capacity Test (Weber, 1986, 1988): Patient counts digit targets in a series and reports the total number at end of task. Conditions for identifying targets increase in complexity (e.g., reporting number of 8s followed by 5s). Eliminates PASAT requirements for adding and rapid verbal response.

Test d2 (Brickenkamp, 1981; see Spreen & Strauss, 1991): A cancellation task with other visual demands. Targets for cancellation are only those "d"s paired with two marks, either above, below, or both.

Alternating

Symbol-Digit Modalities Test (Smith, 1973): Working from a key that associates symbols with numbers, patient writes the digit that goes with each symbol in a long

Table 4–8. *Continued*

list. Written and oral administrations possible; performance on both correlates positively with education.

Trail Making Test, part B (Army Individual Test Battery, 1944; Reitan, 1958; Reitan & Wolfson, 1985): Patient given a series of numbers and letters, and must connect them consecutively by alternating between numbers and letters. Usual cutoff scores misclassify 90% of normal people in their 70s as brain damaged. Davies (1968) provides extended norms for aging people.

Other Aspects of Strategic Attentional Control

Stroop test (see above) as indicator of strategic attentional system's (SAS) function in overcoming the most automatic or habitual form of response (e.g., reading a word rather than naming ink color).

Cognitive Estimations test (Shallice & Evans, 1978) as indicator of SAS function when no routine procedure is available to generate an appropriate response. Patients estimate magnitudes, such as the average length of a human spine, or the speed of a galloping horse. A related task asks for cost estimates of real items represented by toys (Smith & Milner, 1984).

Tower of London (TOL) (Shallice, 1982), also to examine SAS-directed planning and problem-solving. Stacks of blocks must be moved to create a pictured configuration in the minimum number of moves. Designed as an improvement on the Tower of Hanoi, as the TOL includes qualitatively different problems of comparable difficulty (Shallice & Burgess, 1991a).

Composite Attention Measure

Detroit Test of Learning Aptitudes-2, Attentional Composite (Hammill, 1985). Contains 11 subtests in 2 domains, one emphasizing focused concentration and immediate memory functions, the other emphasizing attention in longer-term memory tasks (e.g., comprehension and reasoning).

---

progress in treatment, but its validity, reliability, and sensitivity for assessing component attentional processes have not been established.

5. **Memory.**

   a. Nonverbal memory deficits are prevalent in RHD adults and are frequently targeted in neuropsychological assessment. Some nonverbal memory tests are listed in Table 4–7.

   b. Several other pertinent aspects of everyday memory function (e.g., topographical memory, prospective memory) are tapped by the Rivermead Behavioural Memory Test (RBMT) (Wilson, Cockburn, & Baddeley, 1985). The RBMT is a quick measure of everyday memory abilities, that includes items such as recalling a route, or remembering a name. There are three prospective memory items: remembering to ask for a hidden belonging, remembering to ask about an appointment when a timer rings, and remembering to take and deliver a message on a route traced around the examining room.

Many studies have been done since the test was published that expand on the data provided in the RBMT manual. For example, Cockburn and Smith (1991) documented performance of the oldest-old (from ages 70–93). Periodic supplements to the test manual, and current reference lists, are available upon request from the test publisher (Thames Valley Test Company, 7-9 The Green, Flempton, Bury St. Edmunds, Suffolk, IP28 6EL, England; FAX: 284-728608). One supplement reported that patients who exhibited perceptual problems on the Rivermead Perceptual Assessment Battery (Whiting, Lincoln, Bhavnani, & Cockburn, 1985; see Table 4–7) scored worse on the RBMT than did patients without perceptual impairments, especially on items assessing immediate and delayed route recall, orientation, current date, and face recognition. The authors recommend eliminating these RBMT subtests when assessing memory performance in patients with perceptual impairments.

c. Sohlberg and Mateer (1989b) also describe a Prospective Memory Screening that evaluates a patient's ability to remember to do something after varying amounts of time have passed, or when a specific cue occurs (e.g., when the timer rings, do X).

d. Working memory was emphasized in Chapter 2 as a potentially important correlate of RHD patients' ability to perform many kinds of tasks with high information processing load. Tompkins et al. (1994) report an experimental measure of auditory working memory capacity that taps simultaneous information processing and storage functions. Patients judge the truth value of each sentence in a set as it is heard, while maintaining in memory the final word of each sentence in that set for later spoken recall. The task has been used to study RHD patients' inferencing and discourse comprehension ability and preliminary psychometric evaluation is promising. The "central executive" component of working memory is also believed to be tapped by performance on various tests discussed in conjunction with the Supervisory Attentional System (e.g., Stroop Test; Tower of London) and others to be introduced for assessing planning and problem solving (e.g., the Wisconsin Card-Sorting Test). Although some authors use a simple digit span task as a measure of working memory, forward digit span does not predict either the more complex measures of concurrent information processing and storage, or patients' other cognitive and communicative abilities.

e. Some evidence suggests that metamemory, or one's insight into one's own memory function, may become impaired in the process of normal aging. Some patients will also be unrealistic about their memory abilities, possibly resulting in a reluctance to participate in generating or learning compensatory processing strategies. If this is the case, a metamemory assessment may be in order. Metamemory is usually evaluated with questionnaires about the nature and frequency of memory failures experienced in daily life. Two examples include the Memory Assessment Clinics Self-Rating Scale (MACS) (Winterling, Crook, Salama, & Gobert, 1986) and the Memory Functioning Questionnaire (MFQ) (Gilewski, Zelinski, & Schaie, 1990). Metamemory assessment is very tricky because a valid evaluation assumes the accuracy of self-ratings and retrospective reports (for further discussion, see Harris & Morris, 1984).

6. **Integration processes.** Integration processes are involved in most every cognitive and communicative activity imaginable; accordingly, integrative functions are tapped by many assessment procedures that have already been discussed. Among these are tests of visual integration and anomaly detection (see Table 4–7) that necessitate a synthesis of stimulus information; many discourse measures (section III-C), including aspects of continuity (e.g., cohesion, coherence), inference generation, and the detection and expression of main concepts or themes; and the pragmatic-social skills assessments associated with sensitivity to listener and situation or "seeing the big picture" in the ways discussed in Chapter 2. The Specific Skills Series mentioned earlier in the section on reading comprehension (III-D-3-d) includes graded materials that focus on several discrete processes thought to contribute to higher integration and inferencing abilities, such as seeing relationships and drawing conclusions. And a number of experimental measures could be adapted for clinical purposes from those that have been designed to

examine RHD patients' difficulty integrating stimulus and context information in nonliteral, emotional, and other pragmatic realms (see Chapter 2, section II-A). Insights about factors that facilitate and impede performance on all of these types of tasks can be gained by manipulating or modifying task components, response requirements, or stimulus delivery features in the ways that were noted with the initial presentations of this material. Higher integration processes are also required for planning, reasoning, and problem-solving activities, which form the focus of the next section.

7. **Planning, organization, reasoning, and problem solving.**

    a. Each of these areas involves complex, multifaceted skills. These functions are extremely complicated to assess for some by-now-familiar reasons: The areas themselves are not well defined, performance on measures used to assess these skills may depend crucially on other fundamental abilities, and individual differences are vast in both approaches and aptitudes. In addition, lack of awareness is likely to place severe limitations on a patient's ability to perform and reflect on deliberate problem solving and reasoning activities. Furthermore, planning, reasoning and the like can be hard to measure on formal tests, in part because habitual or automatic routines may be adequate for performing when sufficient structure is provided, and in part because so many component processes are necessary for success. One of the major challenges of assessment is to transfer planning and other decision-making activity to the patient (Lezak, 1983). For all of these reasons, the input and cooperation of a neuropsychologist may be particularly valuable in assessing these areas, and in generating probable attributions for impaired performance.

    b. As noted previously, difficulties in the areas of planning, organization, reasoning, and problem solving are frequently associated with frontal lobe involvement, hence these functions are the focus of much of the literature on traumatic brain injury. Some authors, like Sohlberg and Mateer (1989a) propose that reasoning, problem solving, and other "executive function" deficits rely so heavily on core process areas (e.g., attention, visual processing, memory, language), that treatment for the "core" impairments should precede treatment of, or perhaps even assessment of, the higher-level skill areas. Others, such as Ylvisaker and Szekeres (1994), assert that this sort of hierarchical conception is inexact and perhaps misguided. They emphasize that improvements in some apparently higher level operations (e.g., organizational processes) are essential for effecting positive changes in "lower level" processes like attention (see, e.g., Chapter 7, V-D-5). Further, they note that some reasoning tasks are relatively simple and straightforward, whereas some attentional tasks are quite cognitively demanding. (Similarly, Chapter 2 of this book characterizes "attention" as a multidimensional process that involves some relatively low-level aspects such as "attentiveness" and some higher-level, strategic aspects associated with attentional control.)

c. It is undoubtedly true that a patient must exhibit some minimal processing in fundamental areas (e.g., low level attending and on-task behavior; perceptual ability) in order to take in and profit from information that is presented in assessment and treatment. However, organizing strategies and problem-solving approaches may be integral to improving cognitive processing that occurs beyond the baseline levels, within those same attentional and perceptual domains (see Chapter 7). Thus, this book follows more closely Ylvisaker and Szekeres' line, emphasizing the two-way street between many of the so-called "core" process areas and "higher level" strategic abilities.

d. A number of tasks and measures used to tap these "higher level" thinking skills are listed in Table 4–9.

(1) According to Lezak (1983), some of the formal, standardized measures in Table 4–9 may miss subtle difficulties, because their inherent structure obviates the need for patients to generate their own complex plans, goals, and decisions. Therefore, some of the less structured observations may provide important supplemental information. For example, to assess planning ability, Lezak recommends giving patients a complex task to accomplish without instruction or guidance, such as building something from a set of Tinker Toys. The Multiple Errands Test (Shallice & Burgess, 1991b; and a U.S. adaptation described by Aitken, Chase, McCue, & Ratcliff, 1992) also provides interesting insights into high-functioning patients' ability to plan, organize, and follow a set of rules, in a complex task with greater ecological validity and less inherent structure than other formal tests. Shallice and Burgess reported the task to be sensitive to daily life problems in patients who were above-average in

Table 4–9. Selected measures of reasoning, problem solving, and other "executive functions"

Elements of Reasoning and Problem Solving

Higher Order Inferences

Similarities; Picture Completion subtests of WAIS-R (Wechsler, 1981)

Likenesses and Differences; Verbal Absurdities subtests of Detroit Test of Learning Aptitudes-2 (Hammill, 1985)

Concept Formation; Analysis/Synthesis subtests of Woodcock-Johnson Psycho-Educational Battery (Woodcock & Johnson, 1977)

Nonverbal sorting/classification tasks (see "Flexibility" below)

Strategy Formation

Cognitive Estimates Test (see Table 4–8)

Word Fluency tasks (e.g., Controlled Word Association Test in Benton & Hamsher, 1976)

Tasks involving planning and anticipatory processing or lookahead, such as Porteus Maze (Table 4–7), Tower of London (Table 4–8), and open-ended Executive Function Route-Finding Task (Boyd, Sautter, Bailey, Echols, & Douglas, 1987; described in Sohlberg & Mateer, 1989a).

Observations of planning ability, inferred from tasks requiring patients to describe how they would perform various daily life activities, or by watching their approach to a complex task provided without instruction (e.g., copying a complex figure).

Flexibility

Wisconsin Card-Sorting Test (Table 4–7)

Color Form Sorting Test (Goldstein & Scheerer, 1953; and variations described in Lezak, 1983)

Object Sorting (Goldstein & Scheerer, 1953)

Uses of Objects test (Getzels & Jackson, 1962; a measure of divergent thinking)

Design fluency (Jones-Gotman & Milner, 1977)

Observations of performance when asked to carry out a familiar task in an unusual way

Self-Regulation

Stroop Test (Table 4–8)

Porteus Maze (rule-following; Table 4–7)

Table 4–9. *Continued*

Social Comprehension and Judgment Screening (Sohlberg & Mateer, 1989a)

Observations of social appropriateness

Evaluation of Outcome

WCST (using feedback to shift sets; perseverative errors)

Porteus Maze and similar tasks (rule-following)

Observations of self-monitoring and self-correction attempts

Other Verbal Abstraction and Reasoning

Stanford-Binet Verbal Absurdities (Terman & Merrill, 1973)

Poisoned Food Problems (Arenberg, 1968)

Differential Aptitude Test, Verbal Reasoning (Bennett, Seashore, & Wesman, 1972)

Other "Nonverbal" Abstraction and Reasoning

Stanford Binet Picture Absurdities (Terman & Merrill, 1973)

Raven's CPM (Table 4–7)

Test of Nonverbal Intelligence-2 (Brown, Sherbenou, & Johnsen, 1990)

Other Overall

Executive Function Rating Scale (Sohlberg & Mateer, 1989a; selection and execution of cognitive plans; time management and behavioral regulation; self-awareness and social regulation).

Multiple Errands Test (Shallice & Burgess, 1991b) and United States adaptation (Aitken et al., 1992)

intelligence, and who performed well on conventional neuropsychological assessments. In the U.S. adaptation of the test, patients are taken to a local shopping area, armed only with their watch, a small sum of money, and some written cues about the task. Then they are set out on their own to make several purchases (e.g., a birthday card, a loaf of French bread), while following six rules. They are also given a place and time to meet the examiner during the trip and asked to complete and mail a postcard after gathering some specific information (e.g., the previous day's winning lotto number). However, they are not told how to acquire the information, and some strategies must be inferred (e.g., the need to buy a pen to fill out the postcard; the fact that they could meet with the examiner even if they are not yet finished with the errands). Among the rules to be followed are a stipulation that they cannot go into a store without buying something, they cannot use anything they have not bought to complete any portion of the task, and they must make do with the small sum of money that is given to them. An examiner accompanies them, but waits outside in the square to observe their problem-solving strategies and rule-following activity. Aitken et al. score total completion time, subtask completion accuracy, and efficiency of subtask performance, all of which distinguished their currently small samples of control and cognitively impaired subjects (a mixed group of persons with traumatic brain injury and developmental learning disability). They also score rule breaks and misinterpretations, which did not differentiate the two groups. Aitken and colleagues emphasize the utility of this open-ended context for revealing specific, real life obstacles that were not inferable from their subjects' scores on high level neuropsychological tests.

(2) More generally, careful observations of a patient's approach to any assessment tasks can lead to hypotheses about factors that might be creating difficulty. Clinical probes can examine the influence on performance of the usual kinds of modifications, including familiarity or level of difficulty of the problems or reasoning activities themselves (e.g., nature of inferences required, specificity of goals); rate or pacing requirements; presence and nature of distractions or other competing demands; and extent of structure and specificity of cuing provided.

e. Reflecting more on the measures listed in Table 4–9, several other caveats and recommendations are in order.

(1) A patient who did not use one particular style of reasoning or problem-solving premorbidly should not be expected to demonstrate or adopt it after brain damage.

(2) Even for non-brain-damaged adults, it is questionable whether training on one specific kind of problems (e.g., deductive reasoning) transfers or generalizes to other kinds of problems.

(3) Performance on many of these measures may not reflect RHD patients' daily life difficulties with reasoning and problem solving, though the relevance of some (e.g., Social Comprehension and Judgment Screening; Multiple Errands Test) is more apparent than others.

f. For these reasons, clinical time with brain-damaged patients may be best spent identifying, with the patients and their family members, the daily life problems that are currently causing difficulty or that are expected to pose trouble at some future time, and developing behavioral observations to analyze the source and nature of those difficulties. Ylvisaker and Holland's (1985) guide for real-life problem solving provides some explicit questions that can be used in clinical probes. Their process roughly involves asking patients to identify a problem and state the benefit of solving it, determine what information is needed to solve it, specify strategies for obtaining information that is not available, generate and evaluate possible solutions on the basis of all relevant information, formulate and execute a plan of action, and then to evaluate results. These kinds of questions provide some insight into patients' use of the deliberate, "front-end" aspects of problem solving, noted in Chapter 2 to characterize effective problem-solvers.

IV. OTHER BEHAVIORAL DEFICITS

A. Evaluating Other Behavioral Deficits

Assessments for most of the other behavioral deficits listed in Table 2–12 have already been considered in the material above. Qualitative performance observations will be the primary source of hypotheses about problems in many of these areas (e.g., response delay, poor error awareness). In addition, some measures of attentional control and problem solving may be useful for assessing other difficulties in this list, such as impulsivity, distractibility, and problems switching tasks.

B. Screening for Depression

Depression is not often considered in evaluating RHD adults, perhaps because their condition is frequently associated with unawareness and denial of deficit. However, RHD patients who are aware of their deficits are at least twice as likely as non-brain-damaged adults to exhibit depressive symptoms (Spencer, Tompkins, Schulz, & Rau, in press).

Depression is worthy of attention because it has a variety of negative consequences on cognitive functioning and overall life satisfaction, yet it is frequently missed in post-stroke patients (Spencer, Tompkins, & Schulz, submitted). A quick screening can be accomplished with an instrument such as the Center for Epidemiologic Studies-Depression Scale (CES-D) (Radloff, 1977). The CES-D is a 20-item self-report scale that yields a cutoff score indicating when a respondent is at risk for significant clinical depression and should be referred for further evaluation and recommendations. The scale has strong psychometric properties, has been used in many studies of normally aging persons, and is not heavily weighted with somatic items that can characterize the non-depressed elderly. The Beck Depression Inventory (BDI) (Beck, Ward, Mendelson, Mock, & Erbaugh, 1961) is a similar measure. Gordon and colleagues (1984) provide normative data for a modified version of the BDI, which include separate norms for somatic and nonsomatic symptoms.

V. MEASURES OF TREATMENT OUTCOME

Currently, there is much interest in measures intended to capture broader, and perhaps more relevant, aspects of treatment outcome than do our standardized tests and clinical probes. The notion of levels of outcome, and its relationship to rehabilitation goal-setting, measurement, and documentation, is considered in some detail in Chapters 5 and 6. This section mentions briefly two of the newer trends in outcome measurement.

A. Functional Outcome Measurement

Functional outcome measurement has already become incorporated into the rehabilitation environment. It is intended to document patients' functional status, or the extent to which they can negotiate the world independently in physical, cognitive, and communicative domains. Results of functional outcome measurements are being used by hospital administrators and third-party payers to decide whether treatment is warranted and whether reported treatment gains are manifest in independent daily functioning. At present, many of these measures are designed to capture coarse categories of performance (e.g., seven broad categories for expressive communication ability) and to be applied by professionals without specialized training in each domain being rated (e.g., nursing staff). The idea of documenting the daily life relevance of treatment outcomes is a good one, and it is likely to become more prevalent with recent calls for increased health care accountability. Unfortunately, the measures currently used for this purpose generally fall short in important ways. In most cases, validity and reliability are not well established, raising crucial questions about what is being measured, and how well. In addition, the measures tend to be insensitive to small changes in performance, which may have a number of consequences. For example, important gains in fundamental or prerequisite abilities or processes often will not be sufficient to advance a patient to the next outcome category, or mildly impaired patients who have reached "independence" may have their treatment benefits terminated when there is more room for meaningful improvement. As noted in Chapter 5, section IV-C, ASHA is working on a functional outcome measure that speech-language pathologists hope will remedy some of these problems. It will be a professional challenge to convince administrators and third-party payers to accept a new measure, given that there are now large established data bases for some of the tools currently in use.

B. Quality of Life Issues

Another nontraditional type of assessment is concerned with quality of life (see Birren, Lubben, Rowe, & Deutchman, 1991; and Spilker, 1990, for more information on the areas discussed below).

1. Quality of life (QOL) issues, over and above "functional status," are not yet an integral part of rehabilitation evaluation, but they have been advocated for some time in the gerontology literature (e.g., Birren and colleagues). QOL is a complex and ill defined concept, and there is little agreement on how it should be operationalized or measured. The concept encompasses subjective factors such as life satisfaction, perceived health, and personal autonomy, and more concrete aspects like morbidity and disability, restricted activity days, social networks, and economic status.

2. Two general kinds of instruments are used for assessing dimensions of QOL: subjective measures, focusing on a respondent's self-perceptions, and "objective" measures, which are based on externally dictated or "normative" judgments of QOL. There are problems inherent in each approach (Birren & Dieckmann, 1991).

3. The available instruments are intended to evaluate specific or general aspects for one to four core domains as defined by Spilker: physical condition and abilities, psychological well-being, economic status and factors, and social interactions. Many QOL measures are derived from

a medical model and as such tend to overemphasize physical illness and functional status. Single domain outcome measures may be unsatisfying conceptually because they do not capture the multidimensional nature of QOL, but it can be tricky to interpret multiple domain measures, as different components may yield different results. Spilker's advice is to define beforehand the components that are most and least important for any given question or purpose, and to select instruments and weigh conflicting outcomes accordingly. Both references cited above describe á variety of instruments. One chapter (Arnold, 1991) gives some guidelines for selecting among alternative options depending on the purpose of evaluation (e.g., assessing the effects of various medical, social psychological, or rehabilitative interventions on QOL; evaluating quality of care; conducting needs assessments; or generally improving clinical decisions).

VI. IN SUMMARY: INTEGRATING AND INTERPRETING APPRAISAL DATA

A. The Goals of Appraisal and Evaluation

As noted above (section II), appraisal involves gathering the data that are needed to render a diagnosis, estimate prognoses, and formulate a treatment plan. The diagnostician's job during the appraisal process is one of solving puzzles and includes as its goals:

1. ascertaining patients' behavioral strengths and weaknesses;

2. distinguishing performances attributable to acute neurologic incident from those that more likely reflect pre-existing abilities or strategies, considering age, academic/vocational accomplishments, sensory deficits, cultural factors, social history, and so on;

3. identifying the nature of difficulties that are not consonant with premorbid expectations; and

4. discovering factors that influence performance.

B. The Appraisal Process: Generating and Testing Hypotheses

Potential hypotheses pertinent to each goal are formed as an assessment unfolds, beginning with the record review and patient observations, and continuing through the formal testing and follow up.

1. From direct patient interactions, a clinician's observations of response accuracy, response quality, and strategy or approach to performing a task, can contribute to the generation and evaluation of hypotheses about factors that appear to lead to success or failure, or about the presumed nature of impairments.

2. Strengths and weaknesses, and the nature of difficulties, are also evaluated by inspecting performance on items or tasks that cluster together by virtue of being performed successfully or poorly. These clusters can be analyzed to identify the processing operations or demands that they appear to have in common.

3. Because errors can occur on any test or procedure for a variety of reasons, the diagnostician often will need to entertain several possible explanations for the ways in which performances cluster together. Plausible alternatives need to be examined with relatively "pure" tasks that minimize confounds by focusing as much as possible on a single processing operation or skill at a time.

4. Founded on empirical, theoretical, and/or functional task analysis, probes can be constructed in an attempt to tap the source or level of impairment in any particular task or activity.

C. The Centrality of the Appraisal Process to Other Clinical Efforts

As a final note, a comment that recurs in this book bears repeating here. That is, the inferences derived from integrating and interpreting appraisal data will have important implications for other clinical efforts, including prognosis and treatment planning. It is to those other activities that the next chapters turn.

CHAPTER

5

Prognosis, Recovery, Treatment Efficacy, and Outcome

I. PROGNOSIS

A. Estimating Prognoses: An Introduction

Formulating prognoses involves predicting the future, which is always a tricky enterprise. It is especially so for RHD patients, because we have so little accumulated evidence to guide us. Clinically, to estimate prognoses, we assess biographic, medical, and behavioral variables such as those outlined by Wertz (1985; see Chapter 4, Table 4–1), and align them with our knowledge of the communicative requirements of each patient's everyday environment.

B. Specificity in Prognostication

Global prognostic statements, such as "prognosis is fair," are of little value, since they suggest neither the kind of performance we can expect in various situations, nor when we can expect it. We can be more specific in our forecasts if we ask ourselves the following questions: Prognosis for what level and kind of performance, and at what point in time? Are we predicting the likelihood that an individual patient will change sufficiently to be a rehabilitation candidate after several weeks of spontaneous improvement; to tolerate formal treatment in the first several weeks post-onset; to show meaningful improvement on general measures of communicative functioning after a specified period of treatment; to recognize and correct comprehension errors consistently after treatment; to return to work in some altered capacity within a year post-onset; to return to premorbid status at any time after the stroke; to manage legal and financial matters; to function competently in his or her social environment? Typically, we want to estimate individualized prognoses at a variety of levels such as these. And as indicated in Chapter 3, section III-D, we may need to revise our prognostic estimates periodically.

C. Some Potential Prognostic Factors for RHD Adults

There have been few prognostic studies focusing on RHD stroke patients. Those that are available tend to predict physical outcomes, such as ambulation and self-care ratings, or eventual placements, such as community living or institutionalization. Living at home 1 year after a stroke, with or without assistance, has been associated with the following factors evaluated at 2 weeks post-stroke: absence of neglect, perseveration, confusion, incontinence, or coma; good performance on sensory-motor tasks, mobility assessments, and personal activities of daily living; and relatively positive mood (Henley, Pettit, Todd-Pokropek, & Tupper, 1985). These factors suggest that patients with less severe impairments early on will have more favorable global outcomes. For our immediate clinical purposes, we can also tentatively extrapolate from the aphasia literature, and from some basic research with RHD adults, which has been reviewed in Chapter 2.

1. The aphasia literature suggests that initial severity of language (especially comprehension) impairment is the primary factor influencing later communicative ability. Initial severity is likely to be a potent predictor for cognitive and communicative outcomes after RHD as well. What we should measure to capture initial severity remains an open question. Impairments in selected domains (e.g., motor function) are also likely to predict some outcomes (e.g., ambulation and mobility) better than they predict others (e.g., pragmatic skills).

2. Numerous studies suggest that basic biographical variables are not very useful for predicting how RHD individuals will do on measures of communicative performance. Some results are noted below.

Because this research typically records demographic status and communication performance at the same point in time, we do not know if these biographical variables might predict future outcomes or performance levels.

a. The influence of chronological age is uncertain. It has not correlated with performance in a number of studies in which it has been assessed. In some other studies that have noted an association, large samples of patients have been tested; this allows extremely small correlations, which may be of dubious practical importance, to reach statistical significance. In addition, physical health problems and sensory deficits accompanying advancing age may be more important than age per se, but such variables are rarely accounted for or controlled.

b. Education also appears to be equivocal as a predictor, at least if a certain minimum level of literacy and achievement has been obtained. Some findings suggest that estimated premorbid intelligence (e.g., Barona, Reynolds, & Chastain, 1984; Wilson, Rosenbaum, & Brown, 1979) is a better predictor than the number of years of formal education, perhaps because the composite estimate is a more stable indicator than a single variable. Of course, the importance of literacy skills would depend on the behavior of interest. For example, literacy and premorbid intelligence are not likely to have much influence on the production of prosodic variation in speech or the performance of well-practiced activities of daily living. However, they may be crucially involved in interpreting figurative or implied meanings and in performing complex or abstract language tasks.

c. The influence of gender is also debatable, as gender differences in performance after RHD have rarely been noted. It is possible that some of the pragmatic/social interactional behaviors noted after RHD may interact with gender: Some sociolinguistic research suggests that women as a group are more attuned to social and emotional cues than men. Obviously any generalization of this sort may not fit any particular patient, but it would be important to consider premorbid social attunement when attributing abnormality or predicting outcome in these areas.

d. As indicated in Chapter 1, RHD patients who have communicative disorders have been observed to have a greater incidence of familial left-handedness than RHD patients whose communication is not impaired (Joanette et al., 1990).

3. On the basis of the aphasia literature, a number of medical variables are likely to be important. Generally speaking, prognostic estimates should be more favorable for patients who have smaller lesions, and unilateral lesions; who have not had previous strokes; who do not present with significant cortical atrophy; whose general health status prior to the stroke was good; whose hearing and vision are relatively intact; and whose strokes were more recent. Subcortical right hemisphere lesions have been suggested to be less likely than cortical right hemisphere lesions to result in communicative deficits (Joanette et al., 1990), but attentional disturbances that can accompany subcortical lesions could have profound influences on communicative behavior in RHD adults.

4. Among the behavioral variables that appear to be important is initial severity, as indicated above. Unfortunately, the tests that we can use to generate an index of overall severity have not provided evidence of predictive validity. In terms of more focused deficits, patients with persisting neglect and anosognosia are probably at greater risk for concomitant significant and lasting communication impairments (see Chapter 2). Finally, although it needs further development and validation, the working memory task described in Chapter 4, section III-E-5-d, may have clinical value for predicting RHD patients' performance under conditions of high information load (Tompkins, et al., 1994).

D. Prognostic Treatment

The concept of prognostic treatment, illustrated by Rosenbek, LaPointe, and Wertz (1989), is clinically an important one. These authors suggest that we conduct several treatment sessions to see if our patients will learn, generalize the improvement to untreated stimuli, retain what they have learned, and exhibit a willingness to practice. Patients who achieve all four in a few sessions are enrolled for further treatment, with the expectation of a relatively good prognosis. The book by Rosenbek et al. provides a number of useful examples of this concept and its implementation.

II. RECOVERY

A. The Concept of Recovery

"Recovery" after brain injury can take two forms: spontaneous (natural, or neurologic) and assisted (associated with treatment). "Recovery" is in quotation marks because the term connotes a return to premorbid function which is frequently unattainable after brain injury, particularly for patients who are impaired enough to warrant our services. For this reason, the material below refers to "improvement" rather than "recovery."

B. Spontaneous Improvement

Spontaneous improvement is thought to reflect the resolution of neurologic complications of acute brain damage. For a week or so after a stroke, phenomena distinct from the lesion itself, such as swelling of surrounding brain tissue, widespread release of neurotransmitters, and cerebral hypoperfusion, combine to reduce a patient's abilities in a broad range of functions. As the patient stabilizes and these complications subside, his or her cognitive and behavioral status will change rapidly.

1. There is much debate in the aphasia literature about how long the period of spontaneous improvement lasts; some suggest that its duration is on the order of several weeks, while others argue that it lasts for several months. In any case, the instability of function in at least the initial month following acute brain injury makes it difficult to predict eventual performance levels or to demonstrate intervention effects during that period of time.

2. Patterns of improvement may vary with the type of neurologic event. Change following occlusive stroke tends to be greatest in the first 4 to 6 weeks, whereas patients with hemorrhagic strokes may show little change for the first several months before experiencing a rapid period of improvement that may eventually exceed the level associated with occlusive stroke.

3. Spontaneous improvement has been documented for neglect, anosognosia, geographic disorientation, and prosodic comprehension disorders, and it is likely that it occurs for other deficit areas as well. However, the rate, extent, and sequence of improvement in various functions are unpredictable and unknown. Although these data are essential for prognosis and for treatment planning, they will be very difficult to gather. Early post-stroke intervention, which is becoming the rule, will obscure changes that would occur if a patient were not immediately enrolled in task-oriented communicative therapy.

C. Assisted Improvement

Assisted improvement is that which is assumed to occur as a result of intervention. There is no rigorous evidence on the extent to which treatment can assist RHD patients with communicative deficits. Several reports are available documenting improvements on discrete tasks after interventions for neglect and other perceptual impairments (e.g., Gordon et al., 1985; Weinberg et al., 1977, 1979,1982). In the most controlled of this series of studies, the untreated group caught up to the treated group 4 months after discharge, raising questions about the nature and value of the gains effected in treatment. And for the most part, these studies have neither addressed nor demonstrated long-term maintenance and functional generalization of treatment gains (see Chapter 7, section V-C-6, for more information).

III. TREATMENT EFFICACY AND THE SCIENCE OF CLINICAL PRACTICE

A. The Concept of Treatment Efficacy

The evaluation of treatment efficacy is concerned with the extent to which our clients will benefit from our treatments. The question of efficacy has evolved from "Does treatment work?" to considering as well "What treatments work with what types of patients, and under what conditions?" Most clinicians assume that their treatment is responsible for the progress their clients make. But this remains an assumption unless rigorous evaluation has been done to rule out other possible reasons for change in performance (e.g., see sections III-B-2 and III-C-2, below).

B. The Need for Treatment Efficacy Data

Valid, reliable data documenting treatment efficacy are crucial for several reasons.

1. First, we are professionally responsible for demonstrating that our treatments work. One tenet of the ASHA Code of Ethics (ASHA,1992) is that clinicians must evaluate the impact of their services. In this vein, I concur with Rosenbek et al's. (1989, p. 12) assertion that "untested treatments are immoral, therefore clinical practice must include clinical experimentation." The effects, effectiveness, and efficiency of various assessment and treatment approaches cannot be assumed, and we owe it to our patients to provide them with the most appropriate services.

2. Aphasiologists have struggled long and hard against skepticism from many quarters, including physicians and health-care providers, about the value of our intervention efforts. Our patients' progress is

frequently attributed to spontaneous improvement, or to psychosocial support and attention which, by implication, could be provided
by lots of other people. Thanks to clinical research, we have begun
to accumulate the evidence we need to counter these sorts of claims
for aphasic patients. With the burgeoning of service delivery for
RHD patients, we should anticipate, and be as proactive as possible
about, this same kind of skepticism.

C. An Introduction to Efficacy Evaluation

Clinicians are in a position to contribute meaningfully to the data base
that should form the foundation of our diagnostic and treatment decisions. With some planning and foresight, and some assistance from a
research consultant, many clinicians should be able to provide much-
needed data to the professional literature. Tompkins (1994) puts forth a
number of recommendations for clinicians who wish to contribute to the
scientific data base. At a minimum, clinicians can keep efficacy principles in mind as they plan and evaluate their own interventions (see section III-C, below).

1. **Designs for evaluating treatments.** Single-subject or within-sub-
   ject experimental designs (e.g., McReynolds & Kearns, 1983) are
   probably the most appropriate for clinicians to use in evaluating
   their treatments. In these designs, observable, clearly specified target behaviors (e.g., number of statements that maintain topic appropriately during 2-minute conversations with therapist), are measured
   repeatedly in a pre-treatment baseline phase (designated A) and during treatment (designated B). A variety of sophisticated designs are
   available for a variety of purposes. The two most basic designs,
   reversal and multiple baseline, are discussed below.

   a. The reversal design is also known as a withdrawal or ABA
      design. There are many variations of this design, but in the most
      basic case, baseline (A) and treatment (B) phases are followed
      by a second no-treatment phase (second A), during which treat-
      ment is withdrawn. Treatment effects are demonstrated when
      relatively stable baseline performance is followed by distinctive
      gains in the treatment phase, which recede when treatment is
      withdrawn. Without the reversal phase, it would not be possible
      to separate the gains made during the treatment phase from
      those associated with some extraneous process, like attention,
      social support, or natural improvement. Further evidence of
      treatment effects can be collected by reinstituting treatment

after the reversal phase, creating an ABAB design. If performance improves again, the treatment itself is the most likely agent of change.

Some have suggested that a major problem with reversal designs is that they must be implemented on behaviors that are reversible or that can be turned on and off. For many of our treatment activities, we expect behavior change to be cumulative and long-lasting, and correspondingly we do not expect treatment effects to disappear once treatment is withdrawn. But the effectiveness of treatment can be demonstrated in an ABA design if the target behavior sags somewhat when treatment is withdrawn (although probably not back to pre-treatment baseline level), particularly if a second-treatment phase reverses the trend in the baseline again. ABA designs can also be implemented effectively for behaviors that are expected to change quickly. One can apply a treatment briefly, and after performance has accelerated, withdraw it briefly, before the treatment gains have had time to become consolidated and lasting.

b. Multiple baseline designs incorporate a series of AB designs, staggered in time and typically conducted on the same subject. Different behaviors, settings, or conditions are selected as treatment targets, and performance in each one is measured over time. For simplicity, this discussion refers only to different behaviors.

   (1) Usually, a minimum of three behaviors is targeted, and the same treatment is applied, in turn, to each. This, and other aspects of the following discussion, are illustrated in Figure 5–1, showing one aphasic patient's performance in a multiple baseline study that focused on facilitating requests (Doyle, Goldstein, Bougeois, & Nakles, 1989).

   (2) Before treatment is initiated, baseline data are gathered on all behaviors (requests for information about different topics, in the Doyle and colleagues example), until they demonstrate stability (e.g., a minimum of 3 data points for each behavior, with no more than about 10% variation in performance). Then treatment is applied to Behavior 1 (requests for information about Health Topics, in Figure 5–1), while continuing periodic baseline measurements on the other behaviors. When Behavior 1 has reached the desired (or criterion) level, treatment is discontinued on that behavior and initiated on Behavior 2. While Behavior 2 is being treated, baseline measurements continue on Behavior 3, and measures of mainte-

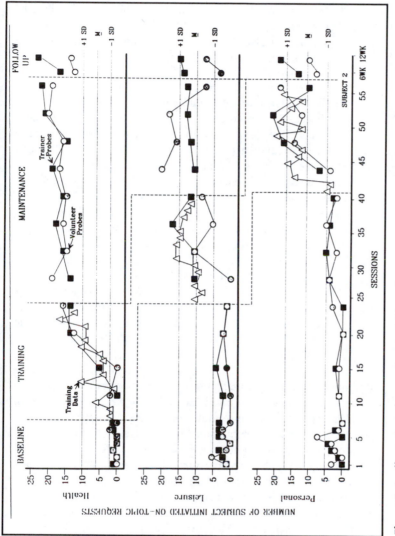
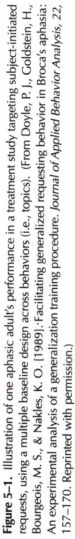

Figure 5–1. Illustration of one aphasic adult's performance in a treatment study targeting subject-initiated requests, using a multiple baseline design across behaviors (i.e., topics). (From Doyle, P. J., Goldstein, H., Bourgeois, M. S., & Nakles, K. O. [1989].·Facilitating generalized requesting behavior in Broca's aphasia: An experimental analysis of a generalization training procedure. *Journal of Applied Behavior Analysis, 22,* 157–170. Reprinted with permission.)

nance are taken for Behavior 1. Finally, the treatment is instituted for Behavior 3, while maintenance data are gathered for the other behaviors. Treatment effects are indicated when each behavior improves over baseline (level or trend) during its treatment phase, while the others remain relatively stable in their untreated phases. Figure 5–1 also illustrates some longer-term maintenance data, taken 6 weeks and 12 weeks after treatment ended for Behavior 3.

(3) To demonstrate treatment effects in a multiple baseline design, the treated behaviors have to be functionally independent, or dissimilar enough, so that treatment applied to one will not generalize immediately to the others. This can strike clinicians as counterintuitive in that our clinical goal is to facilitate generalization. But if all behaviors change when treatment is applied to one of them, the changes cannot be attributed unequivocally to generalization effects of treatment. Some clinician-researchers modify these designs to target several behaviors that they expect to be independent, and several others that they expect to be related to the treated behaviors. This way, they may wind up with the best of both worlds. If each "independent" behavior changes only when it is specifically treated, the treatment can be considered to be responsible for the changes, and if the "related" behaviors change along with the treated behaviors, some generalization is occurring.

c. Single-subject experimental designs are discussed in detail in a number of sources (e.g., McReynolds & Kearns, 1983). Kent (1985) provides a useful table illustrating a variety of research questions together with some of the single-subject designs that are appropriate for addressing those questions. Rosenbek and colleagues (1989) also present a clear discussion of their nature and utility. Examples of studies using these designs with neurologically impaired persons are also available in the aphasiology literature (cf., Bellaire, Georges, & Thompson, 1991; Kearns & Potechin Scher, 1989; Massaro & Tompkins, 1994; Whitney & Goldstein, 1989).

2. **Single-subject designs versus pretest-posttest designs.** Some people mistakenly equate single-subject designs with pretest-posttest case studies. The two are actually quite dissimilar, in that only the former designs incorporate the controls necessary to attribute a change in performance to the intervention per se. In a pretest-posttest design, a tar-

get behavior is measured once prior to treatment, an intervention is applied, and then the target behavior is measured again. This is a weak form of evidence about a treatment's effects because a change from pretest could have resulted from a number of extraneous factors, such as natural improvement in neurologic status; the influence of prior or concurrent other treatments; the patient's emotional adjustment and self-generated compensation; the influence of medication; and/or a general effect of attention and social support. In addition, the single measures taken before and after treatment do not allow inferences about the timing or pattern of change that may be occurring.

Well-conceived single-subject designs are built around components of scientific inquiry, such as operationally defined and replicable procedures, attention to multiple aspects of reliability and validity, and control of confounding variables such as sequence and order effects. Specifically operationalized target behaviors are measured repeatedly in each design phase, with independent verification of scoring for a portion of those behaviors by another examiner (interjudge reliability). Pre-intervention baseline data, ideally at a stable level, are used as reference points for evaluating the effects of well-specified interventions conducted with well-defined subjects. A treatment effect is manifest as an obvious change from baseline in the level or trend of the target behavior, as long as that change cannot be convincingly attributed to extraneous factors. The believability of treatment effects is demonstrated when they are replicated, across patients, across behaviors, and/or across design phases (e.g., baseline, treatment, return to baseline or maintenance).The multiple measures, continuous probing, and replication that characterize single-subject designs allow the investigator, in many cases, to separate extraneous effects from treatment effects with confidence.

3. **Evaluating maintenance, generalization, and clinical significance of treatment.** To supplement the basic information about treatment effects that can be derived from single-subject designs, additional probes are necessary. These are designed and conducted to determine whether treatment effects maintain over time, generalize beyond the training conditions, or reflect meaningful changes.

   a. Short-term maintenance probes are built in to multiple baseline designs, as noted above. Some researchers and clinicians implement follow-up assessments to evaluate longer-term maintenance of treatment gains, but unfortunately it is rare for data to be collected much more than a few weeks after the end of treatment. Evaluating maintenance over extended time intervals should become a priority.

b. If generalized improvement beyond the treated stimuli and tasks is not apparent, treatment effects cannot be considered very meaningful. The previous discussion of multiple baseline designs referred to a limited form of generalization, to responses or tasks related to the treatment targets. For most treatments, more extensive generalization to other situations, conditions, or related abilities does not happen without being carefully planned. Generalization planning involves "comprehensive, multifaceted evaluation; the establishment of generalization criteria; incorporation of treatment strategies that might facilitate generalization; continuous measurement and probing for functional, generalized improvements; and, when necessary, extending treatments to additional settings, people, and conditions until targeted levels of generalization occur" (Kearns, 1993, p. 71). Generalization planning is considered more fully in Chapter 6, section II-F.

c. Direct evaluation of the meaningfulness or "clinical significance" of treatment effects is also important. Goldstein (1990) reviews several approaches for examining clinical significance (sometimes called "social validity"). These include normative comparisons, in which subjects' target performance is measured against a "normal" or "expected" standard; and subjective evaluations of changes by judges unfamiliar with the subjects and their treatment status. Results of these types of assessments have begun to appear in the language intervention literature (e.g., Doyle, Goldstein, & Bourgeois, 1987; Massaro & Tompkins, 1994; Thompson & Byrne, 1984). Another way to assess the importance or strength of a treatment effect is to set a predetermined difference criterion, designating, for example, a change of at least one or two standard deviation units, or a doubling or tripling of baseline performance, as clinically meaningful.

4. Clinicians gathering efficacy data: The potential, and some pitfalls.

a. Despite the value of single-subject designs for examining treatment efficacy, there remain relatively few published examples in the literature on adult neurologic communication disorders. Perhaps the practical difficulty of implementing controlled research in a clinical environment is partly responsible for this situation. The major difference between typical clinical procedure and rigorous study may be the time required to conduct repeated probes of behavior in the no-treatment phases (Warren, Gabriel, Johnston, & Gaddie, 1987). In addition, designing and implementing generalization probes outside the treatment setting take time and planning. Regardless of these barriers, those who have the drive to tackle a research problem, and who consult with knowledgeable investigators, could probably evaluate a number of questions in their clinical settings, particularly if they enlist assistance in scoring, checking scoring reliability, and the like. If several clinicians from one program are interested they can share these tasks, or graduate students from local university programs can be recruited and trained to assist. Some of the kinds of studies which clinicians can probably implement most readily are described by Tompkins (1994).

b. Clinicians who accept the challenge to gather efficacy data should be cognizant of several other possible pitfalls.

    (1) As noted above, documenting progress over the course of treatment does not demonstrate efficacy. There are many things other than treatment that might account for changes in patients' performance.

    (2) The trend toward increasingly early intervention, also noted previously, will make it hard to demonstrate the efficacy of treatment, and particularly so for long-term treatment objectives. In the acute post-stroke period, when neurologic improvement runs its course, pre-treatment performance baselines may be quite unstable, making it difficult to distinguish changes in treatment from improvement that was occurring naturally. In addition, as patients stabilize neurologically and begin to adapt to their altered status, the deficits or skills most appropriate for treatment may change rapidly. Something that looks like a potential treatment target one week may have improved so much by the next week that it does not need to be addressed directly. The tendency to intervene almost immediately after a stroke has other implications for studying treatment efficacy, as well. If, in the immediate post-onset period, we initiate treatment for deficits that would recover on their own, we may use up the patient's rehabilitation allowance before persisting problems are apparent. Patients may not experience the full impact of some of their deficits until they have left the rehabilitation center and returned to the real world. These long-term deficits would be ideal targets for treatment efficacy studies, but if funding has run out, further treatment is unlikely to be provided or evaluated.

D. The Science of Accountable Clinical Practice

Some clinicians will blanch at the thought of doing research, but clinically accountable diagnosis and treatment are based on principles that guide scientific inquiry. An approach, and an attitude, infused by scientific principles should improve the precision and quality of clinical service delivery.

1. According to Silverman (1985), a scientific approach to clinical management involves four principles: specifying clear objectives, posing testable hypotheses and questions, observing and collecting data systematically, and remaining aware of the tentative nature of the findings. Generally, there are many parallels between sound treatment and a research project. For instance, in each session we can and should define a problem, develop and test hypotheses, collect good data, evaluate the results, and then determine the next questions to pursue. Using a hypothesis testing model, we would gather initial information about our patients from a variety of sources, form our best guesses regarding the nature of strengths and weaknesses and what can be done to ameliorate them, and then test and refine our hypotheses.

2. More specifically, single-subject designs and the scientific principles that guide them are important for documenting an individual patient's response to treatment. When used appropriately, they allow us to state with greater assurance whether a change in behavior occurs when we intervene, and whether that change should be attributed to our treatment. The repeated measurement and regular probing associated with single-subject designs can also help to guide day-to-day treatment decisions. When treatment response is not as rapid or as dramatic as we expect, we can make a modification and measure its effect. For example, if performance plateaus on a treatment activity, we can introduce a branch step to help shape our patient's response and resume progression through the treatment program. Ultimately, promising results of efficacy studies will increase our confidence in using a similar approach with other patients resembling our test case.

3. If a full-blown efficacy evaluation is too daunting given day-to-day responsibilities and time constraints, clinicians can make their own treatments more rigorous by incorporating as much as possible the elements of well-designed treatment studies, listed below. The more that we attend to these elements, the more assured we can be in interpreting the results of our interventions, leading to more accountable service delivery (see Tompkins, 1994, for elaboration of these points):

    a. operationally specifying (1) the nature of the client's abilities and deficits; (2) intervention plans, procedures, and decisions; and (3) outcome levels and criteria;

    b. maximizing reliability and validity of measurement for target behaviors and treatment implementation;

    c. collecting an adequate behavior sample, including repeated measurements for assessing stability of baseline performance, pattern of change in treatment, and various levels of generalization;

    d. attempting to account for the effects of extraneous factors like neurologic improvement and premorbid ability/interest;

    e. replicating treatment effects across behaviors and/or conditions;

    f. programming for and measuring generalization to untreated behaviors, abilities, partners, and/or settings;

    g. examining the maintenance of behavior change after treatment ends; and

    h. assessing clinical significance (social validity) to determine whether the changes effected have "made a difference."

4. Finally, a scientific approach is needed to cope with the explosion of professional information on the market today. Many tests and treatment packages are put forward without adequate scientific development or documentation. As suggested earlier, clinicians are well-positioned to collect evidence about the efficacy and applicability of these materials. But minimally, clinicians considering whether or how to use these materials must be aware of their strengths and limitations. Wise consumption of professional information requires critical thinking about the validity of the claims presented in published studies, clinical manuals, advertisements, and continuing education programs. We need to guard against a tendency to accept at face value anything that is published or presented at a conference, especially by someone considered an authority. As noted in Chapter 1, many such materials have flaws that limit their value. Clinicians can consult several sources for guidance in evaluating published material and presentations (e.g., Kent, 1985; Tompkins, 1994).

IV OUTCOME

A. Levels of Outcome and Functional Status

Rehabilitation outcome can be conceptualized and measured on a variety of levels. Clinical significance and meaningfulness of outcome, in particular, have become increasingly important concerns from both clinical and reimbursement perspectives.

1. **Instrumental, intermediate, and ultimate outcomes.** Most of us would agree that our ultimate goal should be to enhance patients' communicative effectiveness in real-life interactions. But we also know that there are typically a number of steps along the way to ultimate, clinically significant outcomes. Campbell and Bain (1991) contrast ultimate outcomes with intermediate outcomes (those believed to be prerequisite for progressing toward ultimate goals) and with instrumental outcomes (those that may lead to other outcomes without further treatment). An example of an intermediate goal for a RHD patient might be to increase time spent attending in rehabilitation tasks, as a prerequisite for improving strategic attentional control. A potential instrumental goal might be to establish a compensatory strategy that is assumed to have broad applicability for functional communication, such as referring to a memory aid. Campbell and Bain note that it is difficult to identify instrumental outcomes in language intervention because we have little information about which cognitive or linguistic abilities would allow other goals to be reached without additional intervention, and that generalization data would be necessary to test the assumption that an instrumental outcome has been achieved.

2. **Impairment, disability, and handicap.** Taking a similar tack, Schwartz and Whyte (1992) discuss interventions in the framework proposed by the World Health Organization (1980), which distinguishes among impairment, functional disability, and related handicap. Impairment refers to specific deficits in psychologic, physiologic, or anatomic structure or function (e.g., neglect). Underlying impairments are often a priority for treatment during the acute phases after stroke. Disability refers to the impact of impairments on specific activities (e.g., neglect may affect the patient's ability to read and write, or to determine the significance and salience of environmental stimuli and cues needed to cross the street safely), and functional disabilities result from lasting impairments. Handicap reflects the effects of disabilities on typical social roles (e.g., neglect mitigates against the patient returning to his job, or contributes to discomfort of friends who subsequently stop including the patient in social activities). Thus, the concepts of "functional disability" and "handicap" in this perspective are related to functional communicative adequacy or ultimate outcomes.

B. Documenting Functional Status

Documenting functional status has recently taken on more practical urgency. Rapidly escalating health care costs and concern about cost accountability have instigated a search for outcome measures that can be used to cut rehabilitation expenditures. A variety of generic rating scales have been proposed to quantify "functional independence" or "functional outcome" (see Warren, Loverso, & DePiero, 1991). These scales are being advocated not only for documenting quality of services and reimbursement rates, but also for determining eligibility for services. Unfortunately, for the most part, issues of reliability, validity, and sensitivity to change have been inadequately addressed in the development and application of these scales (ASHA, 1990; Kearns, 1993). The American Speech-Language-Hearing Association is in the process of validating a more extensive functional communication measure for adults (Fratalli, 1991), an important step in the effort to meld clinical and financial concerns.

C. Conducting Treatment in a Levels of Outcome Framework

1. **Planning the path from impairment and prerequisite goals, to ultimate goals.** Communication intervention for stroke patients has tended to focus much more on impairment than on functional disability or social communication. This may be absolutely necessary, particularly in the early stages after onset, as maximizing performance in areas of basic impairment may be prerequisite to establishing functional interaction in the longer term. But if we do not map out where our prerequisite tasks are leading, we may earn the poor opinion of our professional abilities that is held by some neurologists and other medical personnel. When our treatments are not intended or expected to result quickly in clinically significant gains, it will be incumbent on us to specify the eventual pathway from our treatment focus to the desired end result, indicating why or how our treatment goals should be important steps along the way to more relevant outcomes.

2. **Demonstrating the meaningfulness and durability of change associated with treatment.** Two ways to demonstrate the functionality of outcomes are (1) to achieve generalization to ecologically valid conditions, or settings and tasks more like those the patient faces every day; and (2) to document the social validity of changes. To examine the durability of meaningful change, we can begin to assess clinical significance or social validity using data

from several phases of our treatment programs, including baseline, treatment, and follow-up or maintenance.

D. Melding Functional and Deficit-Oriented Concerns

Although the importance of meaningful outcomes is undeniable, the pressure to document changes in "functional outcome" may have some unintended negative consequences. If clinicians slight intermediate or prerequisite goals in a rush to target ecologically valid conditions such as conversational exchanges, patients may not master, or automatize, some of the "basic building blocks" that would allow them to converse more successfully. And "overlearning," or "training sufficient exemplars," is a frequently advocated principle for enhancing generalization. As suggested previously, functional concerns should be wed with impairment- or deficit-oriented strategies, so that patients can communicate as well as possible at various stages after neurologic insult.

CHAPTER

6

Treatment Principles and Considerations

This chapter focuses first on issues of treatment candidacy, progression, and documentation and ends with a summary of principles to guide clinical management. More basic considerations, such as the general characteristics of individual treatment sessions, are not covered here, as the excellent suggestions provided in other introductory sources on neurogenic disorders (e.g., Brookshire, 1992) are broadly applicable.

I. CANDIDACY FOR TREATMENT

A. The Question of Candidacy

Before considering the when, what, and how of treatment, we must decide the whether of treatment. The question of candidacy is related to prognosis and outcome at both ends of the severity spectrum. At one extreme, a patient with a very poor prognosis, whose impairments were so severe that minimal improvement would be expected with intervention, would be a poor candidate for treatment. On the other hand, someone whose initial symptoms were mild and likely to recover on their own, might not be a treatment candidate, either.

B. Deferring Candidacy Decisions

Due to the rapid physiologic and behavioral changes that follow acute stroke (see Chapter 5, section II-B), candidacy decisions, like prognostic estimates, may be more valid if they are deferred until a patient's condition stabilizes somewhat. Candidacy decisions are best deferred in some other cases as well. For example, when a patient is too weak, ill, distractible, or depressed for an accurate evaluation of his or her deficits and abilities, we are unable to determine candidacy, estimate prognoses, or predict outcomes. In such cases, patients can be followed periodically until their cognitive, physical, and emotional condition allows valid assessment and decision making. Regardless of when the candidacy decision is made, clinicians are usually uncomfortable recommending not to intervene without conducting a period of prognostic treatment (see Chapter 5, section I-D), if a patient has obvious impairments of cognition and communication.

C. Potential Negative Candidacy Indicators for RHD Adults

We have little hard data on which to base candidacy (and related) decisions for RHD adults, but research and intuition suggest that unawareness or denial of deficits that persist after the initial phase of physiologic improvement can be ominous. Patients with these characteristics are unlikely to be active or willing participants in treatment, even if they can be coaxed to attend; patients who do not want to be treated ultimately will not be good candidates for treatment.

II. INITIATING, PLANNING, CONDUCTING, AND TERMINATING TREATMENT

A. Initiating Formal Treatment

How soon to begin treatment after stroke is a question that has long been debated in the aphasia literature. Proponents of early intervention assert that treatment delivered soon after stroke onset may be able to capitalize on the rapid gains associated with physiologic improvement. In addition, early treatment may help avoid the development of mal-adaptive behaviors and strategies. Finally, both patients and families need information, support, education, and referral in the early post-onset phase. Advocates of postponing treatment counter that a patient's performance is too volatile immediately after stroke onset. Some delay is important to allow functions to stabilize so that we can determine more accurately the nature and extent of residual communicative and cognitive deficits. For example, RHD adults whose early attentional-perceptual impairments (e.g., concentration deficits, neglect, anosog-nosia) have improved should be better able to profit from direct inter-vention. It would certainly be possible to provide important supportive services in the immediate post-stroke phase, without initiating formal communication treatment.

There is no easy answer to this question of when to begin treatment, and again, no data to help us decide. My recommendation is for periodic and relatively short evaluative visits during the first few weeks post-onset, depending on a patient's ability to tolerate them. During these visits, the clinician can observe the patient's evolving abilities and self-generated strategies; develop and provide suggestions for coping with immediate communication problems; and offer education and support to patients and families. Any conclusions that are drawn or goals that are set dur-ing this time should remain tentative and should change as performance does. By postponing formal evaluation and treatment for at least the first 3 to 4 weeks post-onset, the clinician will have more accurate infor-mation for guiding treatment plans. Of course, as noted above, formal evaluation and treatment should be deferred whenever a patient is too weak, ill, distractible, or depressed to participate.

B. General Treatment Approaches

1. Two general treatment approaches are most often employed with brain-damaged adults: facilitation and compensation.

   a. Facilitation approaches are based on an assumption that functions previously performed by damaged brain systems can be enhanced, or reallocated, by the treatment process. This assump-tion is usually held when the etiology of damage entails a period of natural improvement, as in the case of stroke and traumatic brain injury. The mechanisms by which facilitation acts on brain systems are presumed to involve restoration or repair of impaired functions (sometimes called restitution), as well as substitution or reorganization by intact parts of the brain. Clinicians who focus on facilitation strategies also frequently assume that knowledge and processing abilities are not lost after stroke. Some of the literature reviewed in Chapter 2 supports that view for RHD adults, although our understanding of the nature of their cognitive and communicative dysfunction is currently minimal.

One problem with designating and developing facilitation techniques is that, even if we were able to pinpoint the cognitive operations underlying specific communicative performances, the exact ways in which those operations were damaged, and the precise nature of their interaction with other processes, we would not know what to do to repair or replace the damaged operations. Certainly, more explicit theories of deficits are needed, together with more specific links between those theories and the characteristics of treatment techniques presumed to be facilitative. Additionally, a theory of treatment is needed that specifies how cognitive systems can be modified by various forms of intervention (e.g., Caramazza, 1989; Holland, 1994).

b. Compensation approaches are based on the presumption that damaged brains do not recover fully. If this is true, we must find ways to help patients circumvent, or work around, their deficits. The purpose of compensatory adjustments is to maximize a patient's (residual) communicative abilities. This usually involves modifying or altering typical means or modes of functioning. For example, a patient whose reading comprehension is compromised by severe visual neglect and restricted scanning could be taught to remind himself to look to the left, and to monitor meaning as he reads. The reading material itself could be structured to reduce scanning problems, and to create obvious discontinuities in meaning when the left-most margin is ignored. The clinician delivering these techniques could sit on the patient's good side to maximize the probability of the patient's profiting from the treatment interaction. Finally, to ensure the severely neglecting patient's comprehension of crucial information, families and staff members could be taught to present the information auditorily, in manageable chunks, while checking regularly for comprehension. These examples illustrate that compensatory adjustments can involve the patient, the environment, or both.

c. The balance between facilitation and compensation approaches often evolves as a patient recovers. Early treatment is likely to focus predominantly on presumed facilitation strategies, while treatment for a more stable patient will likely emphasize compensation. However, even in the early going, a combination of these approaches is often warranted. Treatment should be tailored to try to restore or reroute as much as possible the operations presumed to underlie communicative problems; but at the same time, specific compensations may help an individual to meet immediate everyday needs. Finally, these approaches are not mutually exclusive and often may be interactive. For example, implementing some of the neglect compensations sketched above, especially in the early period post-stroke, may facilitate the allocation of attention for reading.

2. Somewhat related to the contrast between facilitation and compensation approaches is the distinction between focusing on processes versus behavior.

   a. We know that communicative symptoms, or objectifiable behaviors, can arise for different reasons. Much evidence on this point has derived from studies of the multiplicity of factors contributing to word-retrieval difficulties in aphasia. In Chapter 2, we considered how multiple processes may be involved in generating deficient inferences or in difficulties appreciating a variety of intended meanings after RHD, and we noted the multidimensional nature of attention and memory functions. Analyzing the multiple processes that may influence the observable end-point behavior, and selecting some to target in treatment, can be distinguished from focusing treatment solely on the terminal behaviors themselves.

   b. Again, a judicious combination of approaches is appropriate. Intuitively, in many cases, treatment should be most effective if it is directed at component processes or mechanisms identified in task-related cognitive models, rather than at the behavior as a whole. In other cases, it may be efficient to modify certain observable behaviors quickly, even if they could be related to a process model. As possible examples, symptoms such as socially inappropriate remarks, impulsiveness, lack of eye contact, deficient perception of nonverbal cues, poor scanning for functional tasks like reading, and an inability to monitor for discourse errors or conversational signals may respond to behavioral treatments, even while clinicians work on processes presumed to underlie or influence these same behaviors.

   c. As a first step in identifying the component processes potentially involved in communicative and cognitive tasks that are important for RHD stroke patients, clinicians need to review (critically) the relevant literature and continuing education offerings for both brain-damaged and normal adults. Some hypothesized components of specific tasks were discussed in the symptom reviews in Chapters 2 and 4 and will be outlined with potential treatment activities in Chapter 7. Further suggestions for clinicians to follow in designing theoretically based intervention programs, adapted from Sohlberg and Mateer (1989a), are provided in Table 6–1. However, a previously identified caveat remains: Being able to analyze a function and to isolate deficits in process-oriented terms does not directly lead to one "best" intervention strategy.

d. When theoretical foundations for performance are inadequate or unspecified, logical task analysis may help to focus the treat-

Table 6–1. Steps for designing and evaluating theoretically based interventions

Stage	*Action*	*Goal*
Information gathering	Review cognitive psychology literature	Understand nature of cognitive processes
	Review neuropsychologic literature	Understand established scientific processes related to pathology
	Review normal cognitive aging literature	Understand age effects on performance
	Examine clinical practice and efficacy literature	Appreciate successes and shortcomings
Program development	Outline presumed components of tasks and functions	Develop evaluation and treatment model
	Appraise component performance	Identify spared and impaired components
	Organize treatment tasks hierarchically for targeted components	Design remediation program
Efficacy evaluation	Gather baseline and generalization probe data; implement other elements of efficacy study	Assess efficacy (ideally including generalization, maintenance, and social validity)

Source: Adapted from Sohlberg and Mateer, 1989a.

ment process. To develop initial targets and a potential progression for treatment, the presumed steps or requirements for completing specific tasks (usually functional ones) are analyzed and aligned with a patient's abilities. For the example of reading, a clinician would try to identify the perceptual, attentional, and linguistic demands of relevant tasks and to assess the client's performance in each area before targeting specific components or skills.

3. Regardless of one's general orientation, repetition will play a crucial role in treatment. Cognitive processing becomes more efficient, and learning is consolidated, through repeated activation of the targeted systems and operations. It has already been noted that extensive practice makes performance more automatic, presumably reducing demands on limited processing resources (see Chapter 2, section III-D-6-a). Some degree of automaticity may be critical for achieving generalization, or the volitional, self-directed application of target skills and behaviors outside of the clinic room.

4. A note on computers and rehabilitation is warranted here. Software packages are increasingly available that are intended to facilitate skills such as perception, concentration, and problem solving. Testimonials about their effectiveness are also proliferating, despite much evidence to the contrary (see Robertson, 1990, for review).

   a. Computer programs are usually recommended as adjuncts to traditional therapy. A variety of advantages, many of which are procedural and administrative, have been advanced by proponents of computerized rehabilitation programs. For instance, computer packages allow consistent, objective, and repetitive stimulus presentation and efficient administration of practice tasks. They may assist with data collection, data tabulation, and report writing. Further, they may capture a patient's interest, fostering a desire to practice outside of the treatment room.

   b. There are also numerous disadvantages of computerized rehabilitation efforts, many of which were cogently reviewed by Robertson (1990). Efficacy concerns predominate and are the final issues discussed below, after some other problems are considered. Improvements in some of these other problem areas (e.g., flexibility, validity) should enhance the likelihood of obtaining promising efficacy data for computerized treatment programs.

      (1) Some of the disadvantages are due to limitations of the programming itself. For example, flexibility may be a problem (e.g., administering individualized programs of cues,

prompts, or chaining steps for patients contingent on the nature and pattern of their performance, which may change within and between sessions). At present, these kinds of limitations restrict the treatment process, but they may be relatively easily addressed as technology advances.

(2) Other important disadvantages center around concerns of (construct and content) validity. Few computerized treatment tasks are based on models or theories of deficit performance, and few of the programs incorporate sophisticated principles or procedures of treatment progression. A number of packages take a scattershot approach, failing to target distinct and identifiable component processes or skills. As a result, they are rarely focused on patients' specific needs and problems and are likely to be inefficient if they are effective at all. Clinicians should ask themselves whether various computerized treatment packages provide convincing evidence to document that they target what they are intended to target. When that question can be answered affirmatively, clinicians should consider how the programs fit into their treatment models before deciding whether to use them with their patients.

(3) A related issue involves limitations in the kinds of skills that computerized programs can address. Human interaction would seem to be necessary for treating many of the pragmatic and conversational problems affecting RHD adults.

(4) Another issue has to do with patients' reactions. Computers and computer games are not universally motivating, especially for people who have not had prior experience with them.

(5) Finally, insufficient evidence of efficacy is the most crucial concern. In a review of computerized cognitive rehabilitation studies, Robertson (1990) concludes that "no computer cognitive rehabilitation procedures have been shown to generalize to real life, and there is no existing empirical basis for the sale or distribution of any computerized cognitive rehabilitation programmes for nonresearch purposes" (p. 381). Concerns of generalization aside, few of the studies that Robertson reviewed could convincingly assert that changes in patients' behavior were attributable to the treatment provided. He emphasizes that patients and their families are harmed if they buy these packages at high cost and use them for months without benefit.

The evidence for RHD adults is essentially nonexistent. In the few efficacy studies that include some RHD subjects, they are combined with traumatically brain-injured patients and/or aphasic adults. One of the studies with a mixed patient sample demonstrated positive results for a program of activities focused on attention and perceptual speed, that generalized to a range of less-closely related tests of psychomotor function, logical thinking, and spatial reasoning. (Generalization to daily life was not addressed). But as Robertson notes, without evidence of more functional improvement one cannot rule out the possibility that this kind of training simply facilitates patients' ability to increase their arousal, and consequently their performance, in testing and training situations.

C. Setting Treatment Goals and Objectives

1. An ultimate goal of speech-language treatment for neurologically impaired patients is to maximize communicative effectiveness in light of social and vocational wishes and needs. For RHD adults, the major objectives associated with this goal are similar to those for other patient populations: to improve cognitive-communicative functioning (through a mixture of facilitation and compensation techniques); to realize generalization and maintenance of gains in settings and conditions outside the treatment context; and to assist both patient and family in adjusting to their altered cognitive, social, and emotional abilities and situations.

2. As a prelude to proposing treatment procedures, these fundamental objectives are translated to specific treatment objectives aimed at outcomes in both the short-term and in the longer-term. There are several steps involved in setting treatment goals and objectives.

   a. First, we consult with our patients when they can participate in the process, their families, and other rehabilitation staff members to identify their short-term and ultimate concerns. Future plans and placements will be important here, as will the patient's complaints and wishes, if they are realistic.

   b. Next we develop hierarchical goal statements to address the expressed and observed deficits and needs. Hierarchical goal statements flow from general, longer-term objectives to more specific, and measurable, formulations proposed for meeting those objectives. Table 6–2 provides several examples of nested goal statements that might be appropriate for some RHD

Table 6–2. Examples of hierarchical intervention goal statements

1. Basic goal	Increase awareness of deficits
Intermediate goal	Improve awareness of inappropriate social/interactional behaviors and skills
Specific goals	Monitor occurrences of targeted undesirable behaviors (e.g., interruptions; unclear referents; socially inappropriate topics; averted gaze) with 90% accuracy in a 20-minute interaction with an unfamiliar communication partner, for three consecutive weekly probe sessions
	Monitor signals from others (clinician and novel communication partner) regarding occurrence of targeted behaviors, with 90% accuracy in a 20-minute interaction, for three consecutive weekly probe sessions
	Explain reasons for targeting each behavior to family member and novel communication partner, providing 90% of the reasons generated in treatment, for three consecutive weekly probe sessions
2. Basic goal	Increase efficiency of residual attentional control capacities for everyday activities
Intermediate goal	Improve capacity to resist distraction
Specific goals	Identify task-irrelevant signals (distractors) introduced intermittently by the clinician during novel tasks, with 90% accuracy for three consecutive weekly probe sessions
	Maintain task orientation in the presence of routine distractors introduced as above, with 90% accuracy for three consecutive weekly probe sessions [OR decrease interruptions of focal activity from X to Y, maintaining level Y over the same time period]
	Take steps to reduce extreme distractions introduced intermittently during novel tasks (e.g., turn off loud radio or television; close a window; go to a quieter place; request cooperation from person generating the distraction) on 90% of opportunities presented for three consecutive weekly probe sessions
	Identify disruptions in sustained novel task performance that result from internal thoughts, with 90% accuracy over three consecutive weekly probe sessions

patients. The table is organized according to Fey and Cleave's (1990) framework, in which *basic goals* are overarching or general statements of concern; *intermediate goals* represent general areas of weakness that are contained within the basic goals; specific goals reflect operationalized intervention targets considered relevant for achieving the intermediate goals; and *subgoals* specify behavioral objectives and tasks proposed for reaching specific goals. Sample subgoals are not included in the table, as the readers of this book are assumed to be well-versed in writing focused behavioral objectives. Subgoals for the first set of specific goals would focus on identifying target behaviors and their disruptiveness and monitoring them in structured tasks and interactions, with the clinician manipulating context and cues to facilitate goal acquisition. Potential treatment activities and procedures for a variety of communication goals will be highlighted in Chapter 7.

3. Armed with a number of potential intervention goals, we can choose from several methods to help us decide what to treat. Brookshire (1992) has identified three approaches, considered below. Often the core concerns of these approaches are melded to determine the starting points for treatment.

   a. In the "relative level of impairment" approach, clinicians focus on areas of relative strength and weakness in a patient's performance.

      (1) Some clinicians initially choose to target and build on relative areas of success, suggesting that a patient will benefit most from working near the limit of his or her capacities. They choose treatment tasks to capitalize on relatively spared modalities and skills. They design treatment activities so that, initially, most (as many as 70–80%) of the patient's responses meet criterion performance levels (e.g., accurate; communicatively adequate), progressing to 90% or better, maintained over several consecutive sessions. Other clinicians emphasize remediating particular areas of weakness, including behaviors that are absent initially. In either case, it is important for clinicians to structure treatment programs with sufficient steps and cues to elicit successful performance. It has been documented that, in aphasia treatment, errors beget more errors (Brookshire, 1972, 1976).

      (2) Another form of the relative level of impairment approach, originated by Porch (1981), focuses on performance variations within subtests. Porch proposed that a measure of

intrasubtest variability, called "peak-mean difference," would provide valuable information to help identify treatment targets. A peak-mean difference score reflects the extent to which the best, or "peak" response on a single subtest (e.g., correct but delayed), differs from the average or "mean" response on that subtest (e.g., correct with repeated stimulation from the clinician). Porch's idea was that a moderate peak-mean difference suggests good potential for improvement (potential to move from mean performance toward peak ability) in the functions or processes tapped by a particular subtest, making those processes good targets for treatment. The potential for improvement is less when the peak-mean difference is either very low or very high. This is because low intrasubtest variability indicates little room for improvement, whereas an extremely high difference could result from the chance occurrence of a single, atypical "peak" response. When the difference is moderate in size, the "best response" is taken as a good indicator of the nature of information processing that the brain is capable of doing.

(3) Brookshire (1992) reminds us that several requirements must be met to ascertain relative levels of impairment in either fashion. When calculating measures of intrasubtest variability, like the peak-mean difference, individual subtest items must be homogenous in difficulty. And any between-subtest comparisons (e.g., magnitudes of peak-mean difference, or relative success vs. failure) must be based on a common reference value such as percentiles or z-scores.

b. Clinicians who subscribe to a "fundamental abilities" approach target processes that are presumed to underlie a range of deficient performances and to be necessary for eventual communication success. For RHD patients, perceptual skills, attentional/resource allocation mechanisms, and/or inferencing and integration processes might be considered fundamental abilities, as reviewed in Chapter 2.

c. The "functional abilities" approach focuses on daily life competencies and concerns. For example, patients with social communicative deficiencies might be taught to inhibit suggestive and profane remarks, or to regulate eye contact, in order to make their interactions more appropriate.

4. Several factors also influence the order in which to tackle various treatment goals. Among the first to attend to are:

   a. those that would make a rapid positive impact on a patient's daily living situation and interactions;

   b. any felt to be prerequisite to progress in other communicative areas or other treatments, such as basic awareness and concentration deficits;

   c. those for which the patient demonstrates awareness and stimulability;

   d. those that solidify effective patient-generated strategies;

   e. those intended to deter bad habits.

5. As noted earlier, the focus of treatment often evolves with time, from a major emphasis on stimulating component processes and skills that are presumed to underlie communication performance, to a predominant focus on daily life activities.

D. Formulating a Treatment Plan

The initiation and conduct of treatment should be guided by a treatment plan. Of course, initial plans can change during treatment, depending on the patient's progress and circumstances, so flexibility is important. By documenting the results of treatment (see section III), the clinician will be attuned to the need to revise elements of an original treatment plan. The elements of a comprehensive treatment plan are:

1. an outline of the amount and nature of progression expected from initial to ultimate goals. This encompasses:

   a. predicting the extent to which ultimate goals can be achieved with treatment, and

   b. specifying the plans and rationales for linking proposed intermediate tasks and goals with longer term outcomes.

2. an estimate of the time needed to achieve goals at various levels.

3. a treatment program, specifying some of the methods and procedures proposed to work toward focused treatment goals. This aspect of treatment progression is elaborated in section II-E, below.

4. performance criteria that specify the conditions for continuing or altering treatment methods and procedures, and treatment goals. This element is also considered in section II-E.

5. the methods for measuring progress to determine when treatment has accomplished its goals (see Chapter 5, and section III below). This includes a plan for assessing generalization (including maintenance of generalized gains; see section II-F) and clinical significance (section II-G).

6. discharge criteria, which are considered further in section II-H, below.

7. provisions for monitoring, and facilitating, patients' and families' psychosocial adjustment (see Chapter 8).

E. Progression of Treatment: The Treatment Program

This section focuses on planning and implementing a progression from initial (current) responses to terminal (desired) responses for immediate and intermediate goals.

1. Our assessment results, including those from cognitively oriented deficit analysis and functional task analysis, provide the data to identify our patients' strengths and weaknesses. As noted above, this information then assists us in selecting treatment goals. Observations of patients' performance should also lead us to hypotheses about the obstacles they may face in achieving particular goals. We can explore factors that may facilitate or impede performance, given the observed profile of abilities and obstacles, by manipulating some of the variables that are discussed next.

2. After collecting appropriate baseline data, we can endeavor to move a patient's performance along the path from initial to desired responses by selectively building into our treatment tasks some of the parameters contributing to success and failure. Table 6–3 lists a variety of factors that may influence performance after RHD and that, accordingly, can be considered as variables to manipulate in treatment.

    The reader will recognize many of these considerations from the discussion of symptoms in Chapter 2. Some of the other factors are mostly untried with RHD adults, but they are influential in aphasia therapy, and the principles underlying their utility should apply to other neurologically impaired patients. Most of these factors can be manipulated along something resembling a continuum of difficulty. Treatment would begin where the patient first experiences problems, and gradually the facilitators, activities, and requisite processes would be modified to make performance more difficult. The variables in Table 6–3 are categorized, and discussed below, under

Table 6–3. A sample of factors to modify in treatment

Dimension	Attributes
Stimulus characteristics	Perceptual factors (e.g., stimulus clarity, orientation, discriminability, ambiguity); Spatial requirements for location, distance, direction, and memory; number, arrangement of and attention to elements and arrays.
	Central factors (explicitness; redundancy and consistency; predictability; probability, meaningfulness, familiarity, interest, and frequency; computational difficulty).
	Resource factors (requirements for retention, integration, simultaneous processing, coordination, and exact timing, in demanding conditions; automatic versus controlled processing; specific demands for selective attention, resisting distraction, differentiating relevant from irrelevant information, and sustaining, dividing, or switching attention).
	Combinations of the above.
Stimulus modes	Visual, auditory, tactile, combined (but alert to demands for divided attention).
Task characteristics	Performance criteria; level of processing; demands for metacognition; volitionality.
Other facilitators	Procedural factors (practice and demonstration; side from which to deliver treatment). Temporal factors (rate of speech and use of pauses; stimulus-response interval). Cues and compensatory strategies.

the headings of stimulus characteristics, stimulus modes, task characteristics, and other facilitators.

a. The consideration of stimulus characteristics has been organized to focus on four sets of factors: Those that are primarily perceptual; attributes that affect central stimulus processing; resource factors; and combinations of these. This organization is an arbitrary convenience, because these domains undoubtedly interact and influence each other as the patient moves from stimulus to response.

(1) Perceptual factors include mainly visual (especially spatial) stimulus characteristics, but auditory perceptual discrimination ability is also important for tasks involving affect and prosody. In general, perceptual encoding and interpretation are more difficult when stimuli are degraded, embedded, or unusually oriented (e.g., rotated), or when they involve subtle discriminations. Tasks of recognizing and interpreting facial expressions and other subtle social signals may be quite difficult, especially when there is some ambiguity built in to the stimuli. Spatial requirements that necessitate attention to location, distance, depth, and direction may also complicate tasks for RHD adults, and delayed response tasks that tax spatial learning and memory may be particularly problematic. Finally, the number and placement of elements, both in individual stimuli and in stimulus arrays, may be important. Stimuli and stimulus arrays containing fewer elements to be evaluated and integrated are likely to be less difficult to process. And perceptual encoding should be easier when relevant stimuli or stimulus elements are directed to the relatively intact hemifield or hemispace, especially when the patient's attention is drawn to them.

(2) Many factors are presumed to affect more central stimulus processing. Difficulty can be reduced by increasing explicitness or directness, and decreasing abstractness, ambiguity, or nonliteral and inferential stimulus attributes. Redundancy and consistency have also been shown to improve stimulus processing, and heightening the predictability of a stimulus context has been found to enhance emotional, inferential, and figurative language processing. For our purposes, predictability can be construed broadly to capture the extent to which meanings, forms, and functions conform to conventional usages or typical expectations. As for predictability, the positive influence of stimulus probability, meaningfulness, familiarity, interest value, and frequency of occurrence is probably due to the nature of stored mental representations that are built up from frequent exposures to stimuli having these characteristics. When stimuli are high in these dimensions, there is a greater likelihood that patients have available overlearned knowledge and stored routines for processing them. Increasing any of these features may enable patients to contact those relevant sources of knowledge and mental computation, thereby improving performance. Finally, the difficulty of the specific mental computations that are

required in various domains (e.g., problem solving; conceptual integration) will influence success. To exemplify this point in the domain of inferencing, one could contrast the mental operations presumed necessary for generating straightforward inferences that draw on a single source of information (e.g., one character's actions) with those required for integrating information from multiple or disparate sources (e.g., speaker mood, motives, and plausibility) or for retracing and recomputing an interpretation when an initial one becomes implausible.

(3) Resource considerations involve factors that may influence the availability and allocation of limited attentional and working memory resources (see Chapter 2). Generally, the higher the resource demands, the more difficult a task will be. Among the situations in which resource demands can be presumed to be relatively elevated are those that require retention and integration over long chunks of text; essentially simultaneous demands to process, plan, and coordinate various aspects of stimulus interpretation and response; backtracking, or revising existing interpretations; integrating information from multiple or disparate sources; and many computations that have to be completed under time pressure. The distinction between relatively automatic and consciously controlled processing (Chapter 2) is relevant here as well. Tasks that require complex new learning, or conscious control, draw heavily on limited resources, while well-practiced and overlearned skills do not. Repetition and practice of consciously controlled behaviors and skills can move them toward automaticity, freeing resources for other crucial aspects of processing. Demands associated with specific components of attention are also noteworthy. For many patients, tasks will be easier to the extent that they limit requirements for selectively attending, resisting distraction, differentiating relevant from irrelevant material, or sustaining, dividing or switching attention.

(4) Combining attributes of the factors considered above can amplify (and obscure the source of) a patient's stimulus processing difficulty. For example, when tasks that tap slow or otherwise deficient perceptual skills also demand speeded inferential processing in an unpredictable or unfamiliar knowledge domain, the patient's performance may break down for a variety of reasons.

b. The influence of stimulus mode (visual, auditory, tactile, combined) must be analyzed for each patient to determine what is most facilitating. A caveat here: Multiple modality presentation is often recommended to enhance stimulus encoding and comprehension, as well as consolidation of new learning. But for many RHD patients, we must beware of the demands for divided attention when multiple modalities are used. This is especially the case when one of the modalities is particularly deficient (e.g., the visual modality for patients with visual neglect), or when a patient's resource capacity or allocation is especially impaired (e.g., patients with neglect, or with low scores on measures of working memory capacity).

c. Task characteristics considered here include performance criteria, level of processing, demands for metacognition, and volitionality. Performance criteria vary along a number of dimensions; for example, completely accurate and optimally timed responses can be contrasted with those that are acceptable but delayed or those that are approximate without being entirely incorrect. Level of processing refers here to a distinction between recognition and recall (or generation) of criterion responses. The former will always be easier than the latter. Demands for metacognition include those of particular task contexts, such as role playing, and requirements for self-evaluation. Roleplaying, a common clinical activity, demands that patients be able to reflect and report on their knowledge of cognition and social rules, apart from their ability to apply that knowledge. Patients who have just asked relevant conversational questions of a new person in a therapy session have been observed to fail utterly when asked to think about what they could say to someone they have just met. Taking themselves outside of the task requires a level of abstraction that may be quite difficult. Similarly, self-evaluation necessitates an additional level of response monitoring, in which patients consider the extent to which their responses meet established performance criteria. Although crucial for generalization and maintenance of gains, this skill requires insight and divided attention that often make performance more difficult. A final related concern, volitionality, involves the extent to which patients must produce a response or use a strategy spontaneously and on their own, as opposed to relying on cues and structure provided by the clinician (see also next section).

d. Facilitators are the cues, structure, and procedural modifications that clinicians use to enhance a patient's access to available mental knowledge and processing operations and consequently to increase the probability of attaining a criterion response. Broadly speaking, when any of the factors discussed above are manipulated to elicit improved performance, they are being used as facilitators. It is evident when considering all of the possible levels and interactions of these factors that there are an uncountable number of facilitators that can be implemented, and systematically modified, to guide the patient's progress in treatment. Other facilitators that have not yet been discussed are procedural factors, temporal considerations, and cues and compensatory strategies.

(1) Procedural factors include things like the amount of practice and demonstration provided to a patient before initiating a treatment activity, and the side on which the clinician sits to conduct treatment. Providing more structure in the form of demonstration and practice should facilitate performance, as should sitting on and presenting stimuli to the side of the body that is (relatively) unaffected. However, to challenge patients with mild manifestations of neglect, the clinician may purposely conduct treatment from the affected side of the body.

(2) Temporal considerations include, for example, the clinician's rate of speech and use of pauses, and the interval between stimulus and response. A slow normal speech rate, with judicious pauses at natural constituent boundaries, may enhance perception and comprehension, particularly for lengthy or complex stimuli. The nature of the influence of the stimulus-response interval will depend on the patient's characteristics. For patients who often respond impulsively and inaccurately, imposing a delay may enhance success even if it is initially difficult for patients to comply. For reflective patients, reducing response latency may not be easy originally, but can be implemented to facilitate efficiency if accuracy does not suffer.

(3) Cues are like hints, specific or nonspecific, that we provide to elicit success. Cues can be an integral part of a facilitation approach to treatment, or, when patients adopt them and use them intentionally, they can serve as compensatory strategies. Maximal cues might include modeling a specific response or response strategy; minimal cues may involve simply repeating the stimulus or the instruction or asking the patient whether he or she has a strategy in mind.

Moderate cuing may involve outlining response alternatives for a patient, providing partial information, or initiating a response sequence for the patient to complete. Patient-generated cues and compensatory strategies, as opposed to those created by a clinician, should enhance learning and generalization, because they require active information processing and problem solving, and they capitalize on a patient's natural associations.

Self-instruction (e.g., reminding oneself to carry out some process) is one particular form of a self-generated cue or compensatory strategy that may contribute greatly to a patient's success outside of treatment. Another important category of compensatory strategies falls under the heading of "context management" (Davis, 1993) or "anticipatory compensation." Patients learn to anticipate difficult communication situations and to plan ways to handle them. One such strategy might be to alert the others in the situation to some particular modifications that will help the patient comprehend and respond (e.g., providing a theme or cue to orient them before proceeding; phrasing statements and questions directly; arranging visual stimuli for maximum advantage). Some patients will spontaneously generate their own cues or strategies, while others will need to be encouraged or trained to do so.

3. Most often, we want to enhance our patients' success, so we incorporate facilitory elements in our treatment tasks. There are times, however, when we want to challenge patients by making treatment activities more difficult than we might otherwise. This might be the case when performance is at high levels, as noted above for the treatment of a patient with mild manifestations of neglect, or when a patient is approaching discharge from treatment.

4. In any case, it is crucial to foster patients' independence throughout the course of treatment. With respect to implementing facilitators and cues, this means that we should start with those that are least intrusive and most natural so that they are easier to fade or eliminate. And we should continually probe to see if our patients can move along a presumed hierarchy, or sequence, of cues and facilitative strategies more quickly than we originally expected.

F. Planning for Generalization

Generalization planning involves a structured methodology for incorporating elements of natural situations into formal treatment and for introducing patients gradually into situations outside the clinic (Davis, 1993), as well as measuring the effects of doing both. Chapter 5 (section III-B-3-b) quoted Kearns (1993) on the multiple facets of generalization planning. His list of considerations is elaborated here.

1. First, Kearns emphasizes "comprehensive, multifaceted evaluation." This concern is addressed by identifying tasks or contexts that tap performance at varying "distances" from the treatment task (Davis, 1986, 1993), and by designing generalization probes to monitor the patient's performance in those tasks or contexts. The "distance" concept will be elaborated immediately below, but strategies for documenting generalization are taken up later, in the section on documenting progress (section III-A-2).

    a. At the most basic level, gains should generalize from one session to the next, and from treated stimuli to untreated stimuli of the same type (designated "response generalization"). If these levels of generalization do not occur, then something is probably seriously amiss with the treatment plan, the patient, or both.

    b. More often overlooked is the need to document evidence of generalization at higher levels, or in Davis' (1986, 1993) terms, generalization to tasks and contexts that are more distant from the treatment tasks themselves. At an intermediate level, generalization can be evaluated on untrained tasks and activities that are expected to have cognitive requirements similar to those targeted in treatment. For example, to tap functioning that is more distant from the treatment activities than the fundamental level described above, one could give a test or battery that is assumed to measure a dimension for which progress was anticipated, and has been evident, on the treatment tasks. Results of periodic administrations are compared with the (stable) pre-treatment baseline data gathered on the same test or battery, to ascertain whether related, but untreated, gains are occurring. Functional observations and assessments are usually more distant from treatment tasks, depending on the approach adopted in treatment.

    The reader who recalls the discussion of hierarchical goal setting (section II-C-2-b, above) will be able to link the "specific goals" exemplified in Table 6–2 with the concept of intermediate levels of generalization. The "specific goals" presented in the table were formulated to incorporate relevant communication skills in contexts and tasks that, presumably, are fairly distant from typical treatment tasks. Thus, a hierarchical approach to setting intervention goals naturally incorporates some important aspects of generalization planning.

2. Next it is necessary to establish "generalization criteria" (Kearns, 1993). This involves defining the nature, level, and consistency of generalized responding that is desired, along with the contexts in which it should occur. The specific goals in Table 6–2 also exemplify these elements of generalization planning.

3. "Incorporation of treatment strategies that might facilitate generalization" is next (Kearns, 1993). This has also been referred to as programming for generalization. In a review of the aphasia treatment literature, Thompson (1989) suggested that four treatment variables have contributed most consistently to generalized results. These variables, outlined in Table 6–4, are incorporated in Stokes and Baer's (1977) classic recommendations for enhancing the probability of generalization and are considered more fully below. A cogent summary of the Stokes and Baer principles, with examples from aphasiology, has also been provided recently by Brookshire (1992).

   a. Treatment should address a sufficient number of training responses. The original interpretation of this principle focuses on the observation that generalization is more likely to occur when a treatment program targets a number of related types of responses (e.g., different varieties of speech acts; various kinds of nonliteral forms; different ways to reduce distractions). The principle could be extended to encompass as well the importance of providing sufficient numbers of training trials. What constitutes "a sufficient number" is not known, but in the case of treatment trials, more are probably better. It may be necessary to establish some automaticity and overlearning in order to provide patients with the ability to call up trained responses in novel, or stressful, contexts.

   b. Responses should be trained in a sufficient number of conditions. This involves working with a variety of tasks that incor-

Table 6–4. Methods for enhancing generalization

1. Incorporate a sufficient number of training responses: target related types of responses; administer repeated trials to foster automaticity and overlearning.

2. Train responses in a sufficient number of conditions.

3. Incorporate aspects of the generalization environment: use relevant content, apply natural contingencies, vary settings and other contextual factors.

4. Include strategies for mediating generalization: teach self-instruction and verbal mediation, make patients their own clinicians, involve others in transfer activities.

Source: After Thompson (1989).

porate the targeted processes and skills, in a variety of contexts (e.g., with novel partners; in role-playing activities; in other settings or simulated environments).

c. Treatment activities should incorporate aspects of the generalization environment. This principle can be addressed by working with relevant content or topics, exploiting natural contingencies, working in varied settings, and including other salient contextual variables in treatment.

   (1) Relevant topics and meaningful stimuli have been emphasized before. These attributes may enhance the likelihood that patients can activate and draw on well-established knowledge and routines, stored in their brains, to assist them in processing and responding. They can be incorporated profitably into treatment activities as long as they are within the limit of the patient's cognitive capabilities.

   (2) Natural contingencies include reactions or responses, from people in patients' environments, that are likely to reinforce target behaviors when patients produce them. For example, patients who are working on making appropriate eye contact are likely to get attention when they are successful. Attending to the patient, then, may function as a natural contingency that helps to maintain the desired behavior. Natural response contingencies also include those that are similar in schedule, timing, or type to those that are available in the patient's environment. It is a sure bet that patients will not get consistent, immediate reactions or praise in an everyday setting each time they produce a target response or behavior. Reinforcement of this sort does not reflect naturally occurring contingencies and may hamper generalization because it is too distant from the characteristics of the natural environment.

   (3) Settings to enhance generalization might include other treatment areas in a hospital or rehabilitation center; simulated contexts (such as a model living room in the speech-language pathology department, a driving simulator, or a kitchen setting in occupational therapy); a cafeteria or some other on-site common area; and gradually, different real-world settings outside the familiar treatment environment.

   (4) Additional salient contextual variables include communication partners and aspects of social interaction. Patients can extend their communication practice to people who differ from their clinicians in familiarity, shared knowledge, rela-

tive power, affiliation, or social roles. Furthermore, facets of natural interactions such as turn-taking and other regulatory strategies, can be incorporated to simulate more typical communication exchanges. It has been noted that communication may be primarily a vehicle for socialization, rather than for transacting information exchange (Simmons-Mackie & Damico, 1993). If this is so, then strategies for participating in and regulating social exchanges may be at least as important to our patients as a focus on the number of information units that they can convey. Treatment groups may provide another context for transfer; they can present excellent opportunities for patients to practice generalized responding (and for clinicians to document their performance) when faced with variety in partners, purposes and styles of communication, and natural interaction contingencies (although as Thompson [1989] notes, unstructured sessions of this sort may not provide obligatory contexts for producing target responses).

(5) There is some controversy about the extent to which it is necessary for the settings and procedures used in treatment to resemble or replicate natural situations. Brookshire (1992) suggests that it is probably more important for the behaviors and processes targeted to be relevant to daily life communication, but emphasizes that there is little evidence either way.

d. Treatment activities should include strategies for mediating generalization. Such strategies, including self-instruction and verbal mediation, elicit a desired behavior in an atypical way. For example, patients with neglect may be taught to mediate their visual scanning verbally, by instructing themselves to look for the beginning of a line and to read for meaning. Other ways to implement mediating strategies include moving patients toward being their own clinicians (e.g., teaching them to evaluate and modify their own responses; soliciting their participation for planning goals and activities) and involving others (e.g., family members and staff) as practice partners who can elicit generalized responding in carryover activities by reinforcing targeted strategies and skills.

4. "Continuous measurement and probing for functional, generalized improvements" is another facet of generalization planning (Kearns, 1993). The nature and value of regular probe measurements was discussed in Chapter 5 (section III) and is considered again later in this chapter (section III).

5. Finally, Kearns recommends "when necessary, extending treatments to additional settings, people and conditions until targeted levels of generalization occur." This point underscores the fact that, despite our best efforts, generalized responding may not occur. When this appears to be the case, training can be implemented in very salient contexts, to the extent that it is practical to do so.

G. Establishing the Clinical Significance of Treatment Gains

1. Clinical significance refers to the meaningfulness of treatment gains. Clinical significance can be claimed when gains have generalized beyond the treatment settings and tasks and/or when social validation procedures indicate that the patient's performance has changed meaningfully. Two social validation procedures were introduced in Chapter 5 (section III-B-3-c).

   a. In the normative comparison process, we weigh a patient's performance against that achieved by non-brain-damaged adults of similar sociodemographic status, and evaluate progress toward the norm. A conservative criterion for designating performance as socially valid might be that patients should score within one standard deviation of the expected relevant norm in order for their behavior to be considered commensurate with that of their social milieu. A more liberal criterion might specify performance that is two standard deviations from the norm. If neither criterion is met by post-treatment performance, then substantial movement toward the norm from pre-treatment levels would be considered encouraging.

   b. Subjective evaluations involve performance ratings by judges who are unfamiliar with the patients, and their treatment status. Optimally, post-treatment behavior samples will receive reliably and convincingly higher ratings on relevant characteristics than will pre-treatment samples.

2. Many decisions must be made before sound social validity data can be gathered. Some of these concern the choice of behavior samples to evaluate, dimensions to judge, operationalizations for relevant dimensions, rating systems and instructions, and rater characteristics (see Tompkins, 1994, for further discussion of these factors).

H. Terminating Treatment

1. As noted above, a comprehensive treatment plan includes discharge criteria. But, all too often treatment is not ended purposefully and

rationally. Instead, it is continued until a patient's benefits run out or until a training clinic no longer has the resources to see a client. Rather than providing endless treatment, we are ethically bound to discharge patients when they have reached maximum benefit, and/or when their progress is minimal. One exception to this rule might be when patients are enrolled in treatment as training cases for student clinicians; but such patients should be fully informed of our prognostic estimates, and should consent to being treated primarily for training purposes. In any context, we must be careful not to raise or reinforce false hopes through continued intervention; and we must foster independence throughout the treatment period. At some point, patients must rely on themselves and those in their daily environments for continued evaluation of communicative performance and practice of communicative skills.

2. Making a responsible discharge decision requires a clinician to evaluate treatment gains critically (see Chapter 5, and below). Rosenbek and colleagues (1989) suggest that treatment should end when the patient wants it to end, when learning stops, and/or when there is minimal generalization or maintenance despite the clinician's best efforts. I would add a point related to the last one: Treatment should end when the gains being made are of questionable value or relevance to the ultimate goal of making a difference in a patient's daily life. This is a criterion of clinical significance. Of course, the door should be left open for patients to check in periodically, if they desire, for further evaluation or for a therapeutic "tune-up." It is always possible, too, that new developments may suggest a "perfect treatment technique" for a former patient. In such a case, the patient (if willing) can be re-evaluated (with repeated baseline testing to document the stability of target behaviors or skills), and entered into the new treatment protocol, which again should include rational criteria for continuation, modification, and termination.

III. DOCUMENTING RESULTS

A. Measuring Progress

Progress that results from treatment should be evaluated and documented at several levels.

1. Keeping records to document performance on specific treatment tasks is important because the pattern of data affects treatment decisions, as indicated in Chapter 5. In addition, charts of performance

over time may be motivating or educational to patients, families, and other rehabilitation personnel. When a patient, a family member, or a physician inquires about progress, a chart can help make the answer fairly clear. Sometimes clinicians hesitate to show charts of progress to their patients, because they fear that the results are not very encouraging. Gains so minimal should signal a clinician to reconsider the treatment focus, criteria, or procedures.

a. Both quantitative and qualitative dimensions of task performance can be recorded, depending on the specific goals. Quantitative dimensions might include such things as a variety of accuracy measures (e.g., for recognition or detection judgments, the numbers/proportions of "hits" or correct "yes" responses, together with "false alarms" or incorrect "yes" responses, "misses" or incorrect "no" responses, and "true negatives" or correct "no" responses); number/proportion of responses meeting a designated quality criterion (e.g., adequate, appropriate); numbers/proportions and/or types of prompts or cues provided; amount of time on task; and absolute speed of responding. Qualitative dimensions capture other characteristics of accurate or inaccurate responses (e.g., are they impulsive, delayed, self-corrected, incomplete, cued, related to the target, off-target, perseverative, refusals; are they errors of omission or commission; are there patterns of errors or delayed responses, etc). Clinicians can consult several standardized tests, such as the *Porch Index of Communicative Ability (PICA)* and the *Revised Token Test (RTT)*, for examples of qualitative scoring systems.

(1) There are several important cautions about appropriating or modifying these kinds of scoring systems. One involves scoring reliability. The more categories to be scored, the lower the probability of attaining sufficient intra- and inter-judge consistency for applying the scoring system, without specific training. For example, a 40-hour workshop is necessary to use and interpret PICA scores reliably. Clinicians adopting notations of this kind should minimize the number of categories, make those categories as operationally specific as possible, and assess point-to-point agreement with themselves over time, and with other independent scorers, as recommended in Chapter 3 (section V-B-3).

(2) Another caution involves the ways in which the categories are tabulated and interpreted.[1] It is questionable practice,

---

[1] When such scores can be demonstrated to have certain statistical characteristics, like those of the PICA, they can be validly added and averaged, but it would be difficult for clinicians to achieve and document those characteristics in homemade scoring systems.

statistically, to add together, or average, scores that describe categories of responses. Rather, the proportion of trials for which the categories occur, based on a reasonable and consistent number of opportunities, should be recorded.

    b. Whatever dimensions are scored, it is useful to record and organize them on data sheets so that progress (or the lack of it) can be monitored and conveyed to others. LaPointe's Base-10 Response Form (Figure 6–1) provides one example of the infinite number of formats a clinician could adopt. Positive features of this form include provisions for noting baseline data, specifying tasks and performance criteria, recording responses for individual stimuli, and plotting percentage summary treatment data (which can include that for generalization probe data, see III-A-2, below) across sessions. Clinicians can extend the utility of this form, or one like it, by plotting the baseline data and indicating the ultimate and intermediate goals targeted by specific treatment tasks, as well as the nature of any associated generalization measures.

2. It has been emphasized repeatedly, here and in other writings on intervention, that in order to be considered efficacious, treatment must result in gains beyond those achieved on specific tasks. This is the domain of generalization.

    a. Several strategies have been proposed for assessing generalization. Probably most familiar are periodic standardized testing aimed at evaluating intermediate generalization, and the more recently implemented assessments designed to render a global categorization of functional independence. Given the lack of valid, reliable, or sensitive instruments to measure progress in either of these ways for RHD patients, these strategies are of limited value.

    b. Periodic generalization probes, conducted on well-defined stimuli and tasks, offer another avenue for examining generalization. Again, generalization probes assess progress toward intermediate and longer-term goals, beyond the immediate treatment context.

        (1) Probes are structured sets of observations that allow a clinician to evaluate performance trends. Generalization probes incorporate untreated stimuli and tasks, and/or conditions that extend beyond the reach of the treatment environment. Generalization probe stimuli should be delivered using the same methods by which pre-treatment ability is assessed.

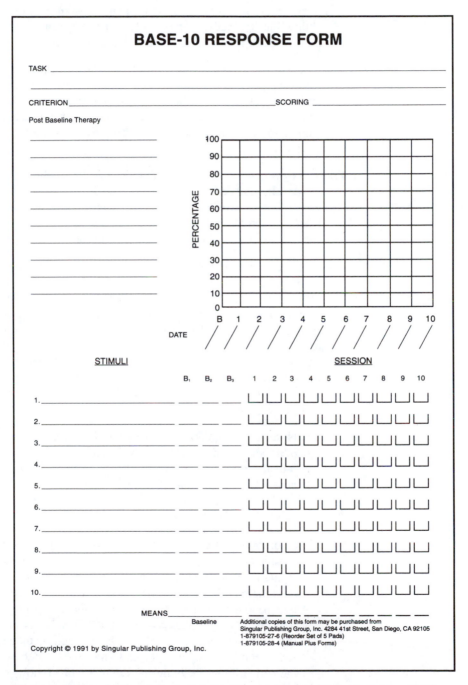

Figure 6–1. Sample data sheet: LaPointe's Base-10 Response Form (LaPointe, 1991)

By definition, this means that the probe data differ from the treatment data. Treatment data reflect the influence of the interventions that we have designed to modify pre-treatment ability, but, typically, in probe situations, we want to see how a patient will do without any assistance or feedback.

(2) To document response generalization, clinicians chart performance for a set of untrained stimulus items. Periodic probes, conducted either before or after the treatment trials, can incorporate subsets of treated stimuli with untreated stimuli so that clinicians can chart progress separately for each set.

(3) To assess generalization at an intermediate level, clinicians can develop and deliver regular (e.g., weekly) probes to chart growth in related behaviors or tasks that have not themselves been exposed to treatment (e.g., a paragraph reading probe can be used to assess progress in treatment for neglect).

(4) Probes can also be developed to evaluate the daily life utility of changes (the domain of clinical significance) outside of the treatment activity or setting. Clinicians can implement such probes themselves, in other therapies, at the bus stop, at home, or in the rehabilitation center cafeteria, for example. Different communication partners (familiar and unfamiliar) can also be incorporated into probe situations. Busy clinicians can also rely on normative comparisons, or structured observations by other people, to provide some of their generalization data.

   (a) Normative comparisons have been introduced as part of a social validation process (Chapter 5, section III-B-3-c; also this chapter, section II-G-1-a). But achieving normatively acceptable performance in functional settings and tasks is also good evidence of the more "distant" form of generalization.

   (b) Additional, but weaker, evidence about generalization outside of the treatment environment (also known as stimulus generalization) can be obtained from the observations and reports of others. Data of this sort will be most valid if the clinician teaches observers how to deliver probes to elicit the target behaviors (e.g., what stimuli to provide and how to deliver them; strict prohibition against trying to help, or to educate, the patient in any way during the probe task); how to record responses (e.g., tape record for clinician's later evaluation and verification); and how to observe in a reasonably structured and consistent way (e.g., at a consistent time, such as the first thing after lunch, or the last 5 minutes of an occupational therapy session). Clinicians who wish to rely on these kinds of observations will want to verify periodically the extent to which stipulated probe conditions are met.

B. Documentation for Reimbursement Purposes

The documentation needed to obtain reimbursement for clinical services is different for different agencies (e.g., Department of Vocational Rehabilitation, private insurance companies, federal government). At the time this book was being written, speech-language pathology intervention for older stroke patients (over age 65) was often covered in part by the federal Medicare program. (General requirements and procedures for Medicare certification and continuation are outlined in Davis, 1993.) However, change is in the wind as Congress and the Clinton administration work to craft a new health care proposal, making it impossible to specify health-care reimbursement policies and procedures here. A general comment to wrap up this section will strike a familiar note: We are more likely to be able to convince third-party payors to cover the costs of intervention if we can provide solid data about treatment efficacy, including documentation of generalized, functional gains. The trend for health care reimbursers to focus on "functional outcome" (see Chapter 5, section IV) is unlikely to change in the foreseeable future, despite the psychometric inadequacy of the measures that are currently used to evaluate it.

IV. SOME MANAGEMENT PRINCIPLES

This section summarizes much of what has come before this point, in this and prior chapters. These principles, which are put forward as general guidelines for approaching intervention, are derived from theory, evidence, and intuition; from professional discussions, and one-to-one clinical interactions. Although articulated in the context of this book on RHD adults, it is my opinion that they apply across populations of neurologically impaired adults.

A. A sound clinical intervention program is planned like a good experiment. Much of Chapter 5 was spent establishing the point of view that sound diagnosis and treatment are based on the principles and methods of science.

B. Clinicians can often focus treatment profitably by attending to the theoretical bases of their patients' deficits and of their treatment procedures. A theoretical focus allows us to identify the nature of performance breakdown and the processes assumed to be fundamental components of tasks or target behaviors.

C. At the same time, when focusing treatment, clinicians should consider a symptom's impact on the daily life of the patient and his or her significant others. As an example, we might consider a patient's speech to be quite aprosodic, but it may not bother the patient or family (even if speech characteristics were different premorbidly). On the other side of this coin, we may judge a patient's post-stroke prosody and other voice characteristics as being within normal limits, but changes related to the stroke may be jarring to patient and family alike. The clinician in the first case would not insist on treating prosodic production, while the second clinician would acknowledge, and look for ways to address, the concerns.

D. Premorbid style should also influence treatment planning. Patients who were never very social, or who never cared to read much, may not need treatment to improve conversational interaction or scanning for reading. At a minimum, performance targets or criteria in areas that were not very important premorbidly would be adjusted downward from the clinician's usual expectation.

E. Among other elements, a comprehensive treatment plan will include the expected progression from initial to terminal goals and the rationales that indicate the (eventual) link between short-term goals and associated activities and daily life needs. This roadmap will be useful for the clinician, and others, to see how the treatment journey is proceeding.

F. Treatment plan notwithstanding, it is essential that clinicians remain flexible. Goals, methods, and procedures will most certainly evolve and change, as the patient does.

G. Clinicians must remain aware of, and assess, the basic abilities required for performing specific treatment or generalization tasks. Consider the example of a RHD patient with perceptual impairments whose treatment activity is focused on higher level inferencing and integration. We would need to examine the extent to which that patient's uncertainty or inaccuracy in processing individual stimulus elements might influence the process of drawing inferences about relationships among them. In this case, slow or otherwise faulty perceptual processes might divert resources from, provide partial or misinterpreted data to, or delay information that is crucial for the operation of, higher cognitive inference and integration processes.

H. Along with cognitive deficit analysis, functional task analysis enable the clinician to identify skills and abilities other than those of primary interest that may be involved in or confound the response to treatment activities. Both procedures also help to provide rationales about where to intervene. A further example of the importance of cognitive deficit analysis can be culled from what we know about comprehending emotion from prosody. In many cases, RHD patients' problems are associated with prosodic discrimination differences, rather than the emotional nature of stimuli. The components of a logical task analysis for reading activities were considered earlier (section II-B-2-d). Similarly, we can try to lay out the steps involved in more complex daily life activities, like driving or crossing a busy street, to match their requirements with the patient's abilities and deficits.

I. Particularly in its initial phases, treatment is generally designed to exploit strengths. As patients progress and gain confidence, the clinician can incorporate activities to bolster or circumvent weaknesses. An exception to this general notion may occur for high-level patients who may need more challenges from the start.

J. It is probably beneficial to incorporate functional and meaningful stimuli in treatment. These stimulus attributes may contribute to generalization of treatment gains, and treatment may be more motivating when stimuli are meaningful. As noted previously, this principle does not imply that treatment tasks and settings need to replicate those in daily life, a cumbersome proposition. Repeated opportunities (when possible leading toward automaticity) to activate and apply targeted knowledge and cognitive processes in a variety of activities and situations, coupled with elements of natural interaction contexts, may go a long way toward inducing generalized responding.

K. Programmed operant constructs and principles have much to offer for structuring and implementing treatment. Among these are the importance of taking careful baseline and repeated probe measures; operationally defining areas to be treated and criterion performance; focusing on antecedent stimuli that influence patients' responses as well as natural contingencies; fading cues and structure as patients move toward performance criteria and goals; implementing small-step progressions in treatment activities; and setting a priori standards for continuing, altering, or ending treatment.

L. Patients should be provided with knowledge of treatment results, in meaningful terms. The value of graphing treatment progress, and a patient's right to know how he or she is doing, have been emphasized above. In addition, learning to gauge his or her own progress is an important element in a patient's journey toward independence from the clinician.

M. Clinicians need to plan for discharge from the day of the initial visit. Just as treatment has a beginning, it has an end. We can prepare patients for this day by previewing it with them and by moving them toward becoming their own clinicians as soon as possible. We accomplish the latter by involving them directly in setting goals and performance criteria, evaluating responses, planning modifications to their responses and to treatment activities, and establishing practice regimens. For more severely impaired patients who cannot contribute in these ways, we need to involve family or other care providers as much and as soon as possible (when their personalities, psychological conditions, and general situations allow), with the goal of providing them the means to facilitate daily life interactions after discharge.

N. Change is not necessarily meaningful. Clinicians should endeavor to demonstrate the importance, or clinical significance, of performance changes by documenting the maintenance, generalization, and social validity of treatment gains.

O. Generalization does not just happen. It must be actively programmed and documented, for situations, partners, and communication activities that differ from those specifically treated.

P. Treatment efficacy must be established, rather than assumed. Clinicians have to begin to accept the challenge of evaluating their own interventions. They can also make important contributions to the clinical data base, as advocated in Chapter 5. Without these sorts of contributions, we will continue to shoot in the dark when we plan treatment programs for RHD adults.

CHAPTER

7

Treatment Approaches and Strategies

I. OVERVIEW CONSIDERATIONS

A. Chapter Organization

The organization of material in this chapter, starting with section II below, follows that established in Chapter 2, review of symptoms, and carried through Chapter 4, assessment. Ample cross-references are provided throughout the treatment material to alert the reader to interrelated considerations and suggestions.

B. Clinical Challenges

Before providing treatment suggestions, several concerns are noted or reiterated here. Some readers may be frustrated by the repeated emphasis on what we have yet to learn. However, it is important that we keep these kinds of challenges in mind so that we continue to be appropriately cautious in planning and documenting our treatments, and to remain alert for, and evaluative of, new developments.

1. There are no data to substantiate the effectiveness of, or the appropriate candidates for, most all of the approaches and strategies discussed below. As a result, this chapter can only offer some educated guesses, and personal biases, for clinical intervention with RHD adults. The creative clinician is urged to modify, extend, and test the ideas below, along with approaches and strategies of his or her own design.

2. Several other factors complicate the process of planning interventions, as well. Some potentially devastating symptoms whose improvement may be deemed logically prerequisite to further treatment (e.g., severe anosognosia) may not be remediable, at least not with the usual amounts of treatment for which patients have insurance coverage. Other ostensible symptoms may reflect premorbid abilities to a large degree and as such may be questionable targets for intervention. As noted previously, the range of normal adult behavior in pragmatic and conversational areas is undocumented, but undoubtedly enormous, as is the potential individual variation in performance for reading, writing, and higher cognitive tasks involving reasoning and problem solving.

3. For similar reasons, designating target performance levels is difficult. What are the "gold standards" for prosodic variation, humor interpretation, conversational relevance, and so forth? How much awareness of deficits or error monitoring ability is enough? The answers to these questions will be highly variable for different patients, performing different tasks, in different situations.

4. Finally, we lack good models, theories, and even evidence about the co-occurrence of and interrelationships among RHD patients' deficits. Some labels like "inference failure" or "integration deficits" have been proposed to describe sets of symptoms that are catalogued in various studies. Some other research indicates that cognitive resource factors are predictive of within- and between-person performance variations, in several pragmatic and discourse areas. But at present the clinical bottom line is this: We do not know what core deficits underlie RHD adults' cognitive-communicative impairments, or what skills or behaviors are prerequisite to attaining others, so we can only guess about how to target our efforts and about the extent to which intervening in one domain may affect performance in another area.

C. Other General Considerations

1. Earlier chapters provided some suggestions about focusing treatment. One primary guideline is to target those areas that emerge from the assessment as hypotheses about the nature of a patient's

impairments. To infer the source or level of a particular deficit, we analyze patterns of performances on various assessment tasks (see Chapter 4) and derive hypotheses from empirical, theoretical and/or functional task analyses (see Chapters 2, 4, and 6). Patients' and families' complaints and concerns, and behaviors presumed important for achieving basic rehabilitation goals, should also receive high priority whenever possible. It is likely to be beneficial, as well, if treatment tasks take into account a patient's premorbid abilities, knowledge, interests, personality characteristics, learning strategies, and communication needs in a variety of contexts (e.g., typical partners and situations; types and complexities of messages processed; family and social roles).

2. It should go without saying that no single approach will be appropriate for every patient, even those whose symptoms are similar on the surface. Any cognitive-communicative symptom can occur for a variety of reasons, and similar symptoms will not be equally handicapping for different individuals.

3. Given the reminders above, a generic caution about treatment workbooks is in order. Most of these provide some useful models of tasks that might be appropriate for some patients and some purposes. But, typically, the exercises are presented without rationales for linking them to the nature or level of patients' deficits or to any particular goals. Clinicians who use workbook materials should pick and choose carefully, being certain to articulate for themselves, and their patients, the rationales for any activities that they use. Published materials also frequently must be modified to make tasks more functional and personally relevant, or to compensate for or circumvent deficits, such as visuoperceptual problems, that clinicians do not wish to target specifically in a particular activity.

4. Finally, when planning interventions for RHD adults, speech-language pathologists should collaborate as closely as possible with other members of the rehabilitation team (see Chapter 8). Cooperation among team members will usually be advantageous for developing and implementing management strategies and procedures to reduce impairment and to minimize disability or handicap, in all areas of concern.

D. Implementing Facilitative and Compensatory Treatment

From the perspective of the impairment-disability-handicap hierarchy, underlying impairments are often targeted for treatment during the acute post-onset phase in an attempt to facilitate recovery (see Chapter

6). As time passes and stable residual impairments become evident, treatment may focus more on compensating for functional disabilities and minimizing social or vocational handicaps. Chapter 6 emphasized the problems of designating and developing techniques that are facilitory and indicated that some compensations, when overlearned and automatized, may actually be facilitative of other behaviors. The treatment sections to follow this overview will describe suggestions for potentially facilitory techniques and compensatory strategies (beginning with section II-C). However, some principles will be summarized first, as they apply across the domains considered below.

1. Regardless of whether approaches are intended as compensatory or facilitative, we aim to vary task difficulty by systematically modifying factors that can lead to success or failure for individual patients (e.g., Table 6–3 and Chapter 6, section II-E-2 regarding stimulus characteristics, stimulus modes, task characteristics, and other facilitators). In general, we want to begin with the fewest, least intrusive, and most natural facilitators and cues that patients can handle while maintaining acceptable levels of accuracy and response time, to make it less difficult to fade or eliminate them.

2. Compensatory strategies may be implemented by the patient or generated by some other person or environmental arrangement.

   a. Much of patient-implemented strategy training involves self-monitoring regimes in which patients learn to identify problem behaviors and situations that call for using some kind of compensation. Examples of internal compensations for RHD adults include monitoring their comprehension or their situational awareness and appropriateness, and initiating the use of functional memory aids, self-instruction, or practical problem-solving guides. (For more about self-monitoring and awareness training, see the end of section I, and II-B-2-d, below.)

   b. Treatment may focus on other-implemented, external strategies under several conditions: while patients are learning to initiate their own strategies, when they are not successful at generating compensations after extended training, or when they are persistently unaware of the need for strategies (see II-B-2-d, below on awareness training). Family members, rehabilitation staff, and others who interact with the patient can be taught to use beneficial strategies whenever the need might arise, rather than waiting for the patient to apply them.

Compensations requested of the patient or generated by those in the patient's environment should match in specificity and directness those that patients practice with their clinicians. Some external compensations might include having those who interact with a patient try to present information in an explicit and consistent form to minimize demands for nonliteral comprehension or reinterpretation; to provide specific verbal guidance; and to cue patients to consult individually tailored problem-solving guides, to initiate self-instructional prompts, or to use socially appropriate behavior. Additional specific examples will be offered in the treatment material presented throughout this chapter.

c. According to Ylvisaker and Holland (1985), ideal candidates for patient-implemented strategy training are aware of their deficits and needs, realistic about their goals, and recognize the value of compensations. In addition, it is critical for patients to have some capacity to distinguish desired from undesired performances (see II-B- 2-d, on error monitoring training).

d. Ylvisaker and Holland also emphasize that strategies should be individually selected, in part by considering a patient's abilities (see Table 7–1), and in part by concentrating on those strategies that are efficient and beneficial, rather than inefficient and maladaptive. To enhance the probability of generalized strategy usage, a clinician should work on solidifying spontaneous, patient-generated strategies that have the potential to be efficient and adaptive, no matter how irregularly used, rather than introducing entirely new strategies. When patients do not use potentially effective self-generated strategies, the clinician can try to guide them toward compensations that may be more generalizable. For instance, self-instruction as a compensation for neglect can be applied in more situations than can an anchor-line in a left margin. Further, compensations that are relatively unobtrusive are more likely to be used outside of the treatment setting. In any case, when targeting strategies for training, the clinician should take care to limit the number that are targeted and to avoid confusions among them.

e. Training patient-implemented strategies often involves some of the following steps (for further information, see Ylvisaker & Szekeres, 1994).

Table 7–1. Variables affecting compensatory strategy selection and training.

Environmental-Social Factors
Pretrauma social, educational, occupational status and interests
Current functional needs and environmental supports

Perceptual-Cognitive Strengths and Weaknesses
Sensory, perceptual, perceptual-motor abilities
Attentional and memory proceses
Language abilities
Organizing, reasoning, problem solving
Level of content knowledge and organization of knowledge
Metacognitive abilities: awareness of strengths, weaknesses; explanation of own
    strategies; prediction of performance
Spontaneous strategies used

Readiness for New Learning
Degree of confusion, disorientation, attentional impairment

Executive Functions
Self-awareness, self-initiation, self-direction, self-monitoring, self-evaluation, and
self-adjustment

Cognitive Style
Impulsive, reflective, persistent, active, passive, flexible, decisive

Situational Discrimination
Ability to distinguish situations that do or do not call for use of a particular strategy

Personality and Social Control
Shy, aggressive, fearful, confident; attitude toward treatment

Motivational Factors
Presence/appropriateness of goals; perceived need for strategies

Source: Adapted from Ylvisaker, M. S., & Holland, A. L. (1985). Coaching, self-coaching, and rehabilitation of head injury. In Donnell F. Johns, (Ed.), *Clinical Management of Neurogenic Communication Disorders* (2nd ed., pp 243–257). Copyright ©1985 by Allyn and Bacon. Used with permission.

(1) Convince the patient of the usefulness of strategies in general. This will not be necessary if a patient has been a devotee of organizers and reminders like schedules, calendars, or post-it notes. Some patients profess never to have used such strategies, but when asked specifically, they may realize that they have relied on devices like shopping lists, address books, timers, bus schedules, putting things in a special place, or asking someone else to remind them to do something. If a patient still denies using or needing strategies, it may help for clinicians, various family members, and/or other patients to describe the strategies that they use and to discuss and demonstrate the benefits of using them as well as the consequences of going without them.

(2) Convince the patient of the usefulness of specific strategies. If a patient occasionally initiates a strategy that could be used more effectively or more often, the clinician can tailor tasks to lead to planned successes and failures, helping the patient to note a contrast in performance with and without that strategy. Similarly, if the clinician selects novel strategies based on assessment and behavioral observation, tasks can be developed to illustrate how they work. The clinician may begin by describing and modeling the strategy and then ask the patient to apply it in contrasting, controlled practice activities. It is useful to video- or audiotape the patient's performance, with and without the strategy, so that clinician and patient can review and discuss the differences together.

(3) From the earliest point in the demonstration process, the patient practices explaining the connection between strategy usage and performance, the ways to implement the strategy, and the behaviors or situations for which it is likely to be needed (developing intellectual awareness, section II-B-2-d). When possible the patient moves toward predicting, from a description of an upcoming task or situation, whether a target strategy may be useful (anticipatory awareness, II-B-2-d).

(4) Strategy acquisition and efficiency building are accomplished through massed practice in a variety of tasks, until the compensations can be generated automatically in appropriate situations. Training tasks and conditions are designed to offer many chances for patients to apply a target strategy and to observe and experience the consequences when it is and is not used. Once strategies are used routinely with the clinician, the patient will probably need extended training to initiate them in a broader range of circumstances.

(5) The clinician continues to record performance, but begins to postpone the tape review as patients learn to monitor strategy usage on-line. On-line monitoring work can start with simple, well-practiced tasks and brief behavior samples. Initially, patients can keep track of appropriate strategy usage and/or missed opportunities, comparing their judgments with those of the clinician. Then clinician and

patient can review performance tapes together to check the patient's analysis and to note remaining problems or discrepancies. Gradually, the patient should practice monitoring longer behavior samples on-line in tasks and conditions that are increasingly novel or complex. Some patients may be more successful initially at monitoring other peoples' strategy usage. This kind of practice can be built into group treatment sessions; or in individual treatment, patients can monitor videotapes of other patients (only with appropriate consent) or track performance of a clinician who deliberately misses opportunities or uses strategies ineffectively.

(6) Training in self-reliance and self-talk accompanies strategy training to enhance the likelihood of generalized responding. Some procedures for self-instruction training (after Ylvisaker and Holland) include: have patients begin every treatment task with verbalized self-reminders, relying on cue cards, lists, or other prompts as long as they are needed; gradually fade clinician-provided cues regarding task performance and the need to initiate self-reminders; make patients' self-instructions more covert; and have patients practice instructing clinicians, family members, and/or other patients in groups. These kinds of activities can begin as soon as patients can handle them without significantly impairing other aspects of performance. The goal is for deliberate activities to become routine again through repeated practice, reducing the need for constant self-instruction. Some patients, however, will continue to need labeled scripts, cue cards, or other organized reminders to prompt and guide their strategy usage.

II. PRAGMATICS DOMAIN

A. General Pragmatic Treatment Approaches and Procedures

1. In their helpful discussion of pragmatic treatment principles and procedures, Newhoff and Apel (1990) recommend that after clinicians select target skills from assessment information, they should determine situations or contexts in which those skills are normally used and then construct or simulate similar circumstances for treatment activities. For example, to work on contingent responses, patients can converse about the main points or most humorous parts of recent movies or television programs, or relate the specifics of an incident from a

family gathering when queried by others. Newhoff and Apel also emphasize that pragmatic treatment settings should provide opportunities for reinforcing effective behaviors, as well as for developing skills to circumvent weaknesses.

2. A number of activities that resemble naturally occurring interactions are well suited as pragmatic intervention contexts.

   a. Referential communication tasks, or barrier tasks, were introduced in Chapter 4 as a method of evaluation, but these kinds of activities can be fruitful treatment tasks as well. In the treatment setting, clinicians develop materials and tasks to target particular pragmatic goals or behaviors, as illustrated in Chapter 4 (section III-B-1-f). To apply these kinds of tasks in treatment, clinicians will define and instruct patients in the use of particular target behaviors and demonstrate or model those behaviors as needed.

   b. Treatment tasks can also be patterned after PACE therapy interactions (Promoting Aphasics' Communicative Effectiveness; see Davis & Wilcox, 1985). The overall goal of PACE activities is similar to that for other referential communication tasks: Clinicians and patients take turns trying, in as few attempts as possible, to convey information that is not known to the other participant, and natural feedback about the adequacy of performance arises from each partner's ability to guess the other's message. One difference from other barrier tasks is that in PACE, clinicians let patients choose any means of communicating their ideas, and clinicians use their own turns to model appropriate behaviors or strategies, rather than directly instructing or restricting the patients' choices. The "unknown information" condition is achieved by having senders select a message to be conveyed from a set of cards that is kept face down and unseen. Alhough PACE therapy is often carried out with picture cards, a wide range of modes and messages is possible. Like other referential communication activities, PACE-type tasks can be structured to provide practice in a variety of pragmatic areas, including emotional or indirect forms, other speech acts, or conversational skills like turn-taking and maintaining relevance (see Chapter 4, section III-B-1-f).

   c. Roleplaying activities are frequently designed for practicing pragmatic communicative skills in situations like those that arise routinely for the patient. Initially, patient and clinician discuss the goal of a planned activity and list possible responses and behaviors. Then roleplaying begins, with opportunities for the patient to use planned responses. Cue cards or other self-instructional devices can be incorporated as appropriate. During this phase of training, clinicians should not to step out of their roles; rather, evaluation and discussion occur after the roleplay is finished. At that time, the patient is asked to describe and analyze successes and problems and to suggest possible alternative strategies, with the clinician's assistance as needed. Videotaped feedback (as in I-D-2, above, and II-B-2-d, below) may be beneficial for this performance review and evaluation, with the clinician fading cues and structure over time. Finally, other familiar and unfamiliar listeners and settings can be integrated with roleplaying activities as the patient becomes more adept with target behaviors.

3. Referential communication, PACE, and role-playing activities are fairly indirect procedures that allow patients a lot of latitude for responding. This is part of their strength as pragmatic intervention contexts. For most patients, however, these kinds of activities need to be supplemented, and often preceded, by more direct intervention procedures. More direct procedures can facilitate acquisition of the well-developed, end-product behaviors and skills that are targeted in indirect activities, and can maximize the number of opportunities for responding appropriately. Some generalities about the possible nature and progression of direct intervention activities are provided below.

a. From an information processing perspective, the least cognitively demanding treatment activities tend to involve identification or recognition, and discrimination tasks. Recognition and discrimination tasks might include separating instances from noninstances (e.g., literal vs. nonliteral interpretations, or topic-related statements vs. unrelated statements), or distinguishing relevant aspects of a stimulus or situation from less relevant aspects (e.g., emphasized words; cues for interpreting indirect requests and irony). At a higher level of processing, activities often focus on association, organization, or appreciation of relationships among instances or aspects. Finally, tasks can call for interpretation, explanation, generation of and contrast between similar or different instances, and so forth. If the nature of impairment has not been pinpointed in the diagnostic evaluation, tasks can be designed to probe performance at the highest levels a patient is expected to be able to handle, stepping back to simpler levels only as necessary. In any case, success is likely to be enhanced when treatment activities draw upon patients' prior knowledge or experience.

b. As needed to facilitate correct responding, direct treatment activities can begin with explicit and clearly interpretable situational contexts that minimize nonessential details, incorporate semantic and inferential redundancy, and specify themes or topics. These kinds of contexts might include titled, verbally conveyed episodes and vignettes with clear and consistent themes. Gradually, contexts can be developed to introduce more nonessential details, implicit main points, and discrepancies that frequently characterize pragmatic interpretations.

c. Because many direct treatment activities for RHD adults build on awareness, association, or integration of multiple aspects of a stimulus context, visual or graphic aids are often beneficial for helping patients to manipulate, and to keep track of various task elements and goals. Diagrams, outlines, and index cards that can be moved about to represent more clearly various stimulus relationships are among the many possibilities. Representations of this sort may be particularly helpful when some elements of a task are ostensibly or actually discrepant or when a task or situation places other heavy demands on patients' working memory and integration processes.

4. Self-monitoring and self-instruction should be incorporated into direct treatment activities as well (e.g., I-D-2, above).

5. Sohlberg and Mateer (1989a) note that many pragmatic treatment activities may require prior training to enhance awareness. Some sample goals for improving awareness of deficits were outlined in Table 6-2, and awareness training is considered below (in II-B-2-d). Sohlberg and Mateer also remind us that training for generalization and maintenance is a must.

a. Generalization is addressed in part by extending training to a variety of extra-clinic settings and partners and by providing opportunities and assignments to use a self-monitoring system (see Chapter 6, II-F, to review suggestions for enhancing generalization).

b. A group treatment context may create a bridge to generalization and maintenance, as well. Pragmatic treatment groups are designed to facilitate appropriate skill usage and monitoring in social interactions.

(1) Ehrlich and Sipes (1985) suggest a procedure for group treatment of nonverbal communication and conversational interaction skills, which can be extended to other targeted areas. Clinicians describe and demonstrate individually targeted skills in videotaped role-play situations that contain appropriate and inappropriate behaviors. These tapes are reviewed and discussed by group members to identify behaviors that lead to communicative successes and failures. Then group members perform role plays of specific social situations, being videotaped for later group evaluation. At this point, the group discusses strengths, weaknesses, and alternatives, as in the roleplay review described above. Each member of the group has individualized goals, and all assist each other in problem solving and evaluation related to their specific goals.

(2) Davis (1993) also describes pragmatics group procedures oriented around PACE therapy for practice generalizing skills from individual treatment. Treatment tasks incorporate the following principles: Patients interact with each other, with the clinician's assistance limited primarily to unobtrusive tasks like taking data, and helping a patient only when necessary; materials are arranged to convey unshared, or "new," information; partners take turns as senders and receivers, with a free choice of communication options; and activities are kept simple and familiar so that interaction is not hindered by task demands. Referential communication tasks are suitable in group treatment as well.

(3) Davis suggests card games as particularly good activities; in a variant of "go fish," patients try to obtain matches between pairs of cards by conveying in some fashion what is depicted on the cards they have been dealt. For RHD adults, a set of cards might be created to portray particular components of communication that cause group members difficulty, such as emotional reactions, figurative versus literal interpretations, or other types of ambiguity. For a focus on prosodic production and interpretation goals, stimulus cards might contain printed stimuli, such as sentences, with large, bold, and/or underlined words serving as cues to emphatic stress placement. In a variation of the matching activity, a deck of cards could include one set of linguistic descriptions (e.g., printed indirect commands or other nonliteral forms; thematic statements) and a linked set of pictured representations or interpretations, or names of events or famous people, with a linked set of descriptions or category instances. Patients attempt to match a stimulus of one form with the other one that expresses the same idea.

(4) Each of these kinds of activities can be performed by paired communication partners, as in a typical game of "go fish."

When skills and personalities allow, creating "teams" also may be beneficial and motivating. Teams can be pitted against each other in terms of the time or number of attempts it takes to reach correct solutions for tasks like those mentioned above, or in activities like "Charades."

(5) Some other possible group treatment activities, which can be tailored according to individualized needs and goals, include:

(a) describing pictures or summarizing media reports, with directions to focus on main themes, to identify the two most salient and most incidental features, and so forth.

(b) recognizing and explaining verbal and visual anomalies and ambiguities.

(c) identifying socially inappropriate comments or reactions and discussing or demonstrating alternatives.

(d) identifying emotional responses associated with specified situations and some nonverbal cues that convey them.

(e) contrasting direct and indirect request forms that can be used to try to get someone to do something and choosing those most appropriate for defined interactions or situations.

(f) deducing speaker intention from a variety of speech acts and signals.

(g) telling a progressive story, with each group member elaborating on the statements of the preceding speaker.

(h) counting inappropriate and appropriate responses of self and others in a variety of tasks; explaining why some are inappropriate; and describing or demonstrating alternatives.

(6) As always, the goals for any such activities should be clearly described and agreed upon by the patients. Of course, any of these kinds of activities can also be used in individual treatment, with patient and clinician working as partners.

6. Some potentially helpful guidelines for structuring pragmatic interventions are also found in interpersonal communication texts. For example, Ratliffe and Hudson (1988) describe learning objectives, skill modules (consisting of orientation, awareness, and demonstration), practice activities, and self-evaluation summaries for a number of skill areas, such as initiating relationships, expressing oneself,

checking perceptions and interpretations, expressing emotions, communicating nonverbally, listening and responding, and managing interpersonal conflicts.

B. Focused Pragmatic Treatment: Principles and Possible Foundations

1. A few additional prefatory remarks are in order here. First, treatment with RHD adults involves ample discussion; explanation, graphic representation, demonstration, and modeling as needed; and self-instruction and self-monitoring on the patient's part whenever possible. Second, one of the principles emphasized in Chapter 6 bears repeating. That is, clinicians need to remain aware of the potential prerequisite abilities for accomplishing any particular treatment task. This principle is important, for example, when pictured materials are incorporated into pragmatic treatment activities with RHD adults. Clinicians must ascertain a patient's ability to select and process key visual information accurately and efficiently, or to interpret the pictured material, before using it as a context for working on other target skills such as appreciating prosody or figurative meanings. Finally, readers are reminded that Table 6–3 and its associated text summarize factors that can be manipulated in attempting to influence the relative difficulty of treatment tasks, depending on a patient's deficits and capabilities, and that Chapter 4 describes referential communication tasks targeting some of the pragmatic behaviors and skills below.

2. Most of the pragmatic communicative skills discussed below (II-C) hinge on several basic abilities, including recognizing ambiguity, appreciating the fact that intended meanings often go beyond literal forms or depictions, and determining what is relevant or important in an interaction. In addition, as noted above, patients' awareness of deficits may need attention before other treatment will be of benefit. Some ideas will be presented next for working on deficits in these potentially fundamental areas.

   a. When patients do not recognize the possibility of alternative interpretations, clinician and patient can start by discussing the fact that many words and phrases have more than one meaning, or can refer to more than one thing. Examples can be taken from areas of high interest or knowledge for the patient; spoken lexical ambiguities that involve names of local sports teams (e.g., Panthers, White Sox) or familiar household products (e.g., Tide) often provide a good starting point. Then patients can practice selecting from a set of possibilities the alternative interpretations for a variety of ambiguous forms (lexical, semantic, syntactic), starting with those that have two familiar meanings. Less impaired patients may begin with tasks that require associating, generating, or explaining alternative interpretations for such stimuli. For recognition and identification tasks, foils can be made more similar as performance improves. In association, generation, and explanation tasks, clinicians can take turns with patients to model the disambiguation process. Clinicians can also generate some less obvious interpretation(s), asking the patient to add others.

b. Some patients who can recognize and identify ambiguity appear to have difficulty understanding that a speaker's intended meaning can differ from what the words actually say. For these patients, it may be helpful to exemplify this notion by discussing some nonliteral utterances that they have used or understood in prior interactions. In addition, their appreciation of the idea of intended meanings is probably better in some domains than in others, allowing clinicians to explain and demonstrate first with forms that patients do understand (e.g., using emphasis, or tone of voice, to convey something; getting someone to do something for them in a roundabout way, without asking directly). Some specific possibilities for introducing the idea of "intended meanings" are included in the discussion of each pragmatic area, below (II-C).

c. Some RHD adults have difficulty determining what is important or central in interpreting situational contexts and conversations or in producing connected discourse. To target the basic concept of "main points," patients can practice identifying them in a number of the vehicles that will be discussed below (II-C), starting with tasks or contexts in which they are most successful. For example, patients can choose the most important elements of emphatically stressed stimuli, the probable intention of indirect requests and other figurative forms, or the likely interpretation of emotional stimuli. They can identify the critical aspects of verbal or pictured contexts, group or rank elements by centrality or tangentiality, or sort according to themes. Graphic representations (section II-A-3-c) may be particularly helpful for these kinds of activities. When necessary, patients can perform these kinds of tasks using elements identified by the clinician before moving on to generating their own lists, groups, or rank orderings. They can select from several choices, or generate if possible, the main ideas and then the details of short discourse contexts, such as those described in Chapter 4 (section III-C). They can identify elements that are essential for different listeners or communication purposes, as suggested in Table 4–5 (Conceptual network level, item 3). In more taxing tasks, they can contrast main points with information that is less essential, explaining why each point is or is not central. Tasks can be made more challenging in a variety of ways noted previously, such as by manipulating explicitness; the number of unnecessary details; the presence of a title or theme; the inclusion of ostensible or real discrepancies; and the salience or predictability of central features, using emphasis, repetition, redundancy, color, and the like. Patients can practice applying their sense of what is central in PACE or barrier tasks, with a goal of minimizing the number of clues or the amount of information needed to get across a message. Clinicians can record performance, or write down the clues that patients provided, for post-task evaluation and review, as suggested in relation to strategy training and roleplay tasks.

d. As noted earlier, awareness training may have to precede more focused pragmatic treatment. Barco, Crosson, Bolesta, Werts, and Stout (1991) describe a number of procedures for training three types of awareness: intellectual, emergent, and anticipatory. Each kind of awareness can be present to different degrees, and it is possible for patients to exhibit different levels or kinds of awareness for different deficit areas.

(1) Intellectual awareness involves some understanding that an aptitude or function is diminished from premorbid levels. To facilitate intellectual awareness, repetitive education is provided to patient and family. Clinicians begin by explaining the nature and potential functional implications of the patient's deficits, relating them to the patient's brain injury. Another technique targets a patient's skills at describing, explaining, and monitoring behaviors. Initially, patients may be more successful identifying and judging the behavior of others, in comparison with their own. If so, this type of treatment can incorporate observation, tallying, description, and discussion of desirable and undesirable behaviors of other patients or clinicians, in groups or videos, before the same procedures are applied to taped samples or written transcripts exemplifying the patient's behavior. When possible, patients participate in labeling their own strengths and weaknesses; but in any case, team members use terminology consistently. The patient and clinician can also cooperate in generating a list of strengths and weaknesses, with clinicians initially providing cues that point to specific areas or examples, as needed, and fading them when possible. As patients begin to make insightful statements about their behavior, it becomes important to demonstrate that particular behaviors or deficits have consequences. This can be approached through videotape review, and, when patients can handle it, by incorporating planned successes and failures into the therapy setting (see I-D, above, on strategy training). Of course, planned failure must be accompanied by emotional support and education. When a patient is persistently unable to describe the nature and impact of problem areas, external, highly structured compensations are in order (e.g., environmental modification or support person training, when realistic and feasible). In such cases, patients should be informed about compensation plans and optimally should agree to them.

(2) At a higher level, emergent awareness reflects an ability to recognize a problem as it is occurring. Some indicators include signs of frustration and self-correction attempts. Generally, treatment aims to move patients from simply identifying and describing behaviors and their consequences, to monitoring or tallying problems and signs of their impact, online (see also I-D, strategy training). To facilitate the development of emergent awareness, clinicians provide specific feedback before and after task performance, with a goal of helping patients realize when they are affected by their problems. Treatment follows procedures similar to those for intellectual awareness, but also involves specifying the observable signs of a problem's impact (e.g., social feedback regarding inappropriate behavior). Some techniques for facilitating emergent awareness include evaluating videotapes, when given cues to focus observations on particular signs or reactions; developing and applying lists of areas to review in videotaped and live interactions; and completing self-rating scales of problem areas such as concentration, with and without the clinician. Some patients may benefit as well from direct work on error recognition. One potential approach involves contrasting actual or simulated errors of the patient's with accurate or more appropriate responses, in discrimination and identification exercises. Such tasks can begin with large discrepancies or logical inconsistencies in short, meaningful stimuli, and move toward subtler distinctions in longer or more complicated examples. Patients whose emergent awareness remains limited will require situational compensations, such as tailored

checklists or other reminders that are used routinely in potentially appropriate circumstances. In such cases, patients, families, and clinicians need to prioritize, because patients can only initiate a limited number of these kinds of strategies.

(3) Anticipatory awareness, or the ability to foresee a problem, requires high level cognitive skills to project the future and to recognize the implications of deficits. Anticipatory awareness is a prerequisite to anticipatory compensation, in which a patient implements a strategy to avoid an expected difficulty. Facilitation of anticipatory awareness involves guiding patients toward predicting and planning how to handle problems. Initially, patient and clinician can review and discuss examples of problem behaviors or mistakes from past interactions and decide how those could be avoided. For practice, patient and clinician think through the skills or behaviors that might create obstacles in an upcoming task or situation and plan appropriate strategy implementation. After carrying out the task, the patient indicates what strategy was used and at what point. This can be done by reviewing videotapes, or if possible, by reflecting on what just happened. When feasible, patients can start to signal as they actually implement a strategy. Eventually, as well, patients can be asked to anticipate independently by stating how they think they will do on specific tasks, and why. Over time, clinician participation and cuing for projecting difficulties and planning alternatives will diminish. Consolidating antici-patory awareness may require extensive practice in a variety of simulated and real situations; much of this practice can be accomplished through independent outside assignments, with patients keeping track of successes and failures for discussion with the clinician. For patients who do not develop anticipato-ry awareness, recognition compensations are appropriate. These involve patients turning to a compensation at the first instance that they recognize a problem occurring (e.g., when given signals from others).

(4) Readers may remember Table 6–2, which exemplified a basic goal of increased awareness of deficits, along with several specific goals. In Barco et al.'s (1991) terms, one of those specific goals ("explain reasons for targeting behaviors") is directed at a high level of intellectual awareness, while the others ("monitor on line"; and "mon-itor signals from others" as a possible subgoal) focus on emergent awareness.

(5) Some other principles for implementing awareness training include the following:

(a) A trusting relationship between patient and clinician is essential for patients to "hear" and benefit from feedback designed to enhance awareness. In some cases, feedback from others who are in a similar situation (e.g., other participants in a group treatment context) may be easier for patients to accept, especially at first.

(b) Treatment should always emphasize strengths as well as undesirable behaviors so as not to devastate self-esteem or to reinforce a fear of failure or specific negative behaviors.

(c) Treatment tasks should use meaningful materials and be relevant to patients' needs.

(d) Self-evaluation should be encouraged at every step as soon as patients can confront their own behavior: after, during, and eventually prior to completing treatment tasks. As soon as possible, modification, repair, or anticipatory compensation should be connected with evaluation and monitoring.

(e) Treatment goals should be clear, and the links between treatment activities and goals should be carefully explained to patients and family members.

(f) Families or other support persons should be involved when possible, as soon as possible, in providing accurate feedback or signals to patients. In addition, family members can be central in developing incentive or contingency programs for patients with fundamental awareness problems that may be manifest in refusal to attend or to participate fully in treatment. Some such patients may be willing to follow through to please a family member or to receive some particular reward. In such cases, the patient should be kept informed and should be involved to the extent that it is possible in setting specific contract agreements and incentives. Some patients who can be induced to attend and work may begin to develop the trust that is essential for profiting from awareness training.

(g) Finally, it must be remembered that denial can serve an important psychological protective function. If it persists, patients should be referred for psychological consultation

C. Focused Pragmatic Treatment: Approaches and Procedures

1. Prosody.

a. Direct, facilitative treatment for RHD adults' *prosodic production impairments* is rare unless diminished prosody is associated with a dysarthria. In this case, clinicians may work to improve speech intelligibility and naturalness by heightening stress and emphasis, using tasks such as contrastive stress drills, query responding, or disambiguation exercises.

(1) For contrastive stress drills, the clinician and patient start with a premise, such as "Bill and Mary bought a pizza." Then, the clinician makes a statement or asks a question that contradicts the premise (e.g., "So, Bill and Mary made a pizza" or "Did Bill and Sue buy a pizza?"). The patient's task is to respond by emphasizing the key element of the premise ("No, they BOUGHT a pizza"). Initially, to reduce memory demands, the premise can be stated directly, and written on an index card. When a more difficult task context is appropriate, the cue card can be removed, the premise can be embedded in a lengthier context, and/or the premise can be one that is implied by a picture or by a figurative or indirect utterance (assuming that the patient can extract the implied meaning). Query responding tasks proceed similarly. For the premise above, the clinician may ask "Who bought the pizza?" or "What did they buy?" Practice is accompanied by discussion of the ways in which stress or emphasis can highlight different aspects of meaning.

(a) When patients do not produce emphatic stress in tasks like these, they should be asked to point to, repeat, or underline the contradictory element of the clinician's stimulus to see if they can identify target stress location,. If patients are not successful it may be necessary to train them first to identify the occurrence, and eventually the location, of differences between the clinician's statements and the given premises, moving from obvious to subtle.

(b) Many patients who do not use emphatic stress can identify the element to be highlighted or the part of the statement that is most important. These patients can be instructed directly in ways to achieve vocal emphasis (e.g., "Say that part louder"). If this fails, patients can be given visual cues to guide their independent production attempts or to accompany trials in which they imitate the clinician's utterance, whether immediately or after a delay. Visual cues include those provided by a clinician's modeled utterance displayed on a Visipitch screen; by written stimuli that incorporate underlining, bold print, or color-coding; or by index cards containing individual portions of the stimulus, arranged on a table or on a musical staff by height, according to the relative amount of emphasis.

(2) In disambiguation exercises, patients can be given ambiguous surface forms and asked to say them in more than one way. Appropriate material is provided by lexical (e.g., "record," "green house"), syntactic (e.g., question vs. statement intonation for simple declaratives like "He left early"), and semantic ambiguities (e.g. literal vs. figurative interpretations). Patients who are poor at demarcating pause boundaries can practice with ambiguous mathematical operations (e.g., $4 + 2 \times 2$) where there are two possible answers, depending on the grouping of elements. Of course, these activities assume an ability to appreciate the various alternative interpretations, an assumption that should be checked for individual patients (see also II-B-2, above).

b. Compensatory strategies for prosodic production may include teaching patients to generate emphasis on particularly important aspects of messages, to minimize the need for emphatic stress by stating explicitly the main points of their messages, or to provide other cues (first letter; topic of conversation) to enhance intelligibility. These kinds of compensations can also be cued by others in the environment, who are taught when and how to request them. Others can be taught as well to check their interpretations with the patient.

c. When diminished speech prosody is rooted primarily in emotional impairments rather than motor control deficits, it is not appropriate to work on prosodic production without attending to the emotional factors. Prosodic and emotional expressiveness can be muted by depression, a potentially serious condition that needs to be identified and managed (VI-B). When family members are concerned about a lack of vocal variation in a depressed patient, the clinician may need to counsel them about the connection between emotional and prosodic expressiveness. When depression has been controlled or ruled out, and patients are aprosodic in the absence of significant speech motor problems, clinicians probably will not target prosody unless patient and family consider it crucially important for the patient to be more vocally expressive. In such cases, compensatory strategies can be explored, depending on the patient's ability to identify in any way his or her attitudes or emphatic intentions. At the same time, such clients and their families may benefit from education about, and training to use, alternative ways to convey attitudes. Treatment activities for nondepressive emotional interpretation and production problems will be considered in the material below.

d. Several approaches are possible for treatment to facilitate *prosodic comprehension.*

(1) Prosodic interpretation skills help to distinguish a variety of intentions. For example, emphatic stress is often used to mark information that is new, or unshared by communication partners (as opposed to that which is commonly known). Intonational cues also serve to disambiguate linguistic forms and functions. Prosodic information signals other discourse or conversational functions as well, such as inviting responses or maintaining speaking turns. Comprehension tasks can use stimuli patterned after those suggested above for production tasks. Clinicians can present stimuli for interpretation and ask patients to select, associate with different contexts, explain, and/or contrast their meanings; to identify central elements or important ideas on the basis of vocal emphasis; or to indicate when it is or is not appropriate for the next speaker to take a turn.

(2) When patients have trouble discriminating nonemotional speech patterns, treatment may be targeted at that level, particularly if minimal progress is being made in the contextualized identification and interpretation activities described above. Discrimination requirements should progress from obvious to subtle, as the duration, number, or extent of differences between critical elements are varied. Fundamental frequency cues tend to be more difficult for many RHD patients to discriminate than durational cues, so stimuli that differ in durational aspects may be appropriate for explaining, modeling, and establishing early success. Meaningful linguistic material may also provide a good starting point, since it tends to be less difficult for RHD patients than nonsense syllable or musical stimuli. Rapid mid-stimulus

changes of pitch direction in nonsense syllables or music, reported to be especially problematic in prosodic imitation tasks (Tucker & Hamby, 1987), may make appropriate higher-level targets.

(3) Prosodic comprehension problems are often linked to difficulties in judging attitudes or emotions as well. Treatment can begin with some discussion about determining moods from prosody, focusing on the way someone's voice can convey something more than their words do. Many patients resonate to the familiar situation of telling their children "Don't use that tone of voice with me!"

(a) In initial activities, patients can be asked to identify or interpret attitudes in phrases and sentences that are linguistically and prosodically congruent (e.g., "She is thrilled about her daughter's graduation" spoken in a happy tone of voice), moving to congruent prosodic stimuli and pictured scenes as perceptual capabilities allow. In such tasks, clinicians ask patients to select from several mood labels, or to explain when possible, "How does that person sound?" If patients have difficulty with this, discrimination abilities should be ascertained. In addition, clinicians and patients can try to generate a list of vocal cues or signals that help to analyze prosodic contrasts, and listen to prosodic stimuli to identify the signals.

(b) Associating emotional prosody with contextual information comes next, with patients initially matching prosodic stimuli to single mood labels (e.g., ecstatic, joyful) or brief verbally described emotional situations (e.g., "You won the lottery") and then moving toward lengthier descriptions and pictured contexts as appropriate. Patients can also be asked to describe personal situations in which they experienced certain moods and then to associate these contexts with prosodic stimuli.

(c) Later, discrepancies can be introduced between explicit emotional contexts or descriptions (e.g., "She was ecstatic") or expected attitudes (e.g., "We won the lottery!") and prosodic stimuli. Discrepancies between positive and negative affective stimuli will be easier to recognize than discrepancies within positive and negative categories or between emotional and neutral concepts. Patients can start by identifying trials in which there are discrepancies. Failing this, the task can be dissected, and patients asked first to predict from the contextual description "How would that person feel?" and then to indicate from the prosody "How does that person sound?"

(d) When discrepancies can be identified, patients can work on reconciling the conflicting meanings, a skill important for revising interpretations. They can be asked how they might change either the context or the prosody to make the two "go together," choosing from clinician-provided alternatives as needed. At a higher level, clinician and patient can discuss together the occasions in which context-prosody discrepancies are common or appropriate, focusing on speech acts like teasing and irony. Then they can work on identifying ironic or teasing comments in which words and tone-of-voice do not match and associating these kinds of remarks with specified situations, both clinician and patient generated.

(4) For prosodic interpretation activities, serious questions have been raised about the validity of prosodic and emotional contrasts that are produced on-line. Although tape-recorded stimuli have practical disadvantages and are less realistic than live voice presentations, they do provide control over intended prosodic contrasts. It is confusing, at best, to work on prosodic comprehension with target stimuli that cannot be unambiguously interpreted by non-brain-damaged elderly adults.

e. Compensations for prosodic comprehension deficits can include patient-implemented strategies such as asking others to be explicit about main points or attitudes or checking interpretations. Patients can also be taught to ask themselves something like "Does this fit with what I know or expect from this situation?" Others in the patient's environment can be taught to initiate or request these kinds of modifications whenever the patient appears to be having difficulty, or routinely, depending on the patient's level of functioning.

2. Emotion and nonverbal communication.

a. Treatment for impairments of emotional interpretation can proceed similarly to that outlined for emotional prosodic comprehension problems, using facial expressions and other visual stimuli in place of vocal ones. Patients who have difficulty interpreting emotion through visual channels usually do better initially when given descriptions of meaningful situations that tend to elicit particular attitudes. When this is true, activities involving identification, association, contrast, and discrepancy identification and resolution, can build from there. For some patients, it may be necessary to work first with nonemotional stimuli in facial and vocal interpretation tasks. In any case, a multimodality approach is probably appropriate, in which strong channels are paired with weaker ones.

b. Diminished nonverbal animation and coverbal behavior can be targeted with explanation, monitoring, and self-instruction activities. Patient and clinician can discuss together the social ramifications of reduced eye contact and back-channel behaviors, such as head nods that indicate interest in a partner's contributions. Patients can work on identifying instances of targeted nonverbal behaviors, both appropriate and inappropriate, in videotaped interactions featuring their clinicians, other people, and finally themselves. When they are successful at this level, monitoring and self-instructional activities can begin. Eye gaze patterns may improve naturally with time or with training for neglect (section V-C-6), but if nonverbal behaviors are highly distracting or inept, a conscious strategy may help to normalize interactions in the meantime.

c. Difficulties of emotional expression may include problems of muted responsiveness, or disinhibition and inappropriateness. Treatment for the former is typically indirect, focusing as appropriate on either emotional interpretation or diminished affect. Compensatory strategies might include, for example, teaching patients to explain their attitudes and reactions or to verify their feelings when others check with them. Treatment for the disinhibited patient may involve discussion, observation, and monitoring of the effects of his or her behavior. Typically, however, these patients will require social skills training more generally (see II-C-5-c, below).

d. Other compensatory strategies include those noted above for prosodic deficits. In addition, when patients have one relatively strong channel for emotional interpretation, they can be taught to base their initial judgments on that channel and to check their interpretations with other people. More generally, patients and their communication partners can learn to clarify their understanding and interpretations of each other's nonverbal behavior.

Patients may also ask others to observe and interpret their non-verbal behavior and to provide cues that are as subtle as possible when the behavior needs to be modified or explained.

3. Speech acts.

a. For RHD adults, treatment in this area tends to focus on indirect commands and requests, which are special forms of linguistic/pragmatic ambiguities requiring a link between context and response. Initially, clinician and patient discuss the fact that people often make requests of other people, without saying exactly what they want. Good examples include the boss's asking "Is that report ready for me?" or a husband commenting to his wife "It's been too long since we had your chocolate cake." Patients can also reflect on different ways to ask someone to do something for them, like running an errand. Along the same lines, patient and clinician can list modifiers that soften requests to make them more polite (see Chapter 2, II-A-3-b). If patients do not appreciate the ambiguity of indirect speech acts, treatment may back up to focus on identifying ambiguities more generally, as described above (section II-B-2).

b. A potential progression of difficulty can be gleaned from data suggesting that RHD adults are relatively adept with direct requests, but have problems with nonconventionally indirect forms, or hints, like the husband's remark above. To facilitate appreciation of hints, clinicians can create tasks in which hints are initially paired with direct requests (e.g., "Will you bake a chocolate cake for me?"). Patients can practice selecting one or more of several direct requests that express the same intent as the hint and then describing or explaining the common meaning. Similar exercises can be done by pairing conventionally indirect requests (like the boss's question) with direct requests or commands and then with hints. For production practice, patients can give one or several more direct forms of a request when presented with an indirect form, or vice versa.

c. Lower-functioning patients may need to step back from these activities, to identify what the speaker might want, and then to discuss and represent the discrepancy between what the speaker wants and what he or she actually says, using techniques such as those noted above for prosodic interpretation tasks. At yet a lower level, some patients may need initial work to discriminate and identify statements and requests.

d. Continuing from the progression of difficulty in (b) above, patients would begin associating various request forms with specified situations and action responses. At this level, some patients will do better imagining other people in these situational contexts, while other patients can relate to their own prior experience to decide what they would say or do. At first, the contexts should be explicit and easily interpretable, such as a verbal description of a woman, visiting a neighbor, who is so cold that she is shivering. Given several options for remedying this situation (e.g., turn up the heat, build a fire, put on a sweater), patients can select or generate direct and indirect requests that the visitor might use (e.g., "Will you turn up the heat"; "Can you get me a sweater"; "I'm freezing.") [As an aside here, clinicians can incorporate everyday problem-solving practice with this kind of activity by asking patients to generate potential solutions to problems posed by the scenarios; for more on problem solving, see section V-G.] Eventually, contextual information can be made more implicit. For example, the visitor could be described as "shivering" without any explicit mention of being cold, or the scene could be set with pictures. To further increase task difficulty, nonessential details can be included in the scenarios.

e. In such scenarios, clinicians can also vary factors that affect request directness, such as the power of the requester, familiarity of requester and requestee, degree of right to make the request, or degree of obligation to comply (see Chapter 2). To target situational appropriateness of indirect forms, patients can be asked to select from several choices a request that is more or less direct, polite, or fitting for a given situation. These judgments can be associated with the factors affecting directness, above. Patients can also practice identifying request modifiers (e.g., "If it's not too much trouble"; or giving reasons for making a request), and associating them with specified contexts and requests.

f. Compensatory strategies again include patients making their intentions explicit and asking others to do the same. Alternatively, patients who do well appreciating one aspect of a situation (e.g., interpreting the contexts or the hints, without associating them well) can be taught to rely mainly on their strong suit, especially when they pair this strategy with one of checking their interpretations with others. As always, others in the environment can initiate or request compensations like these when patients need assistance.

4. Figurative meanings.

a. Treatment for difficulties with figurative meanings more general-ly (e.g., idioms and metaphors) proceeds similarly to that for indi-rect requests and other ambiguities. Initial orientation and discus-sion focus on the multiple potential interpretations for a single statement and on the difference between what the words say and what they mean. Stimuli should include only those that the patient probably knew and used premorbidly. Idioms, which tend to have conventionalized meanings, will generally be more familiar than many metaphors and proverbs, which can be quite abstract and obscure, especially for people with low education or literacy skills. When possible, treatment tasks should build from nonliteral mean-ings that patients currently use or understand.

b. Initially, nonliteral meanings may be better understood in obvious contexts that include an explicit interpretation of the figurative utterance. Using the example, "They are in the same boat," a ver-bal scenario can be presented that describes two people who are in similar, difficult circumstances. At first, these sorts of contexts can be explicit and semantically redundant. Supplied with a set of writ-ten or pictured alternatives (keeping in mind the caveat about the relative plausibility of pictured literal and nonliteral interpreta-tions, see Chapter 2), patients can be asked to provide or select the corresponding figurative utterance, or when given a less explicit context, to choose the appropriate interpretation of the figurative elements. In higher-level activities, patients can contrast literal and figurative meanings, identify discrepancies between presented contexts and either literal or figurative meanings, indicate how they could change the target interpretation so that it would fit the context, and when possible describe situations from their own experience that fit with the figurative interpretation. For lower-level patients, who may more often be literal in interpreting figu-rative utterances, the clinician can initially exclude the literal sense from the alternatives in a recognition task. These patients may also benefit from practice identifying phrases that have both literal and nonliteral interpretations, and selecting both the literal and figura-tive meanings from a recognition set. For most RHD patients, choosing pictured representations for nonliteral utterances will be more difficult than selecting printed or spoken interpretations.

c. Compensations are similar to those that have already been noted. Figurative production and comprehension problems can be mini-mized when speakers use explicit and concrete language, or provide redundant cues to assist with figurative interpretations, and when listeners check and validate their interpretations. Patients or their conversation partners may request these strategies and/or initiate them as warranted.

5. **Sensitivity to listener and environment.**

   a. As noted previously, presupposition involves taking a communication partner's perspective and forming assumptions about what that person already believes or knows to guide one's own contributions. RHD adults' deficits are typically exhibited in conversational and social interactions, in the form of referential or lexical ambiguity, or problems of topic control and conversational repair. Initial discussion and demonstration in a treatment setting can center on the idea that no one's thoughts are transparent and that misunderstandings may arise if the topic or focus of an exchange is not clear. This idea can be demonstrated in barrier tasks or role-play activities, in which the clinician gives insufficient information or uses inexplicit referential devices. Specific situations can vary in the extent of shared knowledge that is made available to, or attributed to, each participant. Prior to each activity, patient and clinician can list or chart together the information that they consider "given" or known by each partner and what each partner is likely to assume. Then they can plan how to make the purpose of the exchange clear. Performance can be videotaped and evaluated, per the sections above on strategy training and roleplaying. When the patient appears to understand the concept of adjusting to a listener, specific problems of presupposition can be targeted in conversational and discourse activities (see section III, below, on discourse and conversation).

   b. A related aspect of listener sensitivity and response involves understanding what the communication partner considers central in the exchange, to avoid inept topic shading and tangential contributions. Suggestions for heightening patients' awareness of the general notion of centrality or importance are presented above (II-B-2-c). In addition, treatment may target the appreciation of centrality in role-played conversations, progressive storytelling exercises, and so forth (for further applications, see sections on discourse and conversation, III-B-1, III-C-5, III-D-3 and -4). Again, videotaped self-monitoring and self-instruction practice are incorporated when possible.

   c. Some recommendations for treating disinhibition and other social interactional problems are found below.

(1) Boake (1991) reviews a number of approaches to social skills training. Videotaped feedback is often a central element, to enhance discrimination and monitoring of targeted behaviors in a variety of activities. Much of the treatment takes place in group contexts. Families are involved early and informed of targeted skills, appropriate responses, and feedback.

(a) One approach follows Ehrlich and Sipes' (1985) model, introduced above (II-A-4-b). Social skills classes are also described, featuring demonstration, explanation, and practice, often in a game setting. In one example, patients are allowed to move their pieces around a game board when they give acceptable responses in a variety of areas (e.g., compliments, social interaction, politeness, criticism, social confrontation). This aspect of training could focus first on recognizing appropriate responses, if generating them was too difficult.

(b) Another approach (Gajar, Schloss, Schloss, & Thompson, 1984) incorporates feedback, provided by clinicians, in the form of lights to signal appropriate and inappropriate responses in discussions and roleplays (but of course, other forms of feedback signals could easily be used). When a feedback light is displayed, patients say why and indicate how they could change their response. If a patient misses an opportunity to comment when a light comes on, another group member can provide a cue or, as necessary, an explanation. Eventually, patients operate their own feedback lights. Other activities, such as written exercises, are also used to enhance patients' appreciation of appropriate conversational contributions.

(c) Several approaches highlight social problem-solving practice, the rationale being that social skills performance depends in part on an ability to recognize situationally acceptable responses. A published, empirically developed program can be used (*Thinking It Through*; Foxx & Bittle, 1989), in which patients practice appropriate responses to common problem situations generated by rehabilitation staff members. Prompts, cue cards, corrective feedback, and coaching are provided as needed and faded systematically. Sohlberg and Mateer (1989a) cite Corey and Sprunk (1987), who pose questions about hypothetical problem situations to work on various aspects of social comprehension. These questions include "What are two good reasons why most people . . .?"; "When is it socially appropriate/inappropriate to . . .?"; "What are two different things that would be good to do (or say) if . . .?"; and "When would it be a good/bad idea to . . .?"

(d) In some cases, behavioral techniques are introduced to extinguish inappropriate contributions and to shape suitable ones. These techniques include systematic ignoring, time out, and verbal correction for inappropriate behaviors, coupled with attentiveness, interest, and praise for desired behaviors. It should be noted here that patients may need direct instruction about acceptable behaviors that can be substituted for undesired ones.

(2) Some other aspects of communicative social skill, and associated treatment activities, have already been discussed (e.g., politeness, in connection with production and response to indirect requests, and with back-channel behaviors that signal involvement and interest). Additional social interactional skills, such as those involved in turn-taking, will be considered in the section on conversation, below.

(3) Potential compensations for impaired social awareness and response include teaching patients to evaluate environmental signals that cue or guide selection of appropriate behavior. Some of these include posted signs, situational formality, facial expressions or body language indicating positive or negative reactions, and other cues signaling desire to continue or end an interaction. Patients who do not process these kinds of cues can be taught that some behaviors (e.g., crude humor, obscenity) are appropriate only in certain situations (e.g., with a good friend and outside the hearing of others), or conversely, that some behaviors should never occur in specified situations. Patients may also benefit from learning to check their appropriateness by asking themselves or other people questions such as "Am I acting acceptably here?" As noted above for emotion and nonverbal behaviors, others can learn to signal patients, preferably subtly, to anticipate and avoid problems or to modify behaviors as necessary.

6. Humor.

a. Humor is particularly difficult to target in treatment, because it is highly individualistic, even in non-brain-damaged people. When a RHD patient exhibits situationally inappropriate humor, social skills training or some other variant of self-monitoring treatment may provide the most fitting avenues for intervention.

b. If a patient is particularly distressed about diminished humor comprehension following a stroke, several treatment approaches are possible, depending on the nature of the deficit. When problems appear to be linked to difficulties interpreting nonverbal cues, treatment can focus on these areas, as described in several of the preceding sections. When problems reflect impaired integration of content across parts of a narrative (see Chapter 2), treatment activities may focus on determining relevance and centrality (II-B-2-c) and eventually thematic coherence (III-B; III-C-5). Patients with such problems might work on associating punchlines with bodies of jokes, or captions with cartoons, by building from areas of strength in other context association activities (see all pragmatic areas reviewed to this point, and general comments on nature and progression of direct treatment in II-A-3, above). Some patients may need to work first on identifying ambiguities, incongruities, or unexpected elements that lead to the component of surprise in humor (see II-B-2, above). Then, through discussion and demonstration, they can move toward identifying, understanding, and eventually describing the ways in which the "surprise" makes sense, in an unexpected way.

c. Spector (1992) outlines treatment techniques that focus on identifying, and explaining dual meanings that can arise from, various linguistic ambiguities, such as those involving emphatic stress, juncture, or meaning. She gives ideas for targeting the two elements of incongruity-based humor: detecting surprise and achieving coherence. Her article also provides suggestions related to finding and applying interpretational strategies for semantic, metalinguistic, and pragmatic aspects of humor comprehension, and an appendix that lists sources of humorous material.

7. Inference.

a. Previously, it was noted that the term "inference" is often used in a rather undifferentiated way in clinical materials and writings. To the extent that inferencing entails gleaning information that is not specifically provided, inferential operations may be involved in interpreting intended meanings in the areas considered above. Various inference processes have also been identified that are central to discourse or conversational comprehension and higher-order problem solving and reasoning. Some treatment suggestions will be provided in each of those areas, in the relevant sections of this chapter. As always, it is important for clinicians to identify the nature and level of breakdown in inferencing processes, as explicitly as possible, in order to focus treatment. It is tempting to assume that many such tasks and processes are related to one another, but we do not yet have sufficient evidence on this assumption. It is not necessarily the case, for example, that treatment targeting low-level, nonverbal inference processes will have an impact on higher-level, language-based inferences or problem solving skills. It will be valuable for clinicians and clinical researchers to begin gathering evidence to test such hypotheses, as well as some of the others reviewed at the end of Chapter 2.

b. With these points in mind, several tasks are listed below that are often suggested for targeting inferencing processes (see also Myers, 1994; Myers & Mackisack, 1990).

   (1) sorting and explaining stimuli by, for example, theme or gist, perceptual or category similarity, category membership.

   (2) demonstrating appreciation, when given verbal or pictured narratives, of a character's motives, an implied outcome, or the story's practical lessons.

   (3) identifying and explaining absurdities that arise from contextual incongruence or inappropriateness.

   (4) appreciating divergencies and alternative meanings.

   (5) recognizing the need for, and eventually drawing, inference revisions from stimuli that support alternate interpretations.

c. As is true of the activities discussed previously in this section on focused pragmatic treatment approaches, most of these tasks require the patient to draw some connection between probable interpretations or judgments and a given context. Contextual factors can range from those that are external, immediate, and concrete, to those that reflect a patient's world knowledge and experience. The challenge of processing contextual cues can be varied along several lines, including modality, perceptual difficulty, number of cues, cue consistency when multiple cues are provided, and salience of the implicit features (related to emphasis, repetition or redundancy, familiarity, color, etc.). Generally, patients are asked to interpret, explain, and/or contrast, in light of their prior experience. If they have difficulty at that level, they can work on associating, organizing, and identifying relationships in the stimulus and contextual material. Stepping back further, patients may work on recognizing and discriminating elements of stimulus and context. As noted several times previously, treatment activities can focus first on that which is familiar and understood, probing and discussing the relationships between some familiar interpretation and its context, and then, when possible, determining the ways in which interpretations can change along with a context. Some patients will need to work first on basic deficits in identifying and understanding the central or relevant aspects of the stimuli to be interpreted, or their associated contexts, as described above (II-B-2-c).

III. DISCOURSE/TEXT LEVEL

A. General Comments

1. The kinds of activities suggested below for discourse and conversation treatment are, as usual, accompanied by ample explanation, demonstration, discussion, and patient self-evaluation. These procedures are intended to facilitate the patient's intellectual awareness of strengths and weaknesses and to set the stage for active self-monitoring, self-instruction, or other compensations to maximize the informativeness, relevance, and appropriateness of the patient's contributions and interpretations. And as emphasized previously, practice in contexts with decreasing amounts of clinician input and increasing amounts of ecological validity (e.g., referential communication tasks, group settings, and structured conversational exchanges) can be important for solidifying patients' monitoring and compensation skills.

2. A number of variables can be manipulated in an attempt to influence performance on discourse and conversational treatment tasks. Some of these are listed in Table 7–2.

3. As always, clinicians must remain alert to the possible contributions of other basic problems to discourse level impairments, including deficits of strategic attentional control or working memory. For example, Davis (1993) notes that selective attention difficulties may interfere with various aspects of discourse comprehension (e.g., drawing inferences, determining antecedents, maintaining coherence more generally) if critical information is not selected and highlighted in a working memory system. Similarly, limitations of working memory capacity or efficiency may cause the premature displacement or de-emphasis of information that is crucial for building an integrat-

Table 7–2. Some potentially influential variables for discourse tasks.

Participant Factors

Patient's comfort and familiarity with the topic, communication partner, and discourse genre (e.g., storytelling vs. exposition vs. open-ended conversation)

Partner's sophistication as an interactant

Extent of partners' shared topic knowledge, along with the patient's awareness of that shared knowledge

Stimulus Factors

Degree of explicitness and inferential demands

Redundancy, internal consistency, or predictability of the stimulus context

Conventionality of stimulus format

Probability and salience of the information

Procedural Factors

Sufficiency of orienting tasks and instructions

Nature of the tasks themselves (e.g., story retelling or summarization tasks can circumvent inadequate visual perception/inferencing)

Number, types of components or skills targeted in a single task

Number, nature of cues or prompts provided to guide performance.

Cues and prompts can vary from the minimal orienting information that is implied by titles, themes, or brief previews to more extensive, and possibly tangible aids such as outlines of essential questions to help patients organize or glean macrostructure (e.g., What is the setting for the story or message of interest? Who is the central character? What is the most important event that occurs? Is there a complication or problem? How does everything turn out? Is there a lesson to be learned?)

---

ed interpretation. Chapter 4 (section III-C-1) describes a potential influence of perceptual impairments on discourse processing. And some other difficulties noted earlier in this chapter, such as problems dealing with ambiguities or other intended meanings, or determining what is important or central (see section II-B-2, above), may also affect discourse level performance.

4. Analyses based on models of discourse processes (see Table 4–5 and accompanying text in Chapter 4, sections III-C-2-g and III-C-3-e) can help reveal strengths and weaknesses and the nature of breakdown that may contribute to observed discourse production and comprehension performance.

   a. Treatment tasks to target various levels of processing that are highlighted in one recent discourse model (Frederiksen et al., 1990) can be derived from the assessment suggestions in Table 4–5. It was noted in Chapter 4 that, even though the model focuses on discourse production, identical or similar tasks can be designed to target comprehension processes and problems.

b. Some examples will be provided here for the conceptual network level of that model, following Table 4–5. In all cases, the stimulus elements can be conveyed linguistically or through pictures. Treatment ideas for impairments at other levels of the model can be generated similarly from the entries in the table and the explanatory text in Chapter 4.

(1) Difficulties retrieving conceptual organizing principles can be targeted in tasks that require patients to group together under designated headings (e.g., main characters; first events that happen to those characters) the elements that make up different discourse frames. Patients can also be asked to unscramble ill-sequenced sets of discourse elements or to identify gaps in incomplete stories or procedure descriptions. For some such tasks, the elements can be narrative episode components: a setting and its subparts of initiating event, main character, and such; a development or complication; a resolution; and perhaps an optional abstract, evaluation, and end signal (see Tables 4–5 and 4–8). For other tasks and purposes, the elements could be the steps involved in scripted situations or procedures that vary in familiarity or complexity, or the salient aspects of a media report, perhaps organized around a WH-question framework.

(2) Problems elaborating or interpreting conceptual discourse frames can be targeted with tasks that involve selecting or sorting, from information provided by the clinician, that which is essential (core), optional, redundant, irrelevant or unrelated, or out-of-sequence, in relation to different themes, titles, or gists (see also suggestions in II-B-2-c, above, for targeting main ideas). Patients who can identify nonessential and unrelated components can also be asked to make appropriate adjustments in recognition, generation, or explanation tasks.

(3) Impairments in selecting and prioritizing the information to convey explicitly, or to focus on in comprehension, can be targeted in activities such as asking patients to identify elements or propositions that are essential for different listeners, themes, or communication purposes (per II-C-5, above); to identify and list or represent graphically their presuppositions about what a particular type of communication partner knows, needs to know, or considers central (also II-C-5); or to recognize and explain differences between surface and intended meanings, or various communicative intentions and purposes (see II-B and II-C, above).

(4) For each of these kinds of tasks, clinicians can assess the effects of varying the specified goals or purposes of the discourse (e.g., to summarize, to introduce a new or unfamiliar idea or experience, to report events, to explain in depth) and the nature of cues or structure provided to guide performance.

B. Discourse Production

1. Some RHD adults have difficulty conveying essential information in a relevant, efficient, and/or socially appropriate way. As noted immediately above (III-A-4), hypotheses about individual skills and deficits can be developed in part with reference to current discourse models, and specific treatment tasks can be designed accordingly. A number of potential tasks to target informativeness, relevance, and efficiency of contributions are provided in Table 4–5. Other tasks to tackle these skills can focus as needed on discourse cohesion and coherence, which did not receive much attention in Chapter 4. Thus, the sections below provide some suggestions. The material presented below is also pertinent to several components of an "appropriateness" dimension, specifically those that are concerned with textual relevance and presupposition. Treatment suggestions for broader aspects of situational appropriateness were considered previously (II-C-5-c).

   a. Cohesion analyses examine lexical and grammatical links between words in a text (see, e.g., Armstrong, 1991). The main lexical relationships include reiteration (through repetition, synonymy, or superordinate/general reference) and collocation (associations conveyed through synonyms, antonyms, and cause/effect relations). The primary kinds of grammatical cohesive devices include reference (achieved with pronouns, definite articles, demonstratives, and comparatives), substitution of words or phrases for other words or phrases, conjunction, and ellipsis (i.e., an already-mentioned element is left out when it can be implied by reference. For example, ellipsis occurs in the reply, "Sally did" to the question "Who made the fudge?").

      (1) Some patients will benefit from self-monitoring regimens that focus on their typical cohesion errors. These may include unclear or otherwise incorrect references, inadequate lexical reiteration (as when an idea or event is reintroduced after quite a bit of time or intervening material), or other vague/indefinite terms.

(2) Referential ambiguity can be targeted like other cases of ambiguity (see sections II-B-2-a, and more generally, II-C). Clinicians can demonstrate in a variety of ways the general idea that the same word or phrase can refer to more than one thing. Working from spoken, written, or pictured narratives, patients might be asked to choose all possible referents for various personal and demonstrative pronouns. Patients can also practice identifying referential ambiguity in the context of barrier activities, in which the clinician's contributions are purposely inexplicit. Written or recorded speech samples that contain a patient's typical errors can be presented as well for recognition and correction, and the consequences of these errors for listeners can be discussed (see II-B-2-d, above). Suggestions for helping patients appreciate the general idea of adjusting to listeners' knowledge and expectations were previously provided in section II-C-5, and some of those ideas would be appropriate here.

(3) Through discussion and demonstration, as in the barrier activity mentioned above, patients can be tuned into the points at which referent activation or specification tends to be important. These might include the original introduction of topics or characters that are not obvious from the context, or the reintroduction of some referent that recurs after a large amount of intervening material. Patients can also work on specifying explicitly the main idea, event, or character at the beginning of a narrative production or after any change in focus (see II-B-2-c, above, for suggestions related to identifying important or central points).

(4) Patients who overuse exact repetition in repeated references to the same person, object, or event, can work on identifying and eventually generating appropriate synonyms, superordinate terms (e.g., "his pet" for "his dog"), or ellipses.

(5) Materials for all such tasks can be designed to minimize referential confusion at first. For example, they can include only one character or central event, or two characters that can be unambiguously identified through pronoun reference, such as a male and a female, or a human and a non-human character.

b. Coherence reflects the topical or thematic continuity of discourse units. As noted in Table 2–2, coherence can be realized locally or globally, and it can be established overtly from elements in the text, or covertly through stored knowledge and inference.

(1) Mentis and Prutting (1991) emphasize the importance of topic introduction and maintenance parameters in establishing coherence, and describe a reliable system for observing and coding these parameters (see Table 7–3). In their coherence analysis for RHD adults, Joanette and Goulet (1990) focused on a subset of the parameters in Table 7–3. Specifically, they were concerned with identifying patients' problems contributing new information that does not contradict, and is clearly related to, that which has come before.

(2) Problems in many aspects of topic management (e.g., ambiguous topic introduction; noncoherent topic changes;

Table 7–3. Parameters of topic coherence analysis.

Topic/Subtopic Introduction

Type of introduction: new, related/unrelated, reintroduced

Manner of introduction: shifts to related topics, topic changes, noncoherent changes (i.e., without obvious termination or transition cue)

Topic/Subtopic Maintenance

Categories of ideational units (propositional contributions)

1. New information units: requests for novel information, provides requested information, unsolicited novel information
2. No new information: agreement/acknowledgment, clarification requests, provides requested information, repeats old information, confirmation requests, passes, clarification statement, summary statement
3. Side sequences (insertions that do not contribute to topic maintenance or development, but do not constitute an independent topic or topic sequence): for example, environmentally triggered, politeness markers, word search
4. Problematic contributions: ambiguous, unrelated, or incomplete.

Note:

Topic = "a clause or noun phrase that identified the question of immediate concern and that provided a global description of the content of a sequence of utterances" (p. 585).

Topic Sequence = sequence of utterances described by any single topic label (e.g., "Halloween"; "watching a basketball game")

Subtopics = elaborations/expansions of some dimension of a topic; contain increasingly specific instances or descriptions of topic information.

Source: After Mentis, M., & Prutting, C. (1991). Analysis of topic as illustrated in a head-injured and normal adult. *Journal of Speech and Hearing Research, 34,* 583–595. Used with permission.

utterances that presuppose too much; unrelated, contradictory, tangential, or rambling contributions) can be targeted with self-monitoring activities, accompanied as necessary by more focused tasks to sensitize patients to the nature, occurrence, and consequences of these kinds of problems (e.g., see II-B-2 for ambiguity; II-C-5 for difficulties of presupposition/listener adjustment; II-B-2 for determining what is central and salient; and III-B-1-a for application to problems of cohesion).

(3) To highlight the idea of "new information," patients can be provided with concurrent or sequential stimuli and asked to indicate when some portion of the second is novel, as opposed to repeated; they can practice discriminating or identifying what is new or adding some novel feature of their own; or they can monitor a clinician's contributions for redundancy or repetition. To concretize the concept of noncontradiction, patients can identify, explain, and possibly correct elements that are incongruous. This can be done within a given stimulus story or picture or between some specified situation (e.g., a person is planning to go to the beach to swim) and an associated stimulus (e.g., a list of his preparations, presented to the patient, includes a step in which he puts on a tuxedo). Such incongruities can be designed to contradict world knowledge, as in the tuxedo example, or to clash with something specified earlier in a stimulus itself (e.g., a character's name, occupation, or stated goal). Activities of this sort can be extracted from a discourse context as necessary to familiarize patients with the relevant concepts, beginning with concrete, simple stimuli such as lists of words, sequences of tones or pictures, series of sentences, or exemplars of familiar categories, and moving from blatant to more subtle contradictions.

(4) When treatment turns to the discourse level, clinicians can introduce devices that may be used to contrast new information with that which is presupposed or given. A general rule is that new information, presumed not to be part of a listener's activated memory, needs to be highlighted rather explicitly, using markers like proper names and other specific lexical labels, contrastive stress, or syntactic clefting (e.g., "It was Mary who made the fudge" places Mary in the focused, new information role). These kinds of markers tend to occur most often upon first mention of a concept; when two competing referents cannot be distinguished in other ways (e.g.,

two characters are of same gender); at points in discourse where there has been a change in character, setting, or topic; or after lengthy intervening material that may have moved the initial referent out of activated memory. Common markers of givenness include pronominalization, ellipsis, and ordinary (noncontrastive) stress, which tend to be used when a referent or topic is presumed already in focus, and has not been interfered with or changed. Definite article use tends to be associated with presupposition, as well, but non-brain-damaged adults often do not use this marker unambiguously, and the connection between presupposition and definite article use is not transparent or easy to capture in a rule. For example, definite articles can be used with nouns that have not been previously specified linguistically or deictically when they refer to concepts that are part of cultural knowledge (e.g., "He joined the army"; "I love the Beatles"); generic concepts (e.g., "The koala lives in Australia"); first-mention referents that are unique in some immediate situation (e.g., "The kitchen in his house was just renovated"); or items associated with a concept in focus (e.g., once "the car" is specified, "the" can be used to describe its steering wheel, engine, etc.).

(5) For patients who have difficulty determining relatedness, clinicians can also try tasks extracted from a discourse context, such as identifying stimuli that represent specific kinds of associations (e.g., categorical, perceptual, or grammatical similarities; causal links), judging or describing the nature of relationships between stimulus items, and/or explaining why certain stimuli are not related. At the discourse level, tasks for appreciating relatedness can focus on recognizing and establishing lexical or grammatical cohesive ties (as immediately above), identifying information that is more or less essential in the context (II-B-2-c, above), and representing graphically the relations between text elements, as suggested next.

(6) A diagram or some other graphic representation may be useful for exemplifying some of the notions related to achieving and maintaining coherence. For instance, to signal centrality, an index card identifying the currently active topic or character in evolving discourse can be placed inside a large circle or atop a tree structure (either of which might be conceptualized as a working memory buffer, e.g., Chapter 2, III-B-3-d, III-E). Additional contributions can be arranged inside or outside the circle, or on other branches of the tree, to represent their relevance to the concept in focus. Depending on their relationship to the central topic, changes of focus can be represented in circles or branches that are connected to or separate from the original center. Divergence from the original, center can provide a focal point for discussing problems of tangentiality, unannounced or unconnected topic switches, and so forth. Representations of this sort can also be used to illustrate the problems of determining how to fit ostensibly discrepant, ambiguous, or otherwise vague contributions into an ongoing discussion.

(7) Some suggestions are provided in the conversation section (III-D, below) for targeting topic manipulation deficits that tend to be observed in RHD adults. A few possible activities for working on topic control at a structured discourse level, in an individual or group context, are listed immediately below. Graphic representations, such as those just described, can be useful supplements to any such tasks.

(a) identifying the main points of a media report, such as a newspaper or magazine article, or an extended documentary; isolating the utterances that introduce each topic or theme; indicating what information is central to a theme, and why; identifying what information can be left out without changing the main points or take home message.

(b) constructing a collaborative story on a specified theme or topic, with each participant providing a new but related contribution as the story advances. Efficiency can be promoted in several ways, such as reviewing the final product to pinpoint less-than-essential information and reconstructing the story to exclude some of it; or specifying, and gradually reducing, the maximum number of contributions allowed for developing and concluding the story. To constrain further the number and kind of possible relevant contributions, patients can be asked to generate a story when given both a beginning and an end.

(c) identifying and revising deviations from a topic or theme, unrelated utterances, and ambiguities, whether they originate from patients' contributions or are injected purposely by the clinician.

        (d) maintaining continuity for describing a process, pro-
        viding a set of directions, or retelling a personal expe-
        rience or news event, when hampered by distractions
        or interruptions.

2. As always, patients may profit from compensatory strategies
designed to maximize their discourse production performance.
Considering the range of potential deficits, and the variability in
types of cuing and structure that are most beneficial for individual
patients, such compensations can be extremely diverse. Some general tactics include cue cards, tailored graphic representations, or
specific reminders from other people to minimize cohesion or
coherence errors; or outlines of essential elements to include when
recounting an experience, an observation, or a set of instructions.
Self- or other-prompted reminders can also be introduced as compensatory rules, as needed (e.g., "Always introduce the topic or the
person that you are going to talk about"; "Ask yourself: 'Is my listener tuned in to what I am about to say'?"). Possible compensations related to social appropriateness were mentioned previously
(section II-C-5).

C. Discourse Comprehension

1. Treatment aimed at improving particular aspects of discourse comprehension can use a variety of auditory or written materials,
including narratives, expository passages of special interest, news
accounts, and everyday stimuli such as telephone messages or
instructions (e.g., for getting to a specified location, for assembling
something, for carrying out a new activity). Performance can be
charted through tasks involving recognition, question-answering,
free or cued recall, or paraphrase and interpretation, with the
caveat that, in some of these formats, formulation or production
difficulties may mask adequate comprehension. A number of performance measures, that can be tailored according to an individual
patient's difficulties, are noted in Chapter 4 (section III-C-3).

2. One of the discourse comprehension deficits that is often mentioned
in connection with RHD in adults is a difficulty synthesizing interpretations or stored knowledge with stimulus contexts (see Chapter
2). Such a deficit may be manifest in, for example, problems resolving apparent ambiguities or discrepancies, discarding or revising
contextually inappropriate or irrelevant interpretations, and generating or evaluating presuppositions or attributions of speaker intent.
These kinds of problems tend to be most pronounced when the stim-

ulus elements, the situational context, and/or world knowledge and plausibility judgment promote or allow competing interpretations. For example, many types of nonliteral interpretations depend on resolving an ostensible conflict between an utterance's surface form and features of the existing context. The Pragmatics section of this chapter (section II) deals extensively with treatment ideas for these kinds of problems, including suggestions for working with stimuli and contexts that at first glance seem incompatible (see also III-6-e on inference revision, below). In a related vein, the Memory section (V-E-4-b) includes some ideas for targeting difficulties that arise when different sources of information compete to determine a response.

3. As noted previously, Table 4–5 and its accompanying text (Chapter 4) also provide some suggestions for assessing discourse performance, which can be translated to treatment activities that correspond to the presumed nature of comprehension breakdown (e.g., in conceptual or propositional processing; see also discussion in III-B, Discourse Production, above).

4. Though some work suggests that they are not particularly prevalent for RHD adults, problems that arise in appreciating cohesive markers can be targeted using tasks similar to those mentioned in the discourse production section, above (III-B). For instance, if patients have difficulty appreciating that cohesive devices signal specific relationships or linkages, they may benefit from practice in locating potential connections among instances of the same concept, such as referents for personal or demonstrative pronouns, superordinate terms, synonyms, and/or elliptical expressions in a stimulus passage. Patients who have difficulty determining the links between referring expressions and their intended referents can designate all references that are made to one particular text element (e.g., person, concept). Or they can practice identifying (or answering questions about) which of several possible referents is most likely, given world knowledge and the current discourse context; or generating possible referents when presented with referring expressions in isolation (e.g., superordinate terms; specific pronouns). For problems with referential ambiguity, patients can locate referring expressions that are inaccurate, vague, or otherwise unclear, and resolve them, again by choosing the most appropriate referent for a particular context or interpretation. As noted above, stimuli for tasks such as these can be developed to maximize referential clarity at first. Barrier tasks also provide an excellent context for patients to practice recognizing, and requesting repair of, a clinician's intentionally vague or inaccurate references.

5. Difficulties with generating coherent interpretations tend to be more frequent and troublesome for RHD patients. Again, some potential treatment ideas are provided in the preceding sections on discourse production.

   a. In general, patients can be assisted in identifying and appreciating main ideas or salient information, as well as recognizing cues that can signal continuity, or a need to shift interpretational gears. As noted previously, diagrams or charts that represent visually the various topics or other elements in a text, making it apparent what is currently in focus, may be useful for discussing and exemplifying the continuity that leads to coherent interpretations (see also III-B-1-b, above).

   b. Numerous suggestions are presented in this chapter for working on distinguishing central information that forms the focus of a discourse stimulus, from that which is less essential, or that which is clearly irrelevant (II-B-2-c, III-A-4, III-B-1 above, and III-D-3 and -4, below). Patients can also be introduced to specific kinds of cues that help to establish the relationship between the active topic and a further contribution. For example, they can be tuned into the notion of "new" information and can practice identifying it in discourse stimuli, designating the various markers that distinguish it from that which is presupposed, and establishing the ways in which a "new" contribution is connected to that which had been communicated previously (III-B-1-b). Similarly, they can be alerted to, and practice identifying, markers that might indicate topic shifts, or that can signify contradiction or intentional discrepancy (e.g., cue phrases like "but" and "however"). Finally, several sections that focus on topic manipulation difficulties (III-B-1-b, above and III-D, below) provide other ideas that would lend themselves to comprehension tasks targeting coherent interpretation.

6. Inference processes are considered separately here, because they can be crucial for coherent interpretations, and because they are accorded a central place in some thinking about RHD adults' comprehension deficits.

   a. Inferencing takes place at various levels, to various degrees, and for various purposes. For example, as noted in Chapter 4 (section III-C-3-f), McKoon and Ratcliff (1992) argue that normal comprehenders are likely to draw some inferences quickly and automatically, while other inferences may be generated only when there are special comprehension goals or strategies (e.g., to learn something new from a text; to glean the three main points of the text; to generate a moral or consequence; to explain the material to someone who is unfamiliar with it; to evaluate the evidence presented in support of certain premises; or to memorize what one predicts an instructor might ask on the next exam). Based largely on this theoretical position, the material below highlights some factors that may affect the likelihood, ease, or strength of inferencing when they are manipulated in treatment tasks, and provides some other general treatment ideas.

b. According to McKoon and Ratcliff, inferences that are likely to be drawn routinely and automatically are those that establish local coherence between propositions (those for approximately one to three sentences that can be represented concurrently in a working memory buffer) and those based on information that is easily available, whether from a text or from general knowledge. Thus, inferences likely to be generated automatically by normal readers of a text include those that link anaphora with nearby antecedents (e.g., connections among instances of the same concept or pronominal reference); those based on propositional argument overlap (that, as such, reflect information that is in focus, or in the foreground of a working memory buffer); and perhaps those that specify local causal relations for propositions that are concurrently in working memory. General knowledge inferences, such as those that predict what should happen next or that generate instances of categories, are most likely to be drawn without special strategies only if they are highly typical or very predictable (e.g., parts of overlearned scripts, familiar schemas, or expert knowledge) and thus based on information that is well-known and easily available to the comprehender.

c. Strategic inferences include most any other kind, such as expectations that are inferred from less typical or predictable events or attributes, inferences that connect global goals to outcomes or consequences, and more generally, those that do not meet the conditions that support automatic inferences. Strategic inferences are clearly important, as they are often necessary for a complete interpretation of text, and they are integral more generally to learning, problem solving, and decision making.

d. McKoon and Ratcliff specify that quick, automatically generated inferences provide the foundation from which slower, more purposeful inferences are constructed. Thus, an appropriate goal for some patients might be to increase the speed and accuracy of the automatic inferences they draw, in an attempt to solidify the knowledge base that is available to strategic inference processes. In addition, accomplishing this goal may result in freeing some mental resources that could be applied profitably for generating goal-directed inferencing and for reconciling any apparent discrepancies that may arise. [Although strictly automatic inference processes would require few mental resources for normal comprehenders, it is probable that for brain damaged patients, these types of inferences may be generated more slowly and effortfully than is usual, even if they are relatively accurate.]

(1) To influence "automatic" inferencing, treatment stimuli could be designed to maximize the probability that inference-relevant information is easily available to the comprehender. One way to do this is to construct stimulus materials that aim to keep key inference-supporting elements together in an active working memory system (e.g., decrease the distance or amount of intervening material between elements to be linked inferentially; foreground inference-relevant concepts through emphasis, repetition, continued reference, etc. to keep them in focus). In addition, or alternatively, automatic inferencing can probably be enhanced by increasing the opportunity for general knowledge to assist in interpretation (e.g., basing inferences on overlearned, predictable, or highly familiar scripts, schemas, concepts, or expert knowledge domains; providing themes or titles prior to presenting stimulus materials).

(2) Providing extensive practice and repetition with the following kinds of activities may be appropriate to solidify automatic inference processes (see also Chapter 6, II-B-3 and II-E-2-a).

    (a) work on identifying and reconciling local linkages, such as those described above for cohesion/local coherence;

    (b) practice using available knowledge, initially in overlearned or familiar domains, to identify, sort, or generate highly predictable consequences of events or actions, typical features of certain situations or categories, and so forth;

    (c) focus on determining local causal relatedness, mapping out graphically how some character or event X leads to Y. Pertinent tasks might require patients to select, rearrange, or generate propositions or events according to causal connections, or to determine whether and how Y could occur without X.

e. For other patients, strategic inferences can be targeted, either concurrently with automatic inferencing, or alone. If automatic inferences are slow or inconsistent, stimuli for strategic inference tasks can be designed to minimize the demands for automatic inferences, by making local coherence links fairly explicit, and/or by mapping them out with the patient in a separate step, before working on strategic inferencing.

(1) Generally, strategic inferences may be enhanced by helping patients to choose, arrange, recall, and/or relate the key elements, propositions, or contextual features needed to generate them. Gradually, patients can be increasingly challenged through task modifications that decrease the proximity of inference supporting elements, in terms of physical distance or number of intervening propositions or first-mention nouns; that reduce predictability, typicality, or plausibility of inferences; that lessen the degree of redundancy or consistency in the text; or that shift away from subjects' special interests or expertise. Patients can also practice making strategic inferences from several perspectives (e.g., the home buyer vs. burglar example from Chapter 4; or from the point-of-view of each of two characters in a narrative) or for different reasons (e.g., to summarize, explain why something occurred, etc).

(2) For many RHD adults, the greatest difficulty may be posed when ostensible discrepancies must be re-evaluated or reconceptualized. If need be, treatment can start with activities in which obvious contradictions are built into a single stimulus, such as the text itself (see also II-B-2, and III-B-1-b, above), and can progress to those in which discrepancies are only apparent, and can be reconciled by consulting world knowledge or other elements of the stimulus context and situation. A number of relevant treatment ideas have already been presented in the Pragmatics section, above. In many cases, RHD patients can, and will, generate plausible connections that could bridge a gap between competing interpretations, but that are not obviously connected with the text and situation. If so, the challenge is to work on linking what patients have inferred with what the text, or world knowledge, implies. As suggested earlier, work on such tasks can

begin with relatively explicit and easily interpretable stimuli and contexts, that capitalize on a patient's special knowledge, interests, or expertise. Potential activities include:

- constructing outlines or diagrams of the various possibilities suggested by the "discrepant" information;

- distinguishing what is plausible and less likely in a specified situation, and if possible, justifying the choices;

- constructing graphic representations of what is possible, or plausible, in a specified situation without any reference to the stimulus itself; and then comparing them to representations of crucial parts of the stimulus, and of the patient's initial interpretation.

7. Again, potential compensatory strategies for discourse comprehension difficulties are many and varied.

   a. Patient strategies can include initiating input controls, such as asking or otherwise signaling someone to speak more slowly, to allow more time for figuring something out, to wait to give more information until the patient is ready for it, to be explicit about their intention or main point, and/or to use a different modality or format to convey their message. Patients can also ask for background information about unfamiliar topics or contexts; consult organizational guides, such as cue cards, outlines, or other graphic representations, to assist with interpretations; and check their comprehension with the original message source, whether a person, a recording, or a written passage, to verify their interpretations or reasoning. As always, self-monitoring and self-instruction may be beneficial as well (e.g. "What do I know about A, and its relationship to B?"; "Do I get the point?").

   b. Strategies implemented by others might include prompting patients to use relevant compensatory techniques; providing structure and cues such as those mentioned above, without being asked; or signaling comprehension breakdowns, indicating where patients went awry, and helping them recover by modifying or representing the input in facilitating ways.

D. Conversation

1. Many of the skills highlighted in the discourse sections above, such as resolving reference and ambiguity or planning contributions with

an awareness of a partner's knowledge, play a large part in conversational competence. But successful conversational interaction also hinges on cooperative topic management and dynamic turn-taking and repair skills. Ideas for treatment in these areas, many of which were adapted from the comprehensive suggestions of Brinton and Fujiki (1989), follow in this section. In general, patients can be oriented to the nature and consequences of their conversational difficulties, with a goal of improving self-monitoring and self-repair, as described earlier in this chapter (I-D-2; II-B-2-d). As always, particular approaches and target behaviors should be selected on the basis of assessment results, in light of a patient's strengths, weaknesses, and communication needs.

2. In some cases, treatment may be aimed at improving the mechanics of topic control. Patients who launch into an interaction without securing a listener's attention can be tuned into the benefits of doing so and supplied with some appropriate strategies, such as calling the listener's name or providing an introductory phrase (e.g., "That reminds me" or "I heard something surprising today"). Patients who do not make their topic clear can be taught to orient the listener explicitly, perhaps by giving openers, somewhat like the title of a story. A classic example like the Bransford and Johnson (1973) paragraph (see Table 7–4), presented first without any topic information, and then with a topic cue, may help to underscore the utility of establishing topics.

Table 7–4. Passage illustrating comprehension benefits of topic knowledge.

"The procedure is actually quite simple. First you arrange things into different groups. Of course, one pile may be sufficient depending on how much there is to do. If you have to go somewhere else due to lack of facilities that is the next step, otherwise you are pretty well set. It is important not to overdo things. That is, it is better to do too few things at once than too many. In the short run this may not seem important but complications can easily arise. A mistake can be expensive as well. At first the whole procedure will seem complicated. Soon, however, it will become just another facet of life. It is difficult to foresee any end to the necessity for this task in the immediate future, but then one can never tell. After the procedure is completed, one arranges the materials into different groups again. Then they can be put into their appropriate places. Eventually they will be used once more and the whole cycle will then have to be repeated. However, that is part of life." (p. 400)

Topic: Washing Clothes

Source: Bransford, J. D., & Johnson, M. K. (1973). Considerations of some problems of comprehension. In W. G. Chase (Ed.), *Visual Information Processing.* Copyright © 1973 by Academic Press. Reprinted with permission of publisher and author Bransford.

3. A number of tactics can be used to work on problems of presupposition and listener adjustment (see also II-C-5 and III-A-4, above), some of which are related to topic management. For example, patients can be taught to establish or verify a shared knowledge base routinely by introducing referents and background information about people or events to be discussed or by checking the listener's familiarity with this background. The importance of doing so can be highlighted in barrier tasks where ambiguity is intentionally incorporated, or in graphic representations, as noted earlier. Other suggestions for enhancing conversational sensitivity follow (and some elements of turn-taking allocation, section III-D-6, are relevant as well to developing an increased sensitivity to listener and situation).

   a. Improve control over the amount/efficiency and relevance of contributions (see also III-B-1-b above, and III-D-3 and -4, below). Windy or rambling explanations can be targeted generally with identification activities, discussion and demonstration of consequences, self-monitoring practice, and corrective feedback as needed. Focused treatment activities to promote conciseness can include asking patients to figure out how someone could say the same thing in fewer words or sentences (see also II-B-2-c regarding main ideas). Patients can also practice limiting their output to a restricted time frame or number of words, perhaps starting with the requirement to give specific, single word or phrase-length responses to questions, and then progressively allowing more latitude.

   b. Decrease socially and situationally inappropriate topics or contributions. Treatment involves establishing awareness (II-B-2-d), providing feedback, and encouraging self-monitoring (I-D-2). Patient and clinician can discuss why some topics are inappropriate (e.g., they are embarrassing, or exclusive of others) and can reflect on the effects on a partner and on an interaction. (See also II-C-5 re: sensitivity to listener and situation).

   c. Balance self- versus other-oriented topics and contributions. Conversational egocentricity can be tackled similarly, by achieving awareness and practicing monitoring skills (see II-B-2-d and I-D-2).

   d. Work on relinquishing topics or turns, or ending conversations appropriately. Treatment can involve heightening awareness of signals that may be used by others to indicate their readiness to take a turn (see III-D-6 below), to establish a new topic, or to end an encounter. For example, patients can observe videotapes or roleplays to identify common termination moves, such as indicating that one needs to be going, providing a reason for wrapping up an interaction, expressing pleasure in the time spent with the other person, wishing the other person well, planning a future meeting, making motions to gather things and leave, and/or starting another activity.

e. Decrease disruptive topic shading. Brinton and Fujiki (1989) suggest that topic shading can best be managed by improving topic maintenance (see section III-D-4, next).

4. Several activities to enhance topic maintenance were described earlier in section III-B-1-b. Some other suggestions include the following.

a. Patients can practice evaluating topic maintenance patterns, given various partners and purposes for interaction. They can identify who set the initial conversational agenda, and select the "main points" or topics during the interaction, the points at which topics changed, the speaker who initiated a shift, whether the shift was signaled or unannounced, whether the other partner was finished with the prior topic, how the other partner responded to the topic change, and/or the general appropriateness of the shift in light of partner, setting, and communication goals. Initially such activities may make reference to prepared scripts and clinician role-plays; later, it may be possible to work from recordings or transcripts of a patient's own interactions.

b. It can be appropriate as well for patients to practice recognizing, and adjusting as necessary, central versus tangential contributions in these kinds of stimuli. Further activities to promote understanding of the notion of centrality or relevance might involve classification, similarity judgment, or association tasks, among others (see also II-B-2-c). Patients can similarly monitor for, and practice repairing, uninformative contributions.

c. Patient and/or clinician can also review the topic periodically by referring to a cue card, some other graphic representation, or any meaningful reminder that the patient selects. Contributions can be monitored by asking, and having the patient explain, "What does that comment have to do with topic X"? A tangible record (written, taped) can be used to help backtrack and re-establish the focus of an interaction. If needed initially for practice of this sort, clinicians can purposely introduce blatant topic shifts.

d.   Patient and clinician, or patients in a group setting, can take turns following each others' lead in topic selection for a specified period of time or number of utterances. Violations, whether intentionally clinician-generated or naturally occurring, should be signaled and repaired. Again, it may be useful for patients to refer to a record of the prior exchange to get back on track.

e.   Patients who can identify topic switches may be able to learn to provide explicit indicators or transitions to mark them.

5.   Some of the suggestions above focus on the intersection of topic maintenance and conversational repair. Some other ideas aimed at enhancing repair skills include:

a.   Work on identifying and responding to requests for clarification. These can include requests signaled more or less explicitly by listeners through verbalizations (e.g., "What?" or "I'm not sure who you are talking about"), facial expressions, intonation patterns, or combinations of these markers. Identification and monitoring activities can follow those suggested previously (I-D-2; II-B-2-d). In addition, patients can practice identifying a variety of sources of communication breakdown, and generating specifically focused adjustments (e.g., reiterating their utterance for someone whose attention has wandered, repeating themselves a bit louder if they were not heard, elaborating or providing background information to establish the relevance of a contribution, explaining to clear up any other form of ambiguity, or defining a crucial term). When the trouble source is not apparent from a listener's clarification request (e.g., "What?" or "Huh?"), some patients may be able to learn to ask the listener what the problem is, specifically. Otherwise, in such circumstances, patients can try applying a strategy that would be appropriate for repairing their most typical source of difficulty.

b.   Enhance self-repair in patients with emergent or anticipatory awareness who can recognize or foresee a potential trouble source. Depending on their particular strengths and weaknesses, patients might practice, for example, adjusting content to be more informative, or making additions to specify or modify. Along with some of the repairs mentioned above, patients could learn to check a listener's comprehension to establish the need for an adjustment ("Is that clear?") or to comment on their own intention to repair ("Wait, that's not making much sense; let me try again").

6. The allocation and regulation of turns can also be a target for intervention.

   a. Referential communication, PACE-type, and progressive or collaborative group discourse or planning tasks (e.g., story generation; deciding what to do to organize and give a party; other everyday problem-solving activities) have already been emphasized as contexts to foster turn exchange. It may also be beneficial to structure games to rely on turn-taking, with a goal of enhancing the salience of other participants' contributions. Games like Password, 20 questions, Charades, or "guess a hidden object" can be modified in several ways to approach this goal. For example, they can be designed so that each member of a team must ask one question or give one clue before any other member can participate a second time. Another game-like activity involves obtaining specific information from someone else, using lists of questions or topics, with the stipulation that the questioner cannot move ahead until he or she has a clear answer to each preceding question.

   b. Turn overlap or other interruptions, and excessively long turns, can be targeted for reduction using identification activities, demonstration and discussion of their consequences, self-monitoring practice, and corrective feedback where needed. Structured devices like intercoms or walkie-talkies, or disruptions intentionally introduced by the clinician into interactive tasks, may help to make turn-taking problems concrete and identifiable.

   c. Patients may also need assistance in responding appropriately to, or producing, turn-taking signals. Patients and clinicians can review the cues that may be used to signal a desire to speak, such as taking a deep breath, producing a transitional comment, (e.g., "That reminds me"), initiating a gesture, and/or shifting eye gaze away from the communication partner. Simultaneous speaking (interrupting) can also indicate the desire to take a speaking turn, especially when used by communication partners of a patient who does not respond to other kinds of signals. As needed, patients can also work on identifying some of the cues that may signal a speaker's intent to maintain or to yield the floor. When a speaker is ready to relinquish a turn, these indicators might include lengthy pauses, a decline in pitch or loudness, completion of a hand gesticulation, and establishment of eye contact with a listener. Conversely, an averted gaze and continuous speech without much pausing tend to signal a desire to maintain a speaking turn. Some patients may need to be reminded, as well, that even when a current speaker has yielded the floor, a speaking turn may not be available to them. The speaker relinquishing a turn may direct a request to another listener, either explicitly or implicitly (e.g., the response to a particular question requires the knowledge or expertise of one specific person). In initial activities, clinicians can interject turn-taking signals that vary in number and explicitness. In later sessions, clinicians can challenge patients by varying the listener-directedness of turn allocation cues or by recreating conditions that tend to precede specific problems (e.g., inappropriate interruptions, failure to allow someone else a turn, difficulty terminating an exchange).

d. The occurrence and appropriateness of within-turn behaviors that contribute to the structure and rhythm of conversation may also require attention in RHD adults. For example, patients can be alerted to the mostly nonverbal signals that punctuate cooperative listening and speaking. For the listener, these include backchannel responses that signal interest or attentiveness (e.g., nodding to indicate agreement; emitting minimal encouragers such as "Hmm," or "Really?"). These tend to be most appropriate when the speaker has finished a clause, shifted his or her gaze toward the listener, or smiled. In addition, conventional eye contact and eye gaze patterns can be associated with both speaker and listener roles, as noted above.

e. Many "hedges" were used above in writing about the kinds of cues that "may" be used and when they "tend" to be appropriate, to remind us that there are no hard and fast rules for conversational signaling. How such indicators are used, or whether they are used at all, will depend on such factors as the nature of the social situation, the relationships between conversational partners, and cultural variation. Thus, when there are questions about the acceptability or impact of various conversational signals and responses, it will be important to solicit feedback from family members or others in a patient's sociocultural circle.

7. Often, it will be profitable to orient communication partners to potential strategies for enhancing conversational exchanges as a supplement to direct work with patients. And, as noted earlier, partner training may be the only alternative for improving interactions when a patient's awareness and other prerequisite cognitive abilities are severely limit-

ed. Of course, partner compensations will be tailored to fit particular patients' strengths and needs, but a partial list of potential strategies, stated in general terms, is provided below. Routinely, or as indicated, conversation partners can:

a. ask a patient for pertinent background information about the subject under discussion and supply the same kind of information when the patient is in the listener role;

b. ask the patient to explain the global connection or relevance of a contribution, and when acting as speaker, provide explicit linkages for the patient;

c. restate, ask questions to re-establish, or otherwise cue the topic of discussion;

d. prompt or signal the patient to focus on main ideas and central information;

e. emphasize essential information using the modalities and utterance forms that the patient can interpret most readily;

f. make turn-taking, topic shifting, or conversation closing signals overt, clear and explicit, and prompt the patient to do the same;

g. provide focused and consistent requests for clarification, specifying the trouble source for the patient;

h. remind the patient to check whether a listener has understood;

i. supply prompts to guide the implementation of target behaviors or strategies, (tailored in terms of structure and subtlety), and/or cue patients to use such prompts;

j. reduce rate and complexity of questions asked or information provided.

IV. OTHER LANGUAGE AND SPEECH

A. Auditory Processing and Comprehension

RHD patients may have measurable deficits, at the word and sentence level, on some standard tests of auditory processing and comprehension for literal language, particularly for decontextualized stimulus materials such as those used in the Revised Token Test (RTT). However, such deficits are likely to be secondary to problems in basic cognitive areas such as perception, attention, or working memory, rather than a result of specific difficulties in retrieving and manipulating stored knowledge about language. Typically, RHD adults' auditory language comprehension is targeted at a higher discourse level (III-C), and/or indirectly, in the context of activities like those described in the sections on pragmatics (II-C) or in treatment for various cognitive impairments that potentially underlie poor interpretation in the auditory modality (section V).

It has been noted that the RTT may provide useful information on patterns of auditory processing difficulty in individual patients, such as problems tuning in on the first few items of a subtest or task, or attentional fatigue that detracts from performance on the last few items. If a patient exhibits problems tuning in, the clinician can design treatment to incorporate alerting signals, thematic cues, clear transitions from one activity to the next, and/or a greater number of examples or practice items to orient the patient to the task. For a patient who appears to fade out over the course of a task, treatment activities can be presented in shorter segments with frequent breaks, and/or alerting signals can be injected at appropriate points later in a task. In either case, these kinds of cues and modifications are gradually faded or normalized, as it becomes possible to do so. And in either case, patients and others around them can be informed about the problems and educated about the benefits of requesting or using such strategies. If one of these problems persists in a form that appears to obstruct daily life understanding, it may be appropriate to train patients or their families directly to implement useful strategies.

B. Word Retrieval

Though measurable on decontextualized tests of naming, word retrieval problems are rarely treated directly in RHD adults. Their word-finding problems tend to be minor relative to other communicative difficulties, and clinically, it appears that RHD adults' word retrieval impairments do not interfere much with communication in context. Additionally, a number of their errors can be linked to deficits of visual perception or integration, making those areas more appropriate points of focus for treatment.

Nonetheless, there may be RHD patients for whom clinicians will provide direct treatment for word retrieval problems: those who are particularly distressed about their difficulties, and for whom there are few other, more pressing goals for treatment time (though when patients are very distracted by a problem, it may need some attention before they will be able to focus on goals that the clinician considers more important). In such cases, it is possible to train traditional compensatory strategies, such as describing what is known about a word, or generally talking around it. The pragmatic ideal of communicating successfully is emphasized over retrieving specific words. In an approach such as this, some symptoms may actually have communicative value (e.g., listing individual members of a category or elements of a collective noun will convey the point to a listener). If so, patients can made aware of their value and encouraged to use the same behaviors strategically when appropriate. However, there may be a delicate balance involved between strategic facilitation of this kind and digressiveness or excess volubility that may detract from social communicative exchange.

C. Reading and Writing

The whether and the how of treatment for reading and writing will depend to a large degree on how handicapping a patient's deficits are, in light of premorbid skills and interests, and the levels of literacy needed for social, vocational, or recreational purposes. Of course, the severity of patients' deficits and the bases of their reading and writing problems will also influence the nature and direction of treatment.

1. Treatment for reading and writing problems that appear to be related to basic impairments of visual processing or attention (e.g., scanning deficits; neglect) will involve primarily activities focused directly in those areas (see section V). Treatment for discourse level problems of reading comprehension and written expression can be focused using the principles and suggestions that are provided in the discourse section, above (III-C).

2. Severity of impairment will interact with handicap to suggest realistic treatment activities and goals. Some functional reading and writing activities may be appropriate even for patients with relatively severe impairments, particularly if compensatory strategies are used to clue them in to relevant points or key information (e.g., highlighting in red, or others as suggested immediately below). Functionality must be individually determined, but some potential tasks include reading letters, recipes, other kinds of instructions, phone books, indexes, bus schedules, and newspapers; or writing phone messages, checks, lists, notes on birthday cards, addresses on envelopes, appointments in a schedule book, or entries in a diary. Using these kinds of tasks, patients can work as appropriate on answering questions, sequencing sets of instructions, following directions, filling in missing steps, clarifying ambiguous information,

summarizing, identifying main points and unstated assumptions, detecting questions that remain to be answered, recording information in a specified place, and so forth. Those patients with moderate-to-mild impairments can work on increasing the rate at which they carry out specific activities that may contribute to discourse comprehension and expression (e.g., identifying central elements of written passages, and others in discourse section above). In addition, they can be taught to use organizational strategies to direct their approach to written materials. One example for written text comprehension is described in Table 7–5. Organizational structures of this sort will probably work best as external aids, rather than as internalized mnemonics, because an external aid will minimize the mental resources that would be required to generate and consult a memorized format. Other self-instructional, self-monitoring, and self-repair strategies can be used to remedy or avoid specific problems as well.

3. A few of the many possible compensatory strategies for reading and writing, some to be implemented by patients and some by others in their environment, include:

   a. tape record instructions, important messages, and so forth, to replace or supplement the written form;

   b. ask for, or provide, more time to look over written materials or repeated opportunities to read them;

   c. focus attention on portions of a text by covering other portions or by using a ruler to keep track of current position;

   d. develop or use organizational guides such as that in Table 7–5, or structured sets of questions for self-instruction and self-analysis;

Table 7–5. An organizational strategy for reading comprehension.

- Preview material to be read to identify themes and/or central ideas
- Generate questions about those themes or ideas
- Read the material carefully to answer those questions
- Make note of the answers and summarize
- Review the material to check comprehension and verify answers

   e. develop or consult a graphic representation of the text (III-B-1-b, above);

   f. provide bold or brightly colored lines and margins on a page to enhance spatial orientation for reading and writing;

   g. use cue cards or other reminders to keep themes or topics in focus.

D. Dysarthria

Treatment for dysarthric symptoms that result from RHD is most likely to focus on improving intelligibility and/or prosodic variation. Some possible methods were described above in the section on prosodic production (II-C-1). Readers can also refer to the work of Rosenbek and LaPointe (1985), and Yorkston et al. (1988) for more information about treatment for dysarthrias.

V. COGNITIVE AND PERCEPTUAL PROBLEMS

A. Anosognosia

Establishing some degree of self-awareness and self-evaluation is critical for implementing many rehabilitation strategies with RHD adults. Intervention aimed at enhancing awareness of deficits was discussed extensively in earlier portions of this chapter (II-B-2-d). Patients who remain uncritical and unconcerned about their impairments are poor candidates for extended direct rehabilitation. In such cases, the most appropriate intervention options will include simplifying goals and modifying the environment. Environmental adaptation may involve training communication partners to prompt or apply compensatory strategies, such as those described throughout this chapter.

B. Orientation

Orientation deficits are often among the first sets of problems that clinicians address in treating cognitive-communicative impairments in RHD adults. Unfortunately, it has not been established that treatment designed to facilitate recovery of orientation is either necessary or effective for RHD adults who manifest confusion about time and place in the period just after a stroke. At least some remission of orientation problems is likely to occur spontaneously, making it particularly difficult to attribute observed changes to treatment. However, postponing or eschewing traditional facility techniques does not mean that a confused patient needs to stay confused, even temporarily. Rather, external cues and strategies may be well suited for dealing with orientation problems. External aids can be used to alleviate temporary difficulties in an acute post-onset stage, and they will be appropriate for patients whose orientation remains limited over the long term. Additionally, early training with external aids may set the stage for using compensatory guides in other areas (e.g., memory; problem solving) and in other stages of recovery. For all of these reasons, external aids and compensatory strategies may be preferable to exercises intended to facilitate orientation, though both kinds of approaches should be submitted to clinical experimentation. Each approach is reviewed briefly, below.

1. A variety of exercises have been used in an attempt to facilitate recovery of orientation (e.g., many such activities are described in treatment materials published by the Rehabilitation Institute of Chicago; Burns et al., 1983).

   a. Burns and colleagues distinguish passive from active orientation. Passive orientation involves recognition of salient environmental features and time concepts. Active orientation involves manipulating time and place information to get along in everyday living (e.g., navigating from place to place; maintaining schedules).

   b. Typically, activities intended to enhance passive orientation to place use objects in the patient's surroundings, beginning with personal belongings and other familiar objects (or pictures when possible), arrayed to minimize perceptual and attentional deficits. Patients work on identifying objects from the array, naming them, describing their purpose, and/or associating them with various features of, or specific places in, the larger setting (e.g., what one finds in a hospital generally; what belongs in the bedside stand, the bathroom, or a treatment room).

   c. Active orientation to place is targeted with activities designed to assist patients in moving from one place to another in their environment, beginning with immediately visible goal locations, and short distances between starting place and goal. Spoken or written plans and cues are incorporated to help guide movements. Patients may also work on drawing or reading maps or floorplans, or describing how to travel to various locations. Active orientation activities such as these are often included in visuospatial training procedures, as well (V-C-5).

   d. Treatment for problems with passive orientation to time can include activities such as connecting environmental cues with particular days, times of day, seasons of the year, or special days or events (e.g., grandchildren visiting on Saturdays; darkness in the evening; people wearing sweaters in winter; and symbols connected with holidays or other special days like birthdays) and anticipating the next unit of time from the current one. One must be careful about establishing associations like these, as some may be tenuous and potentially misleading: The grandchildren may miss or switch a visiting day; it is dark during the daytime when it's stormy (or when it's winter in Alaska) and light in the evening during the summer; sweaters may be worn when the air conditioning is too cold; and so forth. In other activities, patients' attention is directed to calendars or other posted information, and they are drilled on indicating the day, date, current time, and/or times associated with various daily routines (e.g., getting up, having lunch, etc.). For orientation training, temporal information should be associated with meaningful events whenever possible (e.g., activities or schedule for a certain day), rather than simply memorized.

    e.   Treatment intended to facilitate active orientation to time focuses on estimating elapsed time, time needed to perform various activities, or time remaining until something in progress is completed (e.g., a familiar song, a television show, a treatment session, a special project). Prospective memory training (section V-E-3) also incorporates activities for estimating and tracking temporal units.

2. Compensatory approaches for enhancing orientation.

    a.   Some of the facilitation exercises described above utilize external aids such as calendars, posted schedules, signs, and labels in the patient's environment. Immediately relevant information, such as the current day's activities, the nurse on duty, or the specific time, is often highlighted in some way or isolated to set it apart from the visual background. However, a number of other methods are considered below, to maximize the likelihood that patients will actually use the information that is included in such aids (cf., Bourgeois, 1991).

    b.   Simply posting orientation information may not be very helpful; patients will probably do better when they are trained to attend to and read the posted information. Such training might include repeated exposure, with the routine expectation that whenever a patient sees a sign or label, he or she reads it aloud, or identifies and reports the part that is highlighted. Patients can also be given a purpose for consulting posted information, such as being asked to find out for the clinician when a specified activity or event will occur or who is working on the rehabilitation unit on a particular afternoon. This kind of approach can use a game format if that is motivating for the patient. One example might be to have patients locate information to complete a worksheet or to answer a set of questions, with a goal of beating a best prior time or reducing the number of places where the answers are sought. In relatively easy tasks, the necessary information might comprise basic orientation facts, and at higher levels, patients might be given a goal of identifying specified changes in their environments (e.g., note who comes on duty after someone else leaves; note the room number next to the speech-language treatment room).

c. Another limitation of posted signs and labels is that they are stationary and so of little assistance when they are out of sight. To get around this problem, patients can be given an individualized, portable set of information (e.g., cue cards, pocket notebook, written schedule) to consult whenever it might be helpful. The patient can be trained as above to interact consistently with his or her personalized aid, using tasks that rely on the information that it contains (see also V-E-2, for more on external memory aids).

d. Everyone in a patient's environment can participate in drawing that patient's attention to orientation information as needed, and in reinforcing his or her interaction with the information. Such involvement might take the form of reminding patients to read posted signs or nametags whenever they see them, prompting them to consult their pocket notebooks to answer specific questions, and/or praising them when they comply or initiate target behaviors on their own (in a natural way, such as "way to go, you read my name"). Appropriate prompts, cues, and reinforcement can be evaluated and agreed upon by the speech-language pathologist and other members of the rehabilitation team (see Chapter 8). Family members can be trained to become involved in this kind of treatment, as long as the personalities are right (e.g., both patient and family member agree to family member's involvement, neither overwhelms the other or pushes too hard, etc; see also Chapter 8, section II-A-11).

e. Patients with persistent disorientation may benefit from compensations that include establishing familiar surroundings and consistent, unambiguous routines; minimizing noise and other overwhelming stimulation or distractions; or wearing identification bracelets and carrying labelled belongings so that others can direct them if they get lost.

C. Visual/Auditory Perceptual and Related Functions

1. Speech-language pathologists are likely to be involved with treating RHD adults' perceptual problems to the extent that those problems influence communicative functioning. Auditory perceptual impairments related to the appreciation of prosody are among those that may receive attention from speech-language pathologists. Since these deficits were considered earlier in this chapter (II-C-1), the sections below will focus on visuoperceptual, visuospatial, and visual scanning and search functions. Treatment for visual neglect, which may have an attentional basis, is discussed in this section as many interventions for neglect are aimed at improving visuomotor scanning.

2. Reading and writing activities tap the point of interface between visual impairments and communication. Most of the suggestions below will focus on language stimuli, as such stimuli are essential and functional components of reading and writing activities.

3. It is particularly difficult to know when perceptual treatment, using either language or nonlanguage stimuli, might be important to establish readiness for reading and writing goals, or how this kind of treatment should be implemented and evaluated. One reason is that speech-language pathologists tend to have little training in the nature or assessment of normal perceptual and related functions; another is that there is very little evidence about perceptual prerequisites for reading and writing. In the best situation, speech-language pathologists will develop visual-perceptual treatment goals and generalization targets collaboratively with neuropyschologists and/or occupational therapists (who are concerned primarily with the functional impact of perceptual problems in areas such as navigation and safety), and there will a division of remediation labor and efficacy assessment among these team members. If these other specialists are not available in a clinician's treatment setting, referral for outside assessment and consultation is strongly encouraged. Clinicians who address basic visual perceptual and related deficits without consultation from other professionals should have the appropriate expertise (see Chapter 4, I-B) and should monitor related functions (probe for generalization; Chapter 5, III-C-3, and Chapter 6, III-2) particularly carefully, to gather evidence that supports their intervention plan, or points to the need for modification.

4. Activities to treat visual-perceptual difficulties tend to require simple discrimination and matching, closure, figure-ground differentiation, and visual integration. Words, phrases, and numbers make functional stimuli for reading purposes. Typically, patients work to improve the speed and accuracy of their responses, as stimuli are presented in increasingly demanding viewing conditions.

   a. There are many ways to degrade the quality of visual displays or stimulus elements. Among the ways to increase perceptual difficulty are to change the typical perspective in which stimuli are presented; reduce the directness and brightness of lighting in stimulus pictures; present and remove stimuli increasingly more quickly; make them increasingly incomplete by removing more parts, and increasingly less salient parts; obscure them with grid overlays of differing sizes and densities; embed them in a background; and make them more fragmented by increasing the distance between elements or the number of elements that must be integrated (e.g., to form a complete sentence). These kinds of modifications can be applied to any one or several elements of either single or multiple stimuli and can be combined systematically to manipulate task difficulty.

   b. For patients who have trouble with simple discrimination tasks in nondegraded conditions, treatment might begin with three-dimensional or textured stimuli (e.g., letters made from velcro) that patients can feel, trace, or copy to assist in identifying critical elements. Simple closure activities include selecting or generating complete stimuli when given partial ones in otherwise nondegraded conditions, especially when stimuli are familiar and meaningful. For some patients, stimuli will be easier to process when they capitalize on meaning (e.g., real word stimuli for discrimination tasks, that differ by one or two letters; elements for integration tasks that make up a familiar phrase or sentence rather than individual letters of a word). Patients can also be encouraged to call on some of their remaining strengths (talking; itemizing stimulus features) to work through the ways in which pairs of stimuli are different, or partial stimuli are related to wholes.

5. Treatment for visuospatial problems may be farther outside the province of typical speech-language pathology practice than that for other visual disorders, but clinicians can collaborate, and focus on reading- and writing-related stimuli, as appropriate. Treatment

tasks tend to require patients to practice spatial analysis and perception of spatial relationships among elements. Spatial rotation tasks are commonly used, in which patients match, discriminate, or label stimuli that are rotated to varying degrees, often beginning with three-dimensional or cutout stimuli that can be manipulated physically to assist the spatial analysis. A patient's internal representation of spatial relationships is targeted with tasks such as directing someone to a nearby but out-of-sight location, or describing/drawing maps of familiar places (e.g., the route from a patient's home to work; the street corner at the end of their block; their kitchen floorplan). To link these kinds of activities to reading and writing goals, patients can be asked to describe, or to identify from recognition sets, markers along the route such as street signs, addresses, or names of businesses. Other activities, aimed at analysis of external spatial relationships or spatial search, include working mazes (which could be modified to use words or phrases as signals to clear vs. blind alleys); using maps to locate a hidden object or a room in another part of a building; drawing and labeling maps or floorplans of a space that is visible to the patient; giving directions to a visible location to someone who is in another room or whose eyes are closed; or connecting scattered stimulus elements such as letters or words to form as many meaningful larger units (words, phrases, or sentences) as possible. (See neglect section, next, for more on spatial search activities.) As for any treatment tasks, cues and prompts that are sufficient in number and specificity to foster initial success, can be faded over time. Compensations typically involve guiding patients with written or spoken directions, or with an escort, to help them find their way around.

6. The longstanding and continuing confusion about the mechanisms responsible for various aspects of neglect makes it difficult to propose treatment approaches or tasks with much confidence. It is becoming increasingly common to work directly on improving deficiencies in arousal, attentional orienting and selectivity, and attentional control that tend to correlate with symptoms of neglect, and that may underlie its occurrence. Yet the efficacy of directing treatment towards attentional impairments to reduce manifestations of neglect has not been investigated. Most published evaluations of treatment for neglect have centered on improving environmental scanning, primarily to compensate for presumed problems of spatial exploration. The methods and results of a number of these treatment studies will be reviewed briefly below. As a caveat, much of this work does not separate patients with and without visual field cuts, so it is not clear whether reportedly successful

treatments have their effect on compensating for neglect or for visual field deficits. Many of the reports suffer as well from the use of simple pretest-posttest designs, a failure to demonstrate stability of performance before treatment, and/or lack of documentation of test-retest reliability for their outcome measures. Further, unless specifically noted below, little convincing evidence is presented to document maintenance or functional generalization of treatment gains. The review of treatment studies is followed by a description of some relatively untested ideas. Most of the existing programs incorporate systematic, small-step changes in cuing and task elements, and intensive repetition and overlearning to foster habituation and automaticity.

a.   Treatment approaches evaluated in group research studies.

(1) Some extensive early work (e.g., Diller & Weinberg, 1977; Weinberg et al., 1977), was based on the hypothesis that, to a large degree, difficulties associated with neglect after RHD stem from problems scanning the environment spontaneously and completely. Thus, a comprehensive treatment program was developed to enhance the automaticity and systematicity of scanning. Treatment used a variety of visual tasks designed to cause patients to turn their heads leftward and to search the environment thoroughly (e.g., tracking targets that move at various rates around the perimeter of a board; reporting positions of flashing lights on the board) or to make use of information from both visual fields (e.g., reading newspaper paragraphs projected on a wall). Initial cues, gradually faded, included the provision of anchoring stimuli to guide the initiation of scanning and pacing to decrease rapid and impulsive rightward drift. Experimental and control subjects were assessed once before and once after the treatment period, with tasks selected to tap several levels of generalization. Differences between groups were evident on some tasks similar to the domain of training (e.g., "academic" measures including oral reading of words and paragraphs, simple reading comprehension, copying, and simple arithmetic problems) as well as some divergent measures (e.g., face matching), particularly for subjects whose impairments were initially more severe. The functional impact of training was not addressed, and the maintenance of gains was mentioned only anecdotally. Gordon et al. (1986) provide a detailed description of methods, procedures, equipment and training stimuli,

along with clinical notes about commonly encountered problems in training.

(2) This scanning training did not generalize as expected to some measures, including tests of line bisection or location of body midline, so the authors inferred that the patients had a separate disorder of space perception that was impervious to the scanning treatment. Thus a later study was designed in which training in sensory awareness and spatial organization followed a condensed scanning training program (Weinberg et al., 1979). The new treatment tasks required awareness of the locus of an examiner's touch on the back and estimation of the size of objects external to the body. Based on pre-posttest analysis with different groups of subjects, the authors claimed that this combined treatment was more powerful (produced more generalization) than the isolated scanning treatment from the prior study (Weinberg et al., 1977). Again, Gordon et al. (1986) describe methods, procedures, and stimuli in detail sufficient for replication.

(3) The two training components just described, and a third that focused on complex visual perceptual training, were incorporated sequentially into another treatment evaluation study (Gordon et al., 1985). The new training was implemented because it was noted that, after treatment in the first two domains, some RHD patients continued to have difficulty with more cognitively demanding visuospatial tasks and with reading comprehension. The third training component was designed to promote visual exploration and examination, emphasizing attention to stimulus elements in the patient's left visual field. The tasks required patients to utilize orderly search strategies to impose organization on, and to analyze systematically, spatial information in visual stimuli (see details in Gordon et al., 1986). The outcome measures included tasks of basic scanning (i.e., the previously used academic measures), size estimation and somatosensory awareness, complex visual perception (e.g., Raven's CPM, picture matching, and position preference scores; WAIS Block Design), and some nonspecific generalization tasks and measures of mood. All measures were administered before and after treatment, and most were also given at a follow-up assessment four months after discharge from the rehabilitation program. Data analyses controlled for pre-treatment ability and extent of visual field cut. Posttesting immediately after treatment showed differences between experimental and control subjects for 9 of the 21 measures of primary interest, and for 1 of 8 nonspecific generalization measures (however, given the large number of analyses that were run, some of these differences might be expected to occur by chance). At the 4-month follow-up, the control group was equivalent to, or better than the experimental patients on all but two measures of mood. One explanation offered by the authors was that their treatment protocol may have moved prematurely from one type of treatment to another before gains were solidified, an important possibility in light of the fact that Gordon et al. (1986) later recommended the criteria used in this study to determine the pace at which patients move through the various training modules. The authors also speculated that the other rehabilitation therapies given to the control group during the treatment phase had unintended effects that supported their continued improvement after discharge. In any case, the similarity between groups at follow-up highlights the need for maintenance data in evaluations of treatment efficacy.

(4) Robertson, Gray, Pentland, and Waite (1990) reported results of a randomized, controlled trial that compared computerized neglect training with recreational computer training. Twenty patients in an experimental group were trained on a scanning task to look left, and to engage in systematic search and scanning, using voice synthesis and visual cues to orient attention. Further, they were given structured practice in dividing the computer screen mentally before scanning it, and they received some visuospatial reasoning tasks and general attentional training. Control group subjects engaged in computing exercises that minimized scanning, as well as timed attention activities. Neither experimental nor control subjects improved much, and blind assessments at the end of training and 6 months later revealed no differences between groups. In light of earlier reports that severely affected patients benefited most from neglect training (Weinberg et al., 1977), data from a subset of the most severely impaired patients were submitted to separate analysis, but the null result did not change. It should be noted that neither group received anywhere near the amount of training that was provided in the noncomputerized studies reviewed earlier; however, they received more training than several individual cases whose results initially appeared promising (see Robertson, Gray, & McKenzie, 1988, below).

(5) Pizzamiglio et al. (1992) recently investigated another comprehensive treatment program for neglect patients, all of whom had concomitant extensive field cuts (either homonymous hemianopia or superior quadrantopia). Severity of neglect was reportedly stable, either as demonstrated by two pretests given one month apart (though neither the data nor analytic documentation were provided), or as inferred for patients who were greater than 7 months post-onset. The treatment program was based on four tasks designed to enhance spatial exploration. Patients performed visual-spatial scanning tasks in which they identified digits from a large visual field under increasingly difficult viewing conditions; copied and/or read increasingly complex stimuli; copied line drawings onto matrices of dots that varied in size and density; and described the elements in black-and-white drawings. Initial cues included red flashing anchors either under targets or at the initiation of a line of text, and examiner reminders that varied from specific to generic, or that cued patients to carry out both spatial and semantic analysis (e.g., "Look to the left"; "Who said . . .?"). Efficacy evaluation indicated significant improvements on tests of letter and line cancellation and oral sentence reading. In addition, considerable changes were noted for most patients on a functional observation measure of hemineglect that included tasks of serving tea, using common objects for grooming, describing a room full of objects, and describing a painting in which left-sided input is crucial for interpretation. Unfortunately, it is not clear whether this test was given twice to assess pre-treatment stability of performance. The finding that there was little improvement on other tests of visuospatial ability or on a neurological exam is offered as evidence of the specificity of training. The paper refers to follow-up testing, at least 5 months after training, for 7 of the 13 patients. Few data are provided, but the authors assert that there were no consistent differences from the posttest in neurological or neuropsychological function. Five of the 7 patients, who were retested on the functional neglect evaluation, were found to have maintained their post-treatment gains on that measure.

(6) Ladavas, Menghini, and Umilta (1994) treated spatial neglect with the primary purpose of examining some hypotheses about its underlying nature. They conceptualized neglect as an attentional orienting disorder, and designed a treatment to influence voluntary orienting of attention in the visual modality. Twelve patients who had right parietal lesions of at least 6 months' duration, participated in the study. Subjects were described as having stable neglect in visual and tactile modalities (as well as visual and tactile extinction), but the methods, criteria, and data used to establish or document pre-treatment stability were not provided. Nine of these patients also had deficits affecting one quadrant of their left visual fields.

Neglect treatment, based on Posner and colleagues' paradigm (Posner et al., 1984, 1987; see Chapter 2, section III-D-8-b), was provided for 30 1-hour sessions, 1 per day for 6 weeks. Patients were presented with a visual display with a central fixation mark, and 4 empty squares in upper and lower quadrants of the left and right visual fields. An arrow presented at fixation served as a cue for directing attention to an upcoming target, while a cross served as a nonpredictive or "neutral" cue. The arrow signaled a high probability that the target would occur in the cued location, and the cross indicated equiprobable location. The patient's task was to detect and respond to a target stimulus as quickly as possible, regardless of its position in the display, or the validity of the cue (some arrow cues were invalid, in that they signaled one location but the target occurred in another location).

Subjects were divided into 3 groups of 4 patients each. One group received treatment in a covert orienting condition; one group received an overt orienting condition; and one group received motor treatment as a control condition. In the covert attention condition, the patient was told to fixate on the central point throughout the interval prior to target presentation, regardless of the presence of an arrow cue. In the overt condition, patients were instructed to look at the cued box when an arrow occurred in the central position. Although the authors did not demonstrate comparability of the three groups on pre-treatment neglect measures, the results suggest that both neglect treatment groups improved more than the control group on several dependent measures of neglect (e.g., letter, line, and "bell" cancellation, and object pointing). Generalization to tests of reading, writing, and drawing from memory was claimed but not documented. On the attention training tasks themselves, subjects in both treatment groups became more accurate detecting validly cued trials than neutral or invalid trials, with the greater improvement in the left visual field. This finding indicates positive changes in patients' ability to orient attention voluntarily in space.

Probably because Ladavas et al. (1994) were not interested in clinical questions, their study does not address concerns about the functional impact or maintenance of treatment and generalization was not rigorously examined. Although it has flaws and procedural information is sketchy, the study exemplifies an attempt to capitalize on current theory about the nature of neglect, and as such provides a model for further investigation.

   b.   Approaches assessed in single-subject experimental designs.

       (1) In a multiple baseline design, conducted across subjects, Webster et al. (1984) modified Weinberg and colleagues' (1977) scanning program to emphasize navigation and mobility. They reported good results for three RHD patients with homonymous hemianopsia and neglect. All improved in performance on an obstacle course, decreasing direct frontal contacts with left-side obstacles (but not sideswipes). One strength of this study is its use of repeated measurements in the multiple baseline design, allowing stronger inferences about the stability of deficits prior to training and the reliability and magnitude of changes after training. Another strength is the follow-up data. All patients were reassessed approximately a year after training. Each remained above baseline for scanning and obstacle course measures, though hemianoptic deficits did not change appreciably over the course of the study. The authors note that the extent of change after training brought these three patients into the range of performance for RHD patients who do not have visual field cuts. This note raises the question of the mechanisms by which the treatment had its effects. Perhaps the training primarily helped patients to compensate for their hemianoptic difficulties, without having a particular influence on attentional or representational aspects of neglect.

(2) As one part of a larger report, Webster et al. (1988) alluded to data from a total of 13 RHD patients with neglect (11 with field cuts; 3 reported in the prior study) who were trained using the methodology and procedures described in their previous report (Webster et al., 1984). Obstacle course performance data were combined for the 13 patients and analyzed for treatment effects, comparing the last baseline session with that immediately following the first training session on which subjects achieved 90% correct identification of lights on a scanning board. A significant effect was found that was attributable to improvement on direct hits rather than sideswipes. Unfortunately, neither training nor probe data are graphed, tabulated, or appended, so it is impossible to evaluate factors that are essential to judging the rigor of single subject experimental designs, including the stability of pre-treatment baseline performance, or the extent to which experimental control was maintained. The finding that sideswipes are resistant to treatment suggests that more subtle problems with hemifield inattention are not addressed by the scanning training that was employed.

(3) Robertson et al. (1988) explored computerized neglect training for two right CVA patients, in multiple baseline designs, using methods like those described above for their group study (Robertson et al., 1990). Both patients had relatively stable pre-treatment baselines on criterion measures such as word-search, letter cancellation, telephone dialing, and prose reading, as well as a number of unrelated control measures. Both patients exhibited large improvements in the criterion measures with the onset of treatment, and little change on the control tasks. The authors were optimistic about these findings, but following the negative results in the randomized group trial of Robertson et al. (1990), Robertson (1990) argued that apparent improvements in these individual cases could have resulted from practice effects for the neglect tests that did not affect the control measures. Robertson (1990) concludes pessimistically that there is "no justification at present for routine clinical applications of computerized training for neglect or other visuoperceptual disorders . . . in the case of neglect, pessimistic findings emerge as to whether existing types of [computerized] programmes can work" (p. 393).

c.   Approaches described in case reports and clinical observations.

(1) Horner (1980) outlined a number of activities designed to improve scanning and increase active participation in treatment tasks for a chronic RHD patient whose confrontation naming errors appeared to reflect left visual field inattention, impulsive visual exploration, and impaired analysis and synthesis of defining stimulus elements. Analogous reading deficits were noted, involving primarily letter and word omissions and inadequate scanning. A combination of techniques, aimed at enhancing the patient's attention and intention to respond to stimulus elements, were applied in naming, drawing, and reading tasks. Among the primary treatment activities were tracing pictures, focusing on both contour and detail; searching for left-sided anchoring cues; and verbal self-cuing to look to the left. Reading was treated by using horizontal and vertical anchoring, immediate oral rereading after errors were highlighted by the clinician, and reading for meaning. Horner reports quantitative and qualitative evidence of clinically significant changes, with the exception of more difficult reading tasks (e.g., *Reading Comprehension Battery for Aphasia* [LaPointe & Horner, 1979] subtests requiring comprehension of facts and inferences at paragraph level). Techniques such as these deserve further evaluation, in various combinations, in controlled treatment studies.

(2) In a departure from the prevailing methods of the time, which emphasized improving scanning by increasing attention to perceptual cues, Stanton, Yorkston, Kenyon, and Beukelman (1981) reported a program that used patients' language skills to compensate for visual neglect in reading. They trained two relatively acute patients with severe neglect to shift their attention to the left in various reading tasks. Treatment procedures included matching number, letter, and word stimuli arranged in columns on the right and left of a page; reading sentences orally, in which vertical spacing and print size were progressively reduced; and reading printed text orally, working from large-print, double-spaced paragraphs to magazines and books. Initially, patients were trained to use overt self-instruction to remind themselves to look to the left, with the clinician's cues diminishing in frequency and specificity. Changes in omission errors and reading rate were

charted on an oral paragraph reading task. Because the data were not gathered in the context of a controlled experimental design, it is difficult to attribute the reported changes to the neglect treatment itself, rather than some other aspect of the patients' rehabilitation program, neurological improvement, and/or continued practice with the criterion reading task. Although the authors do not provide any evidence on this point, they suggest that early in treatment, patients with neglect will be better able to profit from training such as theirs, which provides concrete reminders to check for all of the material on a page, than from treatment that asks them to modify their reading on the basis of their judgments about whether what they are reading makes sense. This supposition should be tested empirically, particularly in light of recent evidence about various ways in which neglect symptoms can be attenuated with meaning cues (see Table 2–9; though as noted several times previously in this book, patients may benefit from certain kinds of task structure or cues without being able to make related metalinguistic judgments). Stanton and colleagues do indicate that it would be important to move neglect patients gradually toward using meaning cues to guide their reading.

(3) Mackisack designed two related neglect treatment techniques, Edgeness and Bookness, to target patients' problems with exploring and responding in neglected space more broadly than typical verbal cuing and anchoring approaches (see Myers & Mackisack, 1990). The programs focus on spatial search and response both contralaterally and ipsilaterally to a patient's brain lesion (as is true of many other treatment approaches outlined earlier, but not of pure verbal cuing or anchoring strategies). The programs, which are experimental in nature, are designed to place responsibility for visual search on the patient in an attempt to foster internalization of improved search behavior.

(a) In the "Edgeness" technique, patients identify the boundaries of relevant space for a specific task and then perform tasks within those boundaries. First they trace with their fingers and eyes the perimeter of a three-dimensional board or grid. Subsequently, they locate colored cubes on the grid, that are placed singly and then in pairs at systematically varying positions and distances from each other. Among the other manipulations to increase task difficulty are bigger grids, larger sets of cubes to retrieve, and less predictable associations of cube color and location. Patients are encouraged to explore and trace the edges of any relevant surface or area in a similar way.

(b) "Bookness" is an extension of the edgeness technique, applied to reading. First, patients describe a closed book placed in front of them at midline and explain how people go about reading. Then they trace the edges of the book with fingers and eyes, first when it is closed and again when it is open, describing what they see. Reading tasks begin with matching activities, using stimuli on both the left and right sides of the book. A typical progression of difficulty is used, manipulating the types of stimuli, number and nature of response alternatives, and so forth. Patients also continue to trace the edges of the book before each trial until this process seems no longer necessary.

(c) Appealing rationales are provided for these techniques, and the authors suggest that they are clinically effective. Hopefully, these apparently promising ideas will be studied to ascertain their general efficacy and to identify the specific characteristics of patients for whom they are or are not effective. Myers and Mackisack suggest, as well, that warm-up activities with the grid used for Edgeness training may enhance a patient's attention to critical visual information in other treatment tasks, such as those that focus on pragmatic deficits. Again, this is a reasonable hypothesis, and one that should be evaluated empirically. Indeed, if attentional factors lie at the heart of many of communicative symptoms after RHD, then performance on communicative treatment activities may be enhanced by preceding the primary tasks with, or incorporating into a cuing hierarchy, any activity that channels arousal or attentional resources in an appropriate manner for a particular patient (e.g., any of the attention-directing and exploration activities outlined above and in Table 2–9; see also suggestions in the remainder of this section and in section V-D on attention).

d. Other thoughts and considerations regarding neglect treatment.

(1) Table 2–9 lists some potential cues or facilitory procedures that have been shown to modulate neglect in research studies. These kinds of cues can be explored for shaping responses in neglect treatment tasks, whether in primarily restorative approaches for less severely impaired patients, or in training compensatory strategies for patients with chronic and intractable problems. These kinds of cues may also be useful for structuring other treatment activities to minimize neglect symptoms when they are not the immediate focus of treatment, but have the potential to contaminate performance. It should be remembered, though, that it is never clear how well group findings in laboratory conditions will transfer to individual effects in treatment programs.

(2) The cues outlined in Table 2–9, and many of the techniques described in the review above, most likely have their influence on attentional orienting, or task-relevant arousal and readiness to respond. Considering neglect from an attentional perspective, several other treatment manipulations can be proposed, which extend the ideas already presented (see also section V-D, below, on directly targeting attention and arousal). Some of these include:

(a) practice leftward responses initially in more intact hemifield or quadrants, as needed;

(b) practice components of attentional orienting (disengage, shift, engage) in the relatively intact field, initially;

(c) gradually move practice to the more impaired side of space, keeping the relatively intact field free of stimuli while working on components of attentional orienting;

(d) when stimuli are presented in both fields for search activities, facilitate disengagement or shifting by decreasing the perceptual salience of ipsilesional stimuli, in individually determined ways (e.g., varying features such as color, clarity, or size);

(e) include multiple salient features in stimulus elements that fall primarily in the neglected space to facilitate engagement;

(f) systematically move critical elements from relatively intact (usually right-sided or midline) positions toward the primarily affected hemifield or quadrant, at the same time increasing the distance between targets to be matched or retrieved;

(g) use stimuli and tasks that may activate an underaroused right hemisphere (e.g., responding with the left hand, in the left side of space, to nonlanguage stimuli such as shapes and lines, following tonal alerting signals).

(3) Manipulations like those reviewed in Table 2–9 and in the material above can be integrated into a variety of target detection, matching, identification, and tracking activities, including, for example, those outlined earlier for working on spatial search (section V-C-5).

(4) All of the manipulations discussed so far in this section focus on factors external to the patient. Another consideration concerns the potentially facilitating influence of involving patients actively in directing spatial search and exploration. Much evidence suggests that active involvement in generating strategies, associations, or cues will enhance learning, memory, and generalization in various domains, for both brain-damaged and non-brain-damaged adults. Some possible reasons are that active participation helps to increase task-relevant arousal, to channel attentional resources, or to contact familiar stored knowledge and processing routines. With regard to neglect treatment, active involvement is emphasized, for example, in Ladavas et al.'s voluntary orienting treatment and in Mackisack's program, and is incorporated in several of Horner's techniques (e.g., tracing; labelling elements while constructing drawings). This notion can be extended to other techniques, as well, such as the anchoring cues commonly used in reading tasks. For example, it may be beneficial for some patients to choose and place anchoring stimuli themselves before each trial or task, rather than simply looking for those provided by clinicians.

(5) Another potential patient-related variable concerns the motivational value of treatment stimuli or tasks, which may again be related to arousal or attentional focus. Performance may be best when patients have a purpose that interests them, for carrying out treatment activities. For some patients, the motivation and intention to perform may be maximized through game-like challenges (e.g., solving puzzles; locating increasingly more targets to better a previous performance), whereas for other patients, particularly those who are aware of the impact of their deficits, the possibility of regaining some proficiency in favorite recreational pursuits will enhance their drive.

(6) Related to the "meaningfulness" principle in Table 2–9, stimulus materials can be structured to create obvious discontinuities in meaning if left-sided features are overlooked (although as noted earlier, there is some debate about how soon in the course of treatment patients can capitalize on meaning judgments to enhance search behavior). In addition, the familiarity of functional stimuli and tasks may facilitate spatial exploration. Mackisack's "bookness" program, and others that treat scanning in the context of reading, use some functional materials. Other possibilities include calendars, menus, vending machines, telephone keypads, letters, and various types of books (e.g., date book, phone book, dictionary) from which patients are asked to locate and manipulate specific information.

(7) Readers will note that none of the approaches described thus far has focused on representational aspects or forms of neglect. It is difficult to suggest how one might attack deficits that appear to stem from problems of generating or scanning internal representations. One possible cue, and potential compensation, might be to have patients practice imagining objects or scenes from two vantage points (in front of; behind), starting with three-dimensional stimuli that can be manipulated to provide concrete representations of different points of view. Discrimination or matching tasks could be used, requiring patients to take into account the information obtained from both vantage points. Closure activities might also be useful, with patients imagining and then selecting or generating the incomplete portions of visual stimuli. It is also possible that patients with serviceable external scanning and search behavior can be taught to apply, intentionally, similar principles and strategies to imagined stimuli. For example, any exercises in dividing a stimulus space, either physically with grids and overlays, or mentally (cf., Gordon et al., 1986; Myers & Mackisack, 1990; Robertson et al., 1988) could be used as analogies to guide a systematic search of mentally represented information. However, approaches targeting mental representation may be less relevant for speech-language clinicians than for other rehabilitation specialists, as we tend to focus on neglect in the context of externalized communicative activities involving reading and writing, rather than imagined space. Disturbances of environmental scanning and internal space representation

or manipulation can occur separately in RHD neglect patients (Kinsella, Olver, Ng, Packer, & Stark, 1993), suggesting that competence in one of these areas is not prerequisite for functional performance in the other.

(8) More generally, a difficult unresolved issue concerns what levels or kinds of skills may be necessary precursors for training other deficient visual and cognitive functions.

(a) Some work (e.g., Gordon et al., 1985; Weinberg et al., 1979) suggests that, particularly for severely involved patients, treatment for visual disturbances after RHD should be directed initially toward establishing gross scanning skills before moving to subtler requirements like locating words on a printed page and presumably interpreting them. Thus, early perceptual training is considered fundamental for preparing many patients for higher-level applications such reading for meaning (see also Stanton et al., 1981). It is hard to assess this kind of premise, because generalization of scanning or spatial exploration treatment effects has not been evaluated for areas of functional impact, like crossing the street, and, in the communication domain, has rarely been addressed with anything more difficult than simple reading comprehension tasks.

(b) Besides the uncertainty of generalization, there are several other potential complications of targeting gross scanning skills in the hopes of eventually influencing performance in other areas. From a cognitive resource standpoint, any newly trained strategies considered prerequisite to other behaviors should be overlearned and sufficiently automatized to reduce their demands on mental resources. Otherwise, their effortful implementation may divert mental fuel that is critical for carrying out other processes, which for our purposes might include such things as inferencing, integration, and formulation (readers should remember that strategy usage is often effortful even if a strategy has become internalized and self-generated). Potentially large amounts of treatment time would most likely be required to achieve anything like automaticity for using a new strategy, particularly for patients with moderate-to-severe impairments. As a result, the total available funding resources, and concomitant treatment time for higher-level communicative and cognitive activities, might be seriously depleted before other treatments could be initiated and evaluated.

(c) It has already been noted that when neglect is severe, it may be most realistic to implement methods of compensation. It is likely that, in attempting to compensate for their deficits, severely impaired patients would use up more of their limited mental resources than would patients who are less impaired. Thus, projecting further from resource theories, patients with severe neglect may be more successful at carrying out higher level processing operations when provided with structured tasks and cues to minimize the need for self-initiation of compensatory strategies, than when the patients are expected to implement such strategies on their own. If this supposition has any validity, such patients may be better served by allocating treatment time to more diverse activities, including some that target (probably compensatory) higher-level processing and problem-solving skills, than by focusing primarily on overlearning self-implemented compensations for neglect.

(d) To get some idea about the extent to which compensatory strategy implementation diverts resources from other processing operations, it would be instructive to assess the relationship between the availability of attentional or working memory resources and higher level processing skills in patients who have achieved similar outcomes after scanning or search training for neglect. But in any case, it would be less risky to put so many eggs in the "train-to-automaticity" basket, if we were more certain about what behaviors we should be trying to automatize in the treatment of neglect and about how they were related to higher-level communicative and cognitive processing.

(9) A more focused, but still unresolved procedural question concerns where clinicians should sit and place materials during treatment with neglect patients. One common school of thought contends that clinicians should force patients to use the neglected side. There are no data to substantiate or contradict this idea, but it seems appropriate for working directly on neglect with patients who are

not too severely impaired. As noted above, those with severe deficits may need to establish some scanning or attention channeling behavior with clinicians and materials on the good side of space before facing this kind of challenge. In addition, if neglect per se is not the focus of a particular activity (e.g., treatment for conversational problems), presenting materials from the better side may maximize the likelihood that the patient attends to and perceives the crucial aspects of that activity. However, as always, this kind of decision must be individually determined. Treatment activities should always include the fewest cues and procedural contrivances that the patient can handle, while maintaining acceptably high levels of response accuracy and/or speed.

(10) Finally, it is worth noting here that some pharmacologic treatments for neglect are under exploration. For example, Fleet, Watson, Valenstein, and Heilman (1986) reported that 1 month of treatment with bromocriptine, a dopamine agonist, resulted in improved performance on quantitative tests of neglect for a single patient whose neglect had lasted longer than 6 months (see also Whyte, 1992). Speech-language clinicians can offer valuable contributions to studies like these, by helping, for example, to design appropriate assessments to document patients' pretreatment status; to select both sensitive and functional outcome measures; and to highlight important issues of maintenance, generalization, and social validation.

D. Attention

1. This book has repeatedly noted the potential of attentional impairments to contribute to communicative disturbances after RHD. For example, sustained attention may be important for extended listening, or maintaining continuity of discourse production. Attentional selectivity contributes to processes such as maintaining coherent interpretations, resolving reference, and drawing inferences, by helping to manage the information load that is input to a working memory buffer. Effective control of attentional capacity is involved in keeping track of complicated movie plots, resolving ambiguities, revising interpretations, and resisting distractions. And a number of attentional disturbances tend to correlate with the occurrence of neglect after RHD. If diagnostic testing and informal probes suggest that a variety of communicative symptoms appear to result from some underlying perceptual or cognitive problem, such as impairment of attentional capacity or control, we may be able to achieve a larger payoff in therapy by working on the presumed heart of the deficit, rather than proceeding in a symptom-by-symptom fashion.

2. Treatment for attentional functions, as for other potential cognitive and perceptual underpinnings of communicative difficulties, does not have a long history in speech-language pathology. But for those who believe that improving perceptual and cognitive function may help to roll back problems in other areas, there is no time like the present to initiate some good clinical experimentation. As noted in the section above on neglect treatment, it is important for clinicians to gather evidence of dividends beyond the task and domain being treated, to document treatment effectiveness. And, since other professionals such as occupational therapists or neuropsychologists are often involved in this kind of treatment and often have knowledge and insights that complement those of speech-language clinicians, collaborative efforts are recommended to maximize progress.

3. Earlier portions of this chapter covered treatment for problems with the spatial distribution of attention, considering some factors related to attentional orienting or selectivity and task relevant arousal, and some techniques for focusing attention on an entire stimulus array or spatial region (see V-C-6 on neglect). Other sections of this book contain suggestions for communicative treatment activities and procedures that also target various aspects of attentional channeling and control. Among these are:

   a. treatment activities designed to isolate certain aspects of strategic attentional control, such as distinguishing relevant or central information from that which is irrelevant or nonessential (e.g., II-B-2; II-C; III-D-3 and -4); identifying contextually appropriate interpretations or associations (II-C); and determining priorities about what information to convey or to extract, in relation to presupposition (II-C; III-A through III-D), coherence, and topic manipulation (III-B through III-D).

   b. treatment activities that recombine some of these aspects, by focusing and allocating limited attentional resources in multicomponent tasks. Some examples include drawing connections between probable interpretations or judgments and a given context (II-C); synthesizing stored information with context to resolve ambiguities or discrepancies or to discard or revise inappropriate interpretations (III-C); and conveying or interpreting prioritized information as appropriate, in light of presupposition, coherence, and topic management considerations.

c.   suggestions for capitalizing on relatively automatic processing or otherwise reducing demands on limited capacity. Examples include facilitating and solidifying relatively automatic inferencing and enhancing strategic inference generation (III-C); providing cues or facilitators to minimize demands in treatment activities (e.g., Table 6–3 and accompanying text; Tables 7–1 and 7–2); and limiting the cognitive effort associated with implementing multiple novel compensatory strategies (I-D-6-d; V-C-6-d).

4. When problems of attentional selectivity and control appear to underlie communicative symptoms, it may be beneficial to work directly on facilitating aspects of attention apart from the communicative treatment activities that have already been mentioned.

   a.   Facilitation techniques are most likely to be effective in the acute post-onset phase or with patients whose attentional impairments are relatively mild. Much of section D-5, below, provides an overview of activities and procedures that are aimed at facilitating attentional processing, but compensatory suggestions are included as well.

   b   A number of activities will be described from the Attention Process Training (APT) materials of Sohlberg and Mateer (1986). The APT program is based on a theoretical analysis of attentional functions, and on a process specific approach to cognitive remediation, which assumes, in contrast to general stimulation or strict compensatory rehabilitation approaches, that distinct cognitive deficit areas can be facilitated through specifically targeted treatments. An APT kit provides activities for targeting sustained, selective, alternating, and divided attention, along with scoresheets, administration instructions, and necessary materials. Creative clinicians can generate many extensions and variations of these kinds of activities. Some other possible ideas can be gleaned from materials such as those published by the Rehabilitation Institute of Chicago (Burns, Halper, & Mogil, 1983).

5. For convenience, the discussion about treatment for attentional deficits, below, is organized around specific components of attention. However, many activities and recommendations overlap these

organizational boundaries. Performance data can include any relevant quantitative and qualitative dimensions described in Chapter 6 (section III-A-1), such as numbers or proportions of errors and false alarms, time to completion, and descriptions of error patterns.

a. *Sustained attention activities* focus on the duration and consistency of concentration on relatively simple tasks, such as cancellation or target detection activities in visual or auditory modalities. For people with adequate visual processing systems, the transient nature of auditory stimuli may put more demands on sustained attention than visual stimulation. However, any such difference may be offset for patients who have specific visual processing deficits.

   (1) The APT program includes shape and number cancellation activities that are systematically varied in difficulty, by manipulating factors like the size of the stimulus array, the spacing between stimuli, and the number of targets to be canceled. APT also provides 11 tapes for auditory sustained attention treatment. Eight involve target identification activities that vary in speed and complexity of mental manipulations needed to determine the target; three others require solving arithmetic problems. A serial numbers activity involves mental subtraction. As the demands for mental manipulation increase in these tasks, they are likely to tap other elements of strategic attentional control as well, such as dividing or alternating attention.

   (2) A task like Rizzo and Robin's (1990) Starry Night measure of sustained visuospatial attention (Chapter 4, III-E-3-d) could also be used in treatment. Initially, the stimulus array might include fewer elements, more predictable patterns of target appearance and disappearance, and/or spatial orienting cues to facilitate performance as needed. Along with fading or eliminating these supports, task difficulty could be increased by requiring patients to make a discrimination judgment in order to select an appropriate response (e.g., require different responses to target appearance and target disappearance trials, or to different colors or kinds of target elements). Again, these more difficult manipulations would also increase demands on divided attention (and visual processing).

   (3) Sustained attention can be targeted in a general way, as well, by gradually increasing the length of time spent on relevant treatment activities and by incorporating manipulations designed to minimize attentional fatigue (IV-A).

(4) Patients functioning at very low levels may respond to behavioral programs to shape and reinforce "attentiveness" and duration of on-task behavior (e.g., establishing and maintaining eye contact with the clinician, or orienting body and/or eyes toward task materials, for simple activities with familiar stimuli).

(5) Among the many possible compensations for sustained attention problems are the following: organizing tasks and breaking them into short segments; helping patients develop and practice using check-off forms or charts to insure task completion; scheduling breaks as necessary; or arranging the environment to minimize distractions.

b. *Selective attention* is involved in screening out irrelevant information or otherwise focusing on relevant stimuli, thoughts, and actions. Intervention for spatial selective attention problems, in the context of neglect treatment, has already been considered. More generally, treatment for problems of selective attention can focus on processing in the face of distractions or irrelevancies.

(1) The APT program uses distractor overlays to add "visual noise" to the shape and number cancellation tasks described above for sustained attention treatment. Eight audiotapes contain the same target identification activities described above, embedded in background noise. Sohlberg and Mateer (1989a) recommend individualizing the kinds of distracting stimuli used for selective attention tasks (e.g., sports commentary, television shows, conversation between friends) by creating novel audiotapes. They emphasize that tapes offer more control and comparability from session to session than do typical methods of introducing distractions, such as opening a door to the hallway or turning on a radio. Distractor tapes can also be used with a variety of other activities, ranging from simple localization and discrimination tasks to more complex activities. In general, the level of distraction can be manipulated while task difficulty is kept constant and within the patient's ability; then task complexity can be gradually increased. Features of distractors such as their loudness, duration, physical proximity, and personal salience (e.g., wife's voice vs. one that is less familiar) may influence patients' performance.

(2) Selective attention tasks might also involve asking patients to identify designated target stimuli from larger

sets of numbers, words, or phrases, or from discourse passages. Factors such as the size or length of the stimulus set, the similarity between targets and nontarget distractors, the rate of presentation, and the expected speed of response can be manipulated to influence task difficulty.

(3) Selective attention can also be targeted with Stroop-like activities, that require patients to overcome habitual responses to stimuli containing conflicting features (e.g., color terms printed in incongruous ink colors). Some of the set dependent activities included in the APT program for alternating attention treatment (see below) can be used for this purpose, when presented without the requirements to switch or alternate responses. Sohlberg and Mateer (1989a) also recommend several computer software programs that require patients to inhibit responses during target reaction tasks (e.g., Visual Reaction Stimulus Discrimination 1; Auditory Reaction Stimulus Discrimination; both published by Psychological Software Services, Neuroscience Center of Indianapolis, 6555 Carrollton Avenue, Indianapolis, Indiana, 46220).

(4) A time-honored method for trying to deal with distracting thoughts and worries is to have patients write down or otherwise record their concerns and then set the record aside during treatment activities. Patients can also work on monitoring the frequency of intrusions by distracting thoughts, aiming to reduce the number exhibited in a certain task or time interval. Of course, when internal distractions are extremely upsetting, it will be counterproductive to try to work on specific treatment goals. Counseling and/or referral are in order in such situations.

c. *Alternating attention* is involved in reallocating processing resources for changing task demands. Treatment tasks incorporate repeated shifts in responding.

(1) APT activities focus on shifting attention within tasks. Flexible switching is incorporated into shape and number cancellation tasks by having patients change from canceling one target to another when asked by the clinician or when signaled by cues on the activity worksheets. A similar task requires flexible shifting between adding and subtracting pairs of numbers, as signaled. "Set dependent" activities use Stroop-like stimuli and require patients to switch from one response set to another. For example, the

words "big" and "little" are provided in incongruous sizes, and patients switch from reading the words to indicating their size. Similarly, the words "high" "mid" and "low" are presented on a line in incongruous positions, and patients alternate between reading the words and identifying their positions. As noted earlier, some of the basic "sustained attention" tasks may also tap an internal alternation or division of attentional resources, as their demands for mental manipulation and control increase.

(2) Activities for shifting attention between tasks include some such as those described by Burns and colleagues (1983), which involve moving back and forth between two successful tasks that vary in input modality or output requirements, or shifting from a specific task to an intervening activity (such as a conversation) and then back to the initial task. Patients can also practice alternating between communication partners, within a single task or interaction.

d. *Divided attention* treatment activities typically focus on a patient's ability to carry out two or more tasks or procedures at the same time (but see D-5-e, next, for a broader conceptualization of divided attention). Dual task performance may actually involve very rapid shifts of attention, rather than true simultaneity of processing or response. In any case, some possible tasks are as follows.

(1) The APT program includes a task in which patients respond to auditory attention tapes while concurrently performing cancellation activities. Dual tasks can involve any well practiced activities, which are chosen initially from those that are consistently and successfully performed in isolation, in terms of speed and accuracy. To augment the difficulty of concurrent processing, the complexity or processing requirements of either task can be gradually increased.

(2) Another activity requires attention to several kinds of information in a single task. In APT, patients sort a deck of playing cards by suit, while turning over cards whose names contain a target letter. Again, clinicians should ascertain how successfully and consistently patients can perform each element of this kind of activity in isolation, before combining elements.

(3) Baseline information on speed and accuracy of individual tasks or task components is useful for gauging the deleterious effects of combining tasks and for monitoring progress.

It should be noted here that it is difficult to determine on an a priori basis for individual patients what kinds of tasks or task demands will interfere with each other. For non-brain-damaged adults, nonautomatic tasks that tap similar domains (e.g., language; spatial) or modalities (e.g., auditory) tend to compete with each other more than tasks that differ in these dimensions. For patients, some clinical exploration will probably be needed to design suitable competing tasks.

(4) To maximize attentional power and flexibility, we must be able to divide and allocate our mental resources across a range of priorities. For example, we might decide that two concurrent activities are relatively equal in importance or that one of them should take much greater precedence than the other. This kind of "decision" is often made unconsciously by non-brain-damaged adults. But the priorities in either case, and at various points in between, influence the ways in which we distribute our attentional resources. The published treatment activities just described do not specify priorities for sharing attention among the concurrent tasks. However, patients who can divide their attention to reflect differential task importance may build flexibility by performing tasks like those above with the addition of varying priorities for attention allocation. (See section D-5-e, next, for more on targeting strategic attention allocation.)

e. Some *other considerations related to strategic attentional control* are addressed below.

(1) In this book, the capacity to resist distraction was included in the description of strategic attentional control. Thus, treatments for that aspect of attentional control are similar to those discussed above for the related sense of selective attention. Readers are also reminded that Table 6–2 includes "capacity to resist distraction" as an intermediate goal and provides several examples of possible subordinate, specific goals. Some compensations to minimize distraction by extraneous signals or information, whether implemented by patients or cued by others, include: highlighting important parts of a stimulus or activity; covering up all but small amounts of relevant information; isolating the patient in a quiet and uncluttered area; having the patient wear a headset or earplugs; using a step-by-step checklist or task plan to keep the patient on task; or having

the patient initiate steps such as going to a quieter place or modifying the environment (e.g., closing the door).

(2) Impulsive responding can be targeted for reduction in self-monitoring activities (I-D-2; II-B-2-d, above). To reduce the deleterious effects of impulsivity on performing specific treatment tasks, clinicians can require patients to wait before responding. Eventually, if it is necessary and within their capabilities, patients should take on the responsibility for imposing delays. Clinician and patient can choose a means to signal the fact that the patient must wait to react and/or to indicate when it is okay to initiate a response. Gesturing, counting, tracking elapsed time on a clock, or using audible signals such as vocal instructions are among the many possible cuing options. For severe or persistent problems, it may help to manipulate some aspect of the treatment apparatus to shape response delay (e.g., using software or keyboards that can be time-locked). Some other methods for reducing impulsive responding during treatment include implementing verbal or tactile pacing strategies, or interposing extra requirements between a stimulus request and a desired response, such as searching an entire array, or tracing a stimulus configuration. In general, it is preferable to use the most natural signals and strategies possible, as they can more easily be turned into unobtrusive compensatory reminders.

(3) It was noted previously that multiple mental processes operate to generate a final interpretation or response for communicative tasks (and indeed, most all activities in life; Chapter 2, III-D-8-c). Our limited attentional capacities need to be divided up and parceled effectively for performing and coordinating effortful mental operations and for storing the intermediate results that contribute to a final action or a unified interpretation. These ubiquitous demands for internally divided resources should inform the design and conduct of treatment activities.

(a) Numerous cues and manipulations have been suggested for minimizing simultaneous demands on attentional fuel. Some of these include enhancing perceptual clarity, predictability, coherence or thematic consistency; gearing tasks and interactions to areas of interest, expertise, and processing strength; and reducing linguistic complexity, distractions, ambiguity or apparent disparities, requirements for processing in problem domains, demands for effortful control or complex new learning, and time pressure. Manipulations of this sort can be explored as facilitators or implemented as compensatory adjustments, as appropriate to the level and chronicity of a patient's impairments.

(b) With a view to establishing active compensations to assist with the strategic allocation of attention, it is possible that some high functioning patients can learn to distribute their attention consciously, according to perceived or specified task priorities. This skill would be a precursor to using mental resources most effectively, in light of specific strengths and weaknesses. Patients can work on allocating certain amounts or proportions of their effort to the concurrent performance of two tasks, and later, of various elements within a single task. Before trying such an approach, clinicians should provide an appropriate rationale and assess the patient's understanding of it. Initial activities can involve allocating the bulk of effort to one task that is designated as very important, while all but ignoring the other, designated as not very important at all. Clinicians can instruct and demonstrate that, under dual task conditions, allocating a large proportion of effort to one activity may create errors, or reduce response rate, for another task that one normally does easily. Prior to the patient's turn, clinicians should emphasize that it is fine, and in fact expected, for such disruptions to occur on the secondary task; but in the beginning, patients may need a great deal of encouragement and support to be comfortable with making errors. Gradually, a more even split of mental effort can be requested to work toward the flexible allocation of resources. Patients can also move eventually toward determining how much effort they want to allocate in accordance with priorities. At first, priorities can be specified by the clinician. Later, patients can establish their own priorities, initially on the basis of their analysis of the importance of certain tasks or tasks elements. Importance could be related to message significance or to knowledge of certain kinds of situations or mental processing that may create particular difficulty. Later, patients who are able to judge ongoing social and other environmental feedback and cues can work on setting priorities to reflect their interpretations of those signals.

There are several ways to make these kinds of exercises more concrete initially. For example, patients may be able to conceptualize "sense of effort" using visual feedback such as that derived from a pressure transducer that they squeeze with their hands (Somodi, Robin, & Luschei, in press). Any graphic depiction or biofeedback aid that clearly portrays maximum performance and gradations in between, may serve the same purpose. Visual representations of differing degrees of physical exertion can serve as analogues to the notion of cognitive effort, and clinicians and patients can refer to these representations to help link the concepts of selective physical and mental effort. In addition, beginning with two different tasks may be less abstract than trying to allocate attention to various parts of a single activity.

As noted, a goal of implementing some personal control over attentional allocation is probably most appropriate for relatively high-functioning patients. To use this kind of skill most effectively, patients will need to be able to generate priorities in any of the senses considered above. Somewhat lower-functioning patients, who can determine or, at a minimum, appreciate the concept of priorities, may be able to profit from a few compensatory rules that indicate when they should apply one or two different levels of effort to enhance their performance. This is akin to planning situations or activities that may benefit from momentary compensatory arousal, as discussed next.

f. *Hypoarousal* may also have implications for deriving maximum benefits from treatment and for participating in everyday activities. Tonic arousal deficits are sometimes treated with psychostimulants, which may have their effect on self-monitoring and strategic attentional control rather than simple arousal (Whyte, 1992). Encouraging a patient to take naps, and scheduling important or demanding activities at optimal times of day, may help to compensate for tonic arousal impairments. Facilitators and cues to enhance momentary arousal or compensatory effort include increasing the complexity and importance of the task, or the novelty and salience of the stimuli; and providing performance incentives, alerting signals, and rest breaks. Patients who are capable of recruiting compensatory effort should be counseled, along with their families, that it is impossible to sustain for long periods of time. Such patients may benefit from identifying a few significant activities or situations that call for increased transient arousal, and limiting their compensatory effort to those circumstances.

E. Memory

1. A variety of visual and nonverbal memory deficits have been described that may follow RHD in adults. Speech-language clinicians are unlikely to focus treatment in these areas. However, we may be able to assist patients by recommending compensations, usually involving spared verbal abilities, for difficulties that affect their everyday functioning (e.g., section V-C-5 for route finding). In addition, if we are using visual/nonverbal tasks to work on other cognitive and communicative treatment goals, we can structure the tasks to test the influence of some well-established and potentially facilitating modulators of memory (e.g., see Table 2–11).

2. For patients with verbal memory deficits that interfere with long-term episodic or declarative functions, we may be more likely to invest some treatment time in attempting to boost encoding, storage, and retrieval processes, or to train effective compensations.

   a. Encoding operations are paramount, as the adequacy of encoding has obvious ramifications for storage and retrieval. Improving the allocation and control of attention (see V-D-5) should positively influence input processing. A number of other factors that may enhance encoding and storage, such as prior knowledge and expertise, saliency, and processing for meaning, are listed in Table 2–11. Some additional ways to maximize encoding and storage processes are to use a patient's strongest input modality; simplify and reduce the amount of information to be remembered; chunk input into manageable and meaningful units; mobilize familiar frameworks or organizational schemes (e.g., identifying main ideas, or elements of narrative structure; see also section V-G); and translate what is processed into one's own words. Memory retrieval can be enhanced with prompts and cues, whether generated by patients and noted for later use, or supplied by others at appropriate times.

      (1) Higher-functioning patients may be able to exploit the encoding specificity principle, which captures the empir-

ical observation that recall improves when the purpose and conditions of retrieval match the nature and context of encoding. These patients may benefit from focusing deliberately on some salient features of the external or internal encoding context (e.g., what someone was wearing, what music was playing; how they were feeling, what strategy they decided upon) to develop cues to use at the time of retrieval. Maximal benefit is likely when retrieval cues are not dictated by the clinician; that is, when patients generate their own cues, or when they choose from among various types of cues those that are most meaningful and familiar to them.

(2) Other internal association strategies can boost memory retrieval as well, perhaps by increasing the amount and depth of mental activity devoted to encoding the items that are to be remembered or by connecting those items with something that is already known. Such strategies include creating images, developing stories that incorporate the material to be remembered, or generating mnemonic devices (e.g., first letter acronyms, or rhyme sequences, to which the target information is linked). Since some of these strategies, particularly mnemonic approaches, may compartmentalize the material to be learned rather than relating it to what is already known, they may be more useful for short-term than for longer-term purposes.

(3) Despite the reliability of the encoding specificity effect for non-brain-damaged adults, it should be apparent that the need to focus on retrieval cues while processing for meaning may place a heavy burden on mental resources and thus may not be appropriate for many patients who are more than mildly impaired. And internal association strategies in general are probably too mentally taxing to be advantageous for all but a few mildly affected patients, unless those strategies were naturally learned and well-established before the patient's neurological insult and are still familiar and effective afterwards. Studies in which patients have been trained to use internal associations show that treatment effects tend to be short-lived and limited to the stimuli and contexts trained. In addition, the strategies and examples used in training often bear little resemblance to circumstances likely to be confronted in the real world. For all of these reasons, external strategies and memory aids are preferred in many cases (see also Sohlberg & Mateer, 1989a, and Wilson, 1992).

b. External aids include systems for storing or for cuing the retrieval of information, and environmental modifications. Among the devices that can be used to store information externally are lists, calendars, address books, microcassette recorders, notebooks, diagrams, pocket computers, phone dialers, and other electronic memories. External cuing devices include watches and electronic diaries with data banks and alarms, which can be programmed to provide appointment reminders or other instructions, such as telling a patient to consult some other external source of information. For specific domestic, recreational, or vocational tasks, patients may benefit from the structure provided by individualized checklists with steps numbered by priority or in the most efficient sequence, or by computerized programs that provide step-by-step performance prompts. Parente and Anderson-Parente (1990) describe some successful applications of such devices with brain-injured patients, and Wilson (1992) provides helpful guidelines for selecting, evaluating, and training the use of these kinds of external aids (see also Sohlberg and Mateer, 1989a, for training acquisition, application, and adaptation of memory notebooks). As with any compensatory strategy, patients' attitudes are important, and it may be necessary to demonstrate to them the benefits of using external aids (see I-D-2-e on strategy training). For patients with severe and persistent memory impairments, environmental modifications to supplement structured prompting systems may be most appropriate. Such modifications might include posting prominent labels and notes (and systematically directing patients' attention to them, per section V-B-2), or putting others in charge of remembering.

3. Many of the external aids mentioned above can be used to ameliorate problems with prospective memory, or remembering to do something at a future time. Sohlberg and Mateer (1989b) designed a prospective memory training program that involves extending, gradually, the time interval between a target goal and a specified response. Patients are assigned a target task, such as handing the clinician a pencil, and a time cue or an associative prompt that will be used to signal task initiation (e.g., in 10 minutes; when the alarm sounds). At more difficult levels, patients carry out a distractor task during the waiting period. There are some preliminary data regarding this program's effectiveness with a few traumatically brain-injured patients. However, a compensatory approach that allows rapid generalized improvement may be preferable, due to ubiquitous limitations on rehabilitation time, and is certainly possible, given the naturalness and power of many external prompting devices.

4. Working memory capacity or efficiency may be related to a number of RHD patients' cognitive and communicative symptoms. It is not likely that capacity per se can be augmented in brain-damaged patients, but treatment may influence the efficient use of their capacity.

    a. Factors that can influence demands for limited capacity resources have been amply discussed (e.g., Tables 6–3 and 7–3 and their associated text; also this chapter sections V-D-3, V-D-5; etc.) Among the many ways to reduce demands on simultaneous information processing and storage are:

        (1) foster automaticity of mental operations and strategy application, through practice, overlearning, and repeated opportunities to activate and apply targeted knowledge and processes in a variety of activities and situations. Habituated routines, whether or not they achieve the status of automaticity, will require fewer mental resources than less well-established processes and thus will not interfere as much with other cognitive demands when they are implemented.

        (2) provide adequate orienting tasks, prestimulation, and practice. These procedures may help patients to access the generally appropriate neighborhoods in their mental knowledge networks, to figure out how to get started on a new task, and/or to lay an initial foundation for building a coherent interpretation. Some mildly affected patients can be moved toward generating their own orienting processes and practice procedures by drawing analogies with more familiar tasks or processing requirements.

        (3) decrease rate of presentation by providing more time at critical junctures. Increased processing time may allow a patient's working memory system to coordinate the distribution and cycling of resources more effectively, in light of pervasive problems with rapid information processing. If the mental operations needed for certain tasks are consistently accurate when processing time is unlimited, (e.g., drawing certain kinds of inferences), treatment might target speed by incorporating practice in facilitative contexts with gradually increasing time pressure.

        (4) decrease inferential complexity, and the need to backtrack or to integrate initially disparate information (particularly

over long stretches of text); and increase factors such as stimulus discriminability, thematic redundancy, and foregrounding of salient information (to assist with maintenance and integration in a working memory buffer). These modifications, like decreasing time pressure, should reduce the computational load imposed on the patient.

(5) chunk units of text, and implement compensations to assist patients in looking back over what has come before, such as making notes or drawings to represent an unfolding output plan or interpretation. These kinds of procedures may help to decrease working memory storage load.

(6) exploit, and increase when possible, a patient's relevant knowledge. Information from overlearned or expert knowledge domains is likely to be well-integrated in long-term memory and retrieved into working memory as integrated packets. In terms of capacity theories, such packets take relatively little fuel to retrieve and to maintain in working memory, but accessing them brings to light much that may be relevant for constructing interpretations or performance plans. [Be aware, however, that when goals or task demands are not entirely consistent with overlearned knowledge that is retrieved, RHD adults may have some difficulty suppressing that which is less relevant and thus may err by making familiar responses that are not quite appropriate in the task context; see 4-b, next].

(7) compensate to the extent possible for basic processing inefficiencies, or anything that degrades the input signal. Impaired "lower-level" sensory, perceptual, or attentional processing can provide bad data to and/or disrupt the timing of higher level mental operations.

b. As noted previously, Kimberg and Farah (1993) conceptualize "dysexecutive" deficits as problems that arise from impaired connections between various working memory representations that generate competing activations (e.g., environmental stimulus characteristics, stored knowledge, and behavior goals). Thus, potentially incomplete or contextually less relevant sources of activation may not be appropriately modulated and may interfere with or override a contextually appropriate response.

Kimberg and Farah's proposal has intuitive appeal to account for many RHD patients' difficulties with tasks that lend themselves to alternative interpretations or responses, as does Gernsbacher's conceptualization of the importance of suppression mechanisms (see Chapter 2, II-B-5-d). These ideas point us to an intervention possibility that we have considered, in part, several times previously in this chapter. That is, it may be useful to work with patients on identifying the various sources of information (internal and external) that can determine a response and on resolving apparent conflicts among those sources for differing types of stimuli, knowledge, and goals. Treatment could revolve around tasks like those suggested for working on attentional flexibility, ambiguous pragmatic forms, or discourse and conversational coherence (sections V-D-5-c, II-B and II-C, III). Using such tasks, patient and clinician can diagram or represent in some other fashion the possible alternative interpretations or misleading features of the stimuli, the patient's most typical response on confronting such stimuli, and the goals imposed by the task context. Then through discussion and evaluation of the inconsistencies among these elements, clinician and patient can analyze the ways in which routine responses (or familiar stimulus configurations) must sometimes be overridden (or re-evaluated) in light of specific goals. A number of suggestions were made previously for activities that focus on drawing connections between ostensibly disparate sources of information (see, e.g., II-B, II-C, III).

c.   Graphic representations of the sort mentioned earlier (II-A-3-c; III-B-1-b) may also be useful for fostering compensatory allocation of resources (V-D-5-d and V-D-5-e). Such representations would help to concretize the notion of an activated memory with a limited capacity. Discussion and demonstration can focus on the fact that the system can contain or manage only so much information within its boundaries at any point in time. The information that falls within the boundaries of the system is most easily available for drawing connections among competing possibilities and for planning responses. In addition, patients can be tuned into the consequences of various kinds of system overload. For example, when information comes along too fast, or when there is simply too much to interpret at one time, especially when some of it suggests competing interpretations, some critical information may be crowded out. One possibility when crucial information leaves the center of focus in the active system is that it may be irretrievable. Another possibility is that displaced information can be found again. However, searching for it, and trying to reconnect it with other concepts in focus, will divert some attention from those other concepts, potentially to their detriment. Thus, notions like limited capacity and information displacement can be coupled with the idea of strategically allocating attention (V-D-5-d and V-D-5-e) to manage complicated processing tasks. Patients who are metacognitively aware may benefit from a conscious, step-by-step approach to cognitive processing, gleaning one source of information at a time (e.g., context, goal, etc.) and making notes or diagrams to keep track of what they have worked out, before turning their attention to some other processing requirement and finally linking up the various pieces of the puzzle. At first, patients can work with permanent stimulus records, like video- or audiotapes, that allow them to replay and refocus their processing on various components of a task. Stimuli and tasks can be designed initially to minimize the demands for processes other than those involved in successively generating partial information that will contribute to the final interpretation (e.g., by presenting familiar topics, thematic cues, clearly interpretable forms, and brief uncomplicated sentences with little time pressure).

5. The final memory decrement that can be associated with RHD is metamemory impairment. Problems with metamemory can accompany the normal aging process, and may reflect as well the broader awareness deficits frequently exhibited by RHD adults. Treatment can focus on enhancing awareness, as described earlier (II-B-2-d), and particularly on developing some recognition of occasions that call for strategies or compensations (emergent awareness).

F. Integration Processes

1. Various types of integration difficulties also characterize RHD adults, and treatment suggestions for a variety of domains have already been described. For example, visuoperceptual synthesis and integration are discussed in section V-C-4. Linguistic integration at the discourse level is covered in section III (e.g., achieving cohesion and coherence; generating various kinds of inferences; seeing relationships; detecting and expressing main concepts or themes). The social skills aspects of integration, involving sensitivity to listener and situation or seeing the big picture, are considered in sections II-C-5, III-A-4, and III-D-3. And the Pragmatics section more generally (II-B, II-C) describes many activities aimed at helping patients to integrate possible interpretations with contextual constraints.

2. All such tasks require integration processes. However, it is not known for whom, or how often, deficits in these different areas will co-occur, or whether treatment at one level can generalize to another. These are important questions, that call for continued observation and experimentation.

G. Planning, Organization, Reasoning, and Problem Solving

1. As noted previously, these complex, multifaceted, and highly interactive areas of cognition depend on, and influence, multiple aspects of mental processing and behavior execution. In every section of this chapter, various organizing schemes and problem-solving strategies have been endorsed as potential facilitators or compensatory guides. Recommendations to involve patients, to the extent that they are able, in goal-setting, self-monitoring, self-evaluation, and self-instruction, also reflect the key role of the executive system in treatment and transfer.

2. A number of cautions have been raised regarding the assessment of planning, organization, reasoning and problem-solving skills (Chapter 4, III-E-7; Chapter 2, III-G). These caveats apply to designing treatment as well and relate primarily to the influence of premorbid knowledge and style on performance; problems of generalization associated with the domain specificity of abstract planning, organizational, reasoning or problem-solving practice; and the apparent disconnection between decontextualized measures of these functions and their application in daily life situations. Based on caveats such as these, Ylvisaker and Szekeres (1994) argue convincingly for treatment approaches that target practical thinking and reasoning skills, in meaningful contexts, rather than those that aim to "exercise" component abilities in decontextualized activities. All too often, workbook-type exercises form the focus of treatment in these areas. Tasks patterned after available assessment tools (Table 4–9) target, for example, higher-order inferencing, strategy formation, flexibility, self-regulation, evaluation of outcome, and other abstraction and reasoning activities; without connecting target operations and activities to patients' individual processing strengths and weaknesses, or practical needs. The line taken by Ylvisaker and Szekeres, based on theory, data, and experience, is that abstract exercises of this sort are unlikely to effect meaningful and generalizable changes.

3. In addition, it makes sense to integrate treatment for planning, organization, reasoning and problem solving with that for other

cognitive and communicative impairments to the extent that it is possible, in light of the intersections among these functions, and given increasing pressures on rehabilitation time. Many of the treatment activities already discussed in this chapter provide opportunities for demonstrating the benefits of aids to organization, problem solving and the like, and as such create a springboard for more focused work in these areas when it is deemed appropriate. Further, a number of strategies and guides initiated early in treatment may be modifiable for more permanent use as compensatory aids, if necessary.

4. Treatment for organizational and planning difficulties.

   a. Ylvisaker and Szekeres recommend building from patients' knowledge of familiar organizing principles, such as those associated with narrative schema, or common event and procedure scripts. In addition, if overlearned organizing principles are inapplicable or unavailable, patients can work on imposing their own organizational patterns. Treatment tasks should be related to patients' domestic, social, vocational, and recreational goals and activities. Table 7–6 adapts some of Ylvisaker and Szekeres' ideas on organizing schemes and associated treatment activities, and extends some of the questions that they use to prompt patients' self-analyses. Of course, any of the task guides and organizers recommended earlier in this chapter (e.g., graphic representations for discourse organization and coherence; other specifically tailored memory aids) can be presented with probe questions like those in Table 7–6, to encourage patients' reflections, suggestions, and evaluations.

      (1) Clinicians can also create a variety of other possible treatment tasks associated with daily activities such as planning, preparing, and cleaning up from a meal; doing yardwork; or sorting clothes in preparation for doing the laundry. For the laundry example, patients could be given a list of items to be washed, each of which is described in terms of several salient features (e.g., type of fabric, fabric color, colorfastness, amount of dirt). Patients could specify which items might be put together to form loads of laundry, and/or which might be kept out for the dry cleaners, using the salient features as guides. The caveat about premorbid individual differences in approach is particularly salient for this laundry example: This world must contain an uncountable number of originally white

Table 7–6. Some organizational schemes and sample treatment activities.

Scheme: Discourse Structure (e.g., main idea/topic; narrative schema)

Task/goal	Summarize a current event for a pragmatics group.
Activity	Watch/listen to taped news item. Complete forms to identify themes or main ideas, and to indicate Who, What, When, Where, Why, and What happened. Relate to listeners, using the diagram as needed.

Scheme: General Life Scripts (abstracted common life events)

Task/goal	Create autobiographies to keep on track for introducing ourselves to new group members.
Activity	Complete a form with labelled boxes for common life events (birth, school, marriage, job) and other significant personal events (e.g., stroke, other unique information). Use form as a guide to generate organized information to present.

Scheme: Specific Event Scripts (e.g., doctor visit; card game)

Task/goal	Explain to (a child) what a doctor visit is like
Activity	Fill in form with information to convey, such as who will be there, expected events, expected layout of the room, and some variations if possible. Use guide to explain to a small child, or to carry out a role-play activity.

Possible Reflections for All Such Activities

How does the form help you? Should we add anything to it? Can we take something off of the form? How did you choose to organize your explanation or response (e.g., chronologically; by salience)? What other activities would the form be useful for? When wouldn't the form help?

Source: Adapted from Ylvisaker and Szekeres (1994).

Note: This table excludes examples of organizing approaches based on perceptual and semantic similarity, function, and narrative schema, which are also presented by Ylvisaker and Szekeres.

socks that have emerged pink or blue from a mixed load of laundry.

(2) With higher-functioning patients, one might work on combining tasks and elements of the sort included in the table to create an integrated plan. For example, patients could be asked to prioritize, sequence, and plan how much time to allow for various activities in a series of specific event scripts, such as those associated with an afternoon of errands (e.g., buying gas, getting groceries,

shopping for birthday cards, keeping a dentist's appointment, picking up books at the library, making bank transactions). Initially, a few errands could be presented, each associated with only one or two subgoals (e.g., pick up milk and eggs at the store; open a new account at the bank). Potential obstacles to various plans could be introduced gradually, some of which can be anticipated from the situation presented (e.g., typically busy times at the supermarket) and some of which cannot (e.g., a long line at the gas station; the store is out of an item that is needed).

(3) For persistent deficits, or for particular difficulty in marshaling an organized approach in unfamiliar circumstances, individually structured flowcharts, outlines that indicate topic super- and subordination, or other graphic representations may be valuable as compensatory organizing or planning aids. Of course, patients' degrees of independence in using these kinds of aids compensatorily will depend on, among other things, their levels of awareness (see II-B-2-d). But any patients who profit from organizational structure may benefit from work using these kinds of approaches at some level. Their efforts may be relatively passive and cued by others in the environment; or more strategic, invoking organized approaches when they are not provided, or consulting individualized checklists and other guides as external aids.

b. Other types of organizing schemes, such as alphabetizing and categorizing, are often the focus of treatment workbooks. These kinds of strategies may be appropriate for some practical tasks that have personal utility for the patient, such as arranging information in an address book, or organizing recipes, kitchen implements, or workshop tools. In addition, as noted earlier, practice in generating and using various kinds of organizational structure is often incorporated in treatment for other typical communicative and cognitive deficits. To give just a few examples, patients may work on categorizing the kinds of signals that listeners use to indicate their interest in a conversation, as opposed to their desire to terminate it (III-D); sorting relevant or central information from less relevant information about given topics or tasks (II-B-2-c, III-B-1, III-C-5, III-D-3 and -4); or consulting organizational strategies for reading and writing (IV-C). Sorting and categorizing schemes can also be built into the day of errands activity, described just above, by having patients group together the kinds of things that they need to get according to the places where they can be found, or to categorize by locale, those places that are closest to home, closest to the dentist's office, and so forth, as a prelude to planning the most logical or efficient sequence of events.

c. Other practical reasoning and problem-solving activities, as described next, also assist with developing plans and imposing organization on patients' thinking and behavior.

5. Treatment for reasoning and problem-solving deficits.

a. For the treatment of reasoning and problem solving, Ylvisaker and Szekeres emphasize an organized approach to identifying, clarifying, and analyzing relevant problems, as well as exploring and evaluating possible solutions (see Table 7–7). This kind of approach makes deliberate use of the front-end analyses performed by effective problem-solvers. It also involves a variety of reasoning and executive skills, such as convergent and divergent thinking, analogical reasoning, classification, planning, monitoring, and evaluation. Ylvisaker and Szekeres recommend group discussion and practice as a useful way to maximize the potentially helpful input, coaching, and feedback that can flow from peers.

b. Ylvisaker and Szekeres also underscore the need to help patients become aware of their specific strengths and weaknesses in problem-solving activities so that they can capitalize on strengths and minimize their liabilities. For example, in interpreting pragmatic signs and signals, patients may be able to learn to discount their least reliable channels for evaluating nonverbal, emotional, and other social behavior, and rather to rely on their stronger channels, along with checking their interpretations with others (e.g., see II-C). Patients who depend heavily on particularly deficient skills or unproductive approaches can work on self-monitoring and on substituting alternative, less habitual approaches (I-D-2).

c. On the basis of research in cognitive psychology, Ashcraft (1989) summarizes heuristics and strategies that may improve problem solving and reasoning. Some of these are included in the Ylvisaker and Szekeres framework. Among the most important are suggestions to decrease problem difficulty by increasing knowledge in the problem domain, automating parts of the solution, and following a systematic plan. Other potentially beneficial suggestions include:

Table 7–7. Format for organized approach to problem solving.

1. **Problem Identification:** "Briefly, what is the problem?"
   "What do you need to accomplish?"
   "What are some of the differences between the result that you want, and your current situation?" (perhaps diagrammed as Points A and B)

2. **Problem Classification:** "What kind of problem is this?"
   "Is it similar to other situations you have faced?"

3. **Goal Identification** "What will you gain by solving the problem?"

4. **Identification of Relevant Information:** "Do you have any experience with problems like this that could be helpful?"
   "What do you need to know about, or to count on, or to use, to solve this problem?"

5. **Identification of Possible Solutions:** "What things could you possibly do to solve this problem?"

6. **Evaluation of Solutions:** "What is good or bad about each of these possibilities?"
   CONSIDER: Effective? Able to do it? Enough time? Like to do it? Break any rules? Worked in the past? Effects on others? Yourself? The environment?

7. **Decision:** "What is the smartest thing to do?"

8. **Formulation of a Plan:** "How do you plan to accomplish this?"
   CONSIDER: Steps, sequence, potential barriers.

9. **Monitoring and Evaluating the Outcome:** "Did your plan work?"
   "Are you satisfied?"
   "Any new problems encountered?"

Source: Adapted from Ylvisaker, M. S., & Szekeres, S. F. (1994). Communication disorders associated with closed head injury. In R. Chapey (Ed.), *Language Intervention Strategies in Adult Aphasia* (3rd ed., pp. 546–567). Copyright ©1994 by Williams & Wilkins. Used with permission.

(1) draw and examine inferences, such as determining less obvious aspects or properties of a situation to avoid an overly narrow perspective, or identifying unwarranted assumptions that might be interfering with the generation of a solution attempt.

(2) develop subgoals by breaking problems into smaller parts, a process that forms the core of a means-end analysis. Means-end analysis is a common problem-solving approach that involves repeated cycling through the following steps: setting a goal or subgoal, identifying differences between the current circumstances and the goal, and finding ways to reduce or eliminate those differences. For real-life problems with complicated or vague goals, new subgoals may continue to emerge as original ones are being worked on.

    (3) search for contradictions or unalterable obstacles to help rule out potential solutions.

    (4) search for relations, or analogies, to other problems that are familiar or that have been solved previously.

    (5) reformulate the problem representation by thinking about the situation in less habitual ways, or reordering the givens.

    (6) represent the problem physically by diagramming, verbalizing, or moving about the constituent elements.

    d. Readers are reminded that some treatment suggestions for social problem-solving deficits were considered earlier in this chapter (II-C-5-c).

    6. As always when treatment is focused primarily on one set of processes or goals (e.g., reasoning and problem solving), clinicians can manipulate other factors that tend to influence overall cognitive demands in treatment activities, such as rate or pacing requirements, the presence and nature of distractions or other competing demands, the explicitness and coherence of language used in the problem descriptions, and the extent of structure and specificity of cuing provided to the patient.

VI. OTHER BEHAVIORAL DEFICITS

A. Treatment suggestions have already been described for most of the *other behavioral deficits* originally listed in Chapter 2.

    1. For example, impulsivity, distractibility, and difficulty switching sets are covered in section V (part D) on attentional control.

    2. Error awareness is discussed extensively in section II-B-2-d. An apparent lack of motivation may be related to anosognosia (V-A) and poor error awareness (II-B-2-d).

    3. A discrepancy between knowing and doing is considered in the material on emergent awareness (II-B-2-d) and metamemory (V-E-5). If such a discrepancy results in poor judgment, making a patient potentially dangerous (e.g., patients may plan to continue driving despite knowing that they have been advised to give it up), some intervention options include determining and discussing together possible hazards; showing a film or book that highlights potential consequences; establishing a peer counselor or role model; enlisting someone else, who the patient respects, to explain and insist on restrictions; trying behavioral methods of reward and punishment, either tangible or social; and/or increasing supervision and limiting access to dangerous situations. Patients who develop intellectual awareness of such dangers, and who are amenable, can be trained to check their judgment with others.

4. Finally, a focus on rate of processing and responding can be built into any of the activities in this chapter. Indeed, rate variables have been suggested as factors to manipulate as part of a treatment progression, initially to facilitate performance and gradually to make tasks more difficult (e.g., Table 6–3). Generally, slow responding should not be a great concern until patients develop consistently accurate performance. As accuracy stabilizes at any level of task difficulty, efficiency can be targeted in the ways most appropriate for individual patients (e.g., reducing number or duration of pauses; reducing the interval before requiring a response).

B. Post-stroke depression is often treated with medication, though pharmacotherapy should only be part of an overall approach to depression management. Clinicians should be particularly alert for potential cognitive side effects of some antidepressant medications, especially tricyclics. Cognitive therapy, behavioral therapy, and psychotherapy are reported to be promising alternatives to pharmacotherapy, but these approaches tend to require considerable insight on the part of the patient. Electroconvulsive therapy may also be used, particularly for patients who are resistant to antidepressant regimens, and for whom there is high suicide risk. Some authors emphasize that depression may be ameliorated by the enhanced self-esteem that derives naturally from an increasing sense of ability as patients receive post-stroke counseling, support, and treatment to minimize their functional handicaps. Peer support groups may also be valuable for helping patients to accept their new limitations and themselves as people and to learn other ways of coping with obstacles that may confront them. Clinicians who suspect depression, either major or transient, should refer patients to a rehabilitation psychologist or other medical specialist who is particularly versed in post-stroke depression. Appropriate intervention options for individual patients will depend on a variety of factors, including the nature of the diagnosis, its expected course, and potential side effects of treatment. However, it is probably safe to say that clinicians who observe signs of evident discouragement and frustration in their patients would not often err in exploring and acknowledging the clients' feelings, and in helping them to focus on their remaining skills and abilities.

CHAPTER

8

Other Roles in Patient Management

I. INTRODUCTION

Speech-language pathologists are responsible for much more than the direct communication assessment and treatment activities that have been discussed thus far. Brain damage has a variety of physical, medical, behavioral, and psychosocial consequences, each set of which may amplify the others. These multiple and interacting problems necessitate a coordinated and comprehensive plan of care to maximize each patient's quality of life. Clinicians in rehabilitation settings typically function as central members of an interdisciplinary patient care team. Clinicians in any setting invariably take on educational and counseling functions as well. This chapter reviews briefly our involvement in these important activities.

II. THE INTERDISCIPLINARY TEAM

A. Team Composition and Team Members

The composition of the patient care team will vary for each patient. The team should include the patient and his or her significant others in goal-setting and evaluation, whenever possible. The responsible physician (typically a physiatrist) often leads the team, which may also include representatives from the disciplines of occupational therapy, physical therapy, social work, nursing, psychology (clinical psychology, rehabilitation psychology, neuropsychology), therapeutic recreation, vocational rehabilitation, audiology, and speech-language pathology.

1. A physiatrist is a specialist in rehabilitation medicine. Occupational, physical, and recreation therapists work under a physiatrist's supervision and orders.

2. The occupational therapist (OT) is typically responsible for training to maximize patients' performance of the activities of daily living (ADLs), such as dressing, grooming, eating, or cooking. OTs have special training in sensorimotor and perceptual functioning and in the design and use of adaptive tools and appliances. In some facilities, OTs provide cognitive therapy and vocational consultation.

3. A physical therapist (PT) is involved with evaluating and training muscle strength and range of movement, posture, gait, balance, and ambulation. PTs also provide consultation for outfitting a patient's home with adaptive equipment for special needs.

4. The social worker acts as a liaison between patients, families, facilities, and community agencies and services. The social worker takes charge of evaluating social support and recommending discharge options; arranges for in-home therapies, ADL assistance, or social service programs like Meals on Wheels; and assists with financial inquiries and arrangements. Some social workers also provide patient and family counseling.

5. In an inpatient setting, nursing staff have direct responsibility for implementing and monitoring day-to-day care. Because nurses are so intimately involved with each patient's care, they may be the first to observe changes in functioning, either positive or negative, that are of interest to the rest of the team.

6. A clinical psychologist or rehabilitation psychologist may be involved when the patient and/or family requires help with psychosocial consequences of the stroke, such as depression, grief, fear, frustration, embarrassment, and anger. Psychologists may also be able to assist patients and families in adjusting to the disruptions in established role performance, activity, and social involvement that can antedate stroke.

7. Neuropsychologists are trained to assess cognitive and perceptual abilities. Neuropsychologists and rehabilitation psychologists con-

tribute information to the team about the cognitive and perceptual bases of impaired functioning and about estimated premorbid abilities. They may also play a role in estimating prognoses for employability, learning potential, and independent living ability. Some neuropsychologists and rehabilitation psychologists provide cognitive rehabilitation services as well.

8. Recreation specialists focus on maximizing social interaction and productive use of leisure time. They work with patients and families to increase awareness about the importance of social and leisure pursuits, and teach them how to use community and personal resources to optimize social and leisure participation.

9. Vocational rehabilitation experts will be involved in team planning when returning to work is a viable goal. They are responsible for assessing work tolerance, identifying vocational skills that are compatible with current abilities, recommending appropriate vocational goals, conducting job analyses, and arranging and evaluating job placements.

10. Audiologists are responsible for evaluating all aspects of hearing function and for recommending rehabilitative strategies, where appropriate. The correspondence of advancing age with hearing loss, as well as stroke, means that stroke and hearing impairment will often co-occur, necessitating the services of an audiologist.

11. Patients and their families should be integral members of the team, to the extent that it is possible.

    a. As emphasized previously in this book, patients should contribute to rehabilitation goal setting, when they are sufficiently aware of their deficits to do so. Patients and families can be valuable sources of information about problems and solutions that may not be obvious on testing, or in the rehabilitation environment. Patients should be consulted periodically about their satisfaction with the services they are receiving as well. And it is particularly important that they are involved in planning for discharge so that there are no surprises when the time comes.

    b. Similarly, patients' family members have a great stake in determining goals and plans for their relatives. As noted in Chapter 3 (II-F), family members' concerns need to be addressed in some manner, whether or not they form appropriate rehabilitation goals.

    c. In consulting with a patient's family, professional team members need to be cognizant of the potential importance of prior relationships and personality characteristics. When relationships between patient and family are positive, family members can serve valuable roles as, for example, resources for information about patients' preferences and abilities, advocates for patients' rights and needs, incentives for patients' rehabilitation efforts, and generalization agents. Much more tricky to handle are dysfunctional relationships between patients and family members, many of which exist long before a stroke occurs. Poor prior relationships may result in family members feeling burdened and resentful when asked to participate in the patient's rehabilitation program, or in emphasizing their own best interests rather than the patient's when they do contribute. Family members' personality characteristics are important, too, because some (e.g., extreme overprotectiveness or hypercritical nature) may inhibit a patient's progress. When personalities or relationship issues might impede learning, generalization, or optimal adaptation, patients and/or family members should be referred for appropriate counseling.

B. Contributions of Speech-Language Pathologists to the Rehabilitation Team

The speech-language pathologist (SLP) contributes to the team by providing information about current and expected levels of cognitive-communicative functioning, intermediate and immediate goals, and specific strategies or compensations that other team members should note and reinforce in other contexts. The SLP can also assist other team members in interacting with patients, by making recommendations about effective ways to structure instructions and treatment materials (in terms of, e.g., explicitness, modalities, processing time, attention and memory demands) based on each patient's information processing capabilities. In long-term care settings, SLPs may need to provide diplomatic advice about the adequacy of the communication setting (see Lubinski, 1991, for discussion of the communication-impaired environment found in some long-term care settings).

C. Contributions of Other Team Members to Speech-Language Pathologists

The other team members provide SLPs with useful information about how patients function in different environments and tasks. For instance,

OTs and PTs can note a patient's ability to sustain attention during ADL or ambulation training, or whether that patient initiates compensatory strategies that SLPs have targeted in treatment. Similarly, family members can observe performance on targeted skills in functional interactions. Other team members can also assist in promoting generalization of treated skills, when guided by the SLP. For example, recreational specialists may take patients on community outings. These may provide generalization training opportunities, as well as contexts for evaluating transfer. Furthermore, team members' knowledge of a patient's skills and abilities may contribute to a thorough communication needs assessment. For instance, the vocational counselor's job analysis, or the family member's information on leisure interests, can help us select functional training contexts and tasks.

D. Discrepant Reports from Team Members

Discrepant reports from various team members are possible, and these require further analysis. If differences between team members' evaluations are based on valid and reliable assessments of a particular patient's abilities, we will want to change something about our own treatment, or to suggest appropriate modifications to other team members, to optimize that patient's performance in all contexts.

1. Discrepancies can occur that do not reflect valid or reliable performance differences, when, for example, different team members provide information based on (a) unreliable rating scales, (b) identification of poorly defined behaviors, (c) performance in insufficiently controlled elicitation tasks or contexts, or (d) observations of target behaviors made without adequate instruction and training. Subjective biases and hopes can also affect ratings and judgments and may result in discrepancies between team members. For example, it may be difficult for family members or treating clinicians to provide ratings that are uninfluenced by a desire to note improvement after treatment has begun, whether or not that desire is conscious.

2. Valid discrepancies often occur because team members simply cannot evaluate patients' performance in all relevant contexts or tasks. When team members reporting discrepancies can minimize or rule out invalid influences such as those noted above, they should try to analyze context differences that may suggest what factors are facilitating or impeding performance in various situations.

III. PATIENT AND FAMILY EDUCATION AND COUNSELING

A. Major Adjustments for Patients and Families

Stroke can necessitate major adjustments for patients and families alike, as it has many potential effects on daily life. Because stroke is an unpredictable, uncontrollable event with an uncertain outcome, it is especially stressful, and adjustment is particularly difficult. The patient and each person in the patient's circle must often make unplanned and unwanted changes in many aspects of life.

1. If patients are aware of their condition, they may feel perplexity about what has happened to them, fear about a brush with death, worry that they are losing their minds, embarrassment over physical changes, frustration at being less quick or less able in other ways than before the stroke, grief over lost abilities, anxiety about returning to former levels of functioning, or anger with God for letting this happen or with the world in general (including therapists) for perceived and real indignities. Depression is also a frequent problem when patients are aware of their deficits. Fatigue is common, as activities that were once automatic may take much planning and effort to accomplish. Patients may cope unproductively, as well, by withdrawing from social contact with others, refusing to participate in treatment, and/or relying on one particular person to meet all of their needs.

2. Family members may experience many of these same reactions, with the patient usually at the center of their concern. If they do feel resentment or anger about the sudden or drastic changes in their own lives, these feelings are often associated with guilt for having such uncharitable thoughts. For RHD patients who lack insight into their deficits, though, family members can face a special kind of anxiety and frustration. These patients may refuse to give up activities like driving and may resist supervision in other areas, even when the family is extremely concerned about safety. These patients, believing that nothing is wrong with them, also frequently refuse to attend evaluation, treatment, or counseling sessions. So in addition to their concerns about safety and judgment, family members may worry that the patient will not receive the necessary help.

3. Some family members wrap themselves up in the stroke patient's problems, neglecting to look out for their own mental health. Rehabilitation professionals can unwittingly reinforce this behavior by looking to the family to assist with the patient's adjustment,

without considering that the family members may be having adjustment crises whether or not they are admitting to them. Of course, individuals cope in different ways, so the professional members of the rehabilitation team should not judge any particular coping style as maladaptive without assessing its relationship to psychosocial or physical distress.

4. It is always important to keep in mind that psychosocial responses to a condition like stroke can be exacerbated by preexisting problems (e.g., marital discord; difficulties adjusting to retirement or to the death of someone close). Some premorbid problems, especially those with relationships, are not likely to diminish without counseling intervention, whereas some of the stroke-related adjustment difficulties may improve with time.

B. Ongoing Processes of Education and Counseling

Education and counseling are ongoing processes for both patient and family.

1. Early on, we need to provide information about the nature of the patient's impairments and the recovery process; to make clear our best guesses about meaningful prognoses; to indicate whether or not treatment is warranted and if so, what kinds of changes we expect to be able to effect to improve communication performance; and to estimate the timeframe anticipated for effecting those changes. It is also important to emphasize that "normality" or "the way I did it before" is not a realistic goal after a stroke that is serious enough to warrant cognitive-communicative treatment. We need to be attuned as well to patients' and families' concerns, sometimes expressed only indirectly, so that we can calm their fears or direct them to useful information. However, we also need to be sensitive to the fact that people can absorb only so much at any one time, especially in periods of stress, and that they will filter what they hear according to their own experiences and fears. Patients and families often need to "hear" the "same" information on a number of different occasions before they begin to understand or to accept it.

2. Some educational concerns will be specific to families of patients with RHD. For example, when patients deny obvious deficits, family members need to be advised that they cannot force the patients into awareness through argument or confrontation. That will only increase frustration for the one doing the confronting. For particular-

ly troubling behavioral consequences of RHD, such as crude humor, other inappropriate remarks, or egocentricity, family members may also be educated about the application of behavior modification techniques (e.g., time out or redirecting strategies). And if neglect or poor judgment raise concerns about safety (e.g., for driving, crossing the street, or using the stove), families need to be so informed.

3. As time passes, some symptoms will clear, others will become more obvious, and patients will move from an inpatient setting to the challenges of their usual daily life tasks and environments. New concerns and problems will arise accordingly, and SLPs and other team members must be prepared to respond. We must observe patients' and families' reactions closely to decide when or whether it is necessary and appropriate to initiate certain discussions, such as a realistic talk about what to expect in terms of future stresses and adaptations. Some patients and family members will want to have as much concrete information as possible, as soon as possible, whereas for others, more information and advice will only generate more unproductive anxiety.

4. As indicated above, a central goal from the time of the earliest contacts with patients and families is to help them accept the patient's altered communication status and strategies. Fostering successful communication, and demonstrating or discussing together what the patient still does well, should contribute to acceptance and self-esteem.

5. It is never easy to impart negative information, but that is also an important part of our job. Cognitively and communicatively impaired stroke patients will not return to the way they were before their strokes, and some of their problems may not be amenable to treatment. We need to be professionally accountable enough to inform patients and families, honestly, when our best opinion is that we cannot help them—at all, or any longer. When a candidacy decision is negative, a prognosis is unfavorable, and/or discharge looms, some patients and family members may "shop" for a more favorable opinion. If they tell us that they are going elsewhere to be treated despite our best judgment, we should not insist that we are right. At that point, we can only wish them good luck.

C. Clinicians as Counselors

Clinicians should strive for unconditional positive regard and empathy in their interactions with individual patients and family members, putting aside any stereotypic notions or feelings of discomfort they might experience. In such a welcoming environment, clients with sufficient insight can feel comfortable talking about their wishes and their problems. This may help clinicians to identify when psychosocial responses are getting in the way of progress. Symptoms of depression and other psychosocial concerns that occupy mental resources can interfere with performance on specific treatment activities and with generalizing targeted skills and strategies. Of course, some bad days and bad moods are inevitable. The clinician can help a patient to clarify feelings and to identify whether and how those feelings are interfering with daily activities. The clinician can also discuss the fact that the patient's reactions are normal in the circumstances. But when a patient appears to be bogged down, or when there is any question of clinical depression, it is important for us to refer that patient for medical work-up, counseling, and/or evaluation for psychological or pharmaceutical intervention.

D. Clinicians as Referral Agents

Regardless of the accepting atmosphere we create in the clinic room, we cannot, and should not try to, handle all psychosocial issues on our own. As noted above, we should remain alert for the need to refer patients for workup and treatment of depression and other lasting or potentially serious adjustment problems. The same holds for family members, whose adjustment is not only important in its own right, but may influence and sustain the patient's goals and motivation. In addition, we should not try to deal with common concerns about the risks of incurring another stroke, activity or health practices, or financial options; similarly, we are not trained as marital counselors, sex therapists, or vocational specialists. But we can act as referral agents, interacting as appropriate with those who are trained to carry out these functions. We can also inform patients and families about existing stroke clubs and support groups where they can socialize, share their experiences with similarly affected people, and learn more about dealing with the challenges they face.

E. "The Door is Always Open"

Our education and counseling role often continues after discharge from treatment. Patients and families frequently develop trusting relationships with their clinicians, and they may want to consult us periodically for advice or referral. For most patients and families, we should leave the metaphorical door open upon discharge, so they feel comfortable contacting us as their lives evolve.

References

Adamovich, B. L., & Brooks, R. L. (1981). A diagnostic protocol to assess the communication deficits of patients with right hemisphere damage. In R. H. Brookshire (Ed.), *Clinical aphasiology: Conference proceedings* (pp. 244–253). Minneapolis: BRK Publishers.

Aitken, S., Chase, S., McCue, M., & Ratcliff, G. (1992, November). *An American adaptation of the Multiple Errands Test: Assessment of executive abilities in everyday living.* Paper presented at the National Academy of Neuropsychology, Pittsburgh, PA.

Albert, M. L. (1973). A simple test of visual neglect. *Neurology, 23*, 658–664.

Allport, A. (1989). Visual attention. In M. I. Posner (Ed.), *Foundations of cognitive science* (pp. 631–682). Cambridge, MA: MIT Press.

American Speech-Language-Hearing Association. (1990). *Report of the advisory panel to ASHA's Functional Communication Measures project.* Rockville, MD: American Speech-Language-Hearing Association.

American Speech-Language-Hearing Association. (1992). Code of Ethics. *ASHA, 34*(Suppl. 9), 1–2.

Apel, K., Van Dyke, P. M., & Fedorak, A. (1992, November). *Right-hemisphere-damaged patients' production and comprehension of figurative terms.* Paper presented at the American Speech-Language-Hearing Association Annual Convention, San Antonio, TX.

Ardila, A., & Rosselli, M. (1993). Spatial agraphia. *Brain and Cognition, 22*, 137–147.

Arenberg, D. (1968). Concept problem solving in young and old adults. *Journal of Gerontology, 23*, 279–282.

Arguin, M., & Bub, D. (1993). Modulation of the directional attention deficit in visual neglect by hemispatial factors. *Brain and Cognition, 22*, 148–160.

Armstrong, E. (1987). Cohesive harmony in aphasic discourse and its significance in listener perception of coherence. In R. H. Brookshire (Ed.), *Clinical aphasiology* (Vol. 17, pp. 210–215). Minneapolis: BRK Publishers.

Armstrong, E. (1991). The potential of cohesion analysis in the analysis and treatment of aphasia discourse. *Clinical Linguistics and Phonetics, 5,* 39–51.

Army Individual Test Battery. (1944). *Manual of Directions and Scoring.* Washington, DC: War Department, Adjutant General's Office.

Arnold, S. B. (1991). Measurement of Quality of Life in the frail elderly. In J. E. Birren, J. E. Lubben, J. C. Rowe, & D. E. Deutchman (Eds.). *The concept and measurement of quality of life in the frail elderly* (pp. 50–74). New York: Academic Press.

Arvedson, J. C., McNeil, M. R., & West, T. L. (1985). Prediction of the Revised Token Test overall, subtest, and linguistic unit scores by two shortened versions. In R. H. Brookshire (Ed.), *Clinical aphasiology* (Vol. 15, pp. 57–63). Minneapolis: BRK Publishers.

Ashcraft, M. H. (1989). *Human memory and cognition.* Glenview, IL: Scott, Foresman.

Baddeley, A. (1986). *Working memory.* Oxford, England: Clarendon Press.

Baggs, T. W., & Swindell, C. S. (1993, November). *Narrative modification in right-hemisphere-damaged stroke patients.* Paper presented at the American Speech-Language-Hearing Association Annual Convention, Anaheim, CA.

Ball, M., Davies, E., Duckworth, M., & Middlehurst, R. (1991). Assessing the assessments: A comparison of two clinical pragmatic profiles. *Journal of Communication Disorders, 24,* 367–379.

Barco, P. P., Crosson, B., Bolesta, M. M., Werts, D., & Stout, R. (1991). Training awareness and compensation in postacute head injury rehabilitation. In J. S. Kreutzer & P. H. Wehman (Eds.), *Cognitive rehabilitation for persons with traumatic brain injury: A functional approach* (pp. 129–146). Baltimore: Paul H. Brookes.

Barona, A., Reynolds, C. R., & Chastain, R. (1984). A demographically based index of premorbid intelligence for the WAIS-R. *Journal of Consulting and Clinical Psychology, 52,* 885–887.

Beaton, A., & McCarthy, M. (1993). "Auditory neglect after right frontal lobe and right pulvinar thalamic lesion": Comments on Hugdahl, Webster, and Asbjornsen (1991) and some preliminary findings. *Brain and Language, 44,* 121–126.

Beck, A. T., Ward, C. H., Mendelson, M., Mock, J., & Erbaugh, J. K. (1961). An inventory for measuring depression. *Archives of General Psychiatry, 4,* 561–571.

Beeman, M. (1993). Semantic processing in the right hemisphere may contribute to drawing inferences from discourse. *Brain and Language, 44,* 80–120.

Bellaire, K. J., Georges, J. B., & Thompson, C. K. (1991). Establishing functional communication board use for nonverbal aphasic subjects. *Clinical Aphasiology, 19,* 219–227.

Bennett, G. K., Seashore, M. G., & Wesman, A. G. (1972). *Differential Aptitude Tests. Manual* (5th ed.). New York: Psychological Corporation.

Benowitz, L. F., Moya, K. L., & Levine, D. N. (1990). Impaired verbal reasoning and constructional apraxia in subjects with right hemisphere damage. *Neuropsychologia, 28,* 231–241.

Benson, D. F. (1979). *Aphasia, alexia, and agraphia.* New York: Churchill Livingstone.

Benton, A. L. (1950). A multiple choice type of the visual retention test. *Archives Neurology and Psychiatry, 64,* 699–707.

Benton, A. L. (1974). *The Revised Visual Retention Test* (4th ed.). New York: Psychological Corporation.

Benton, A. L. (1977). The amusias. In M. Critchley & R. A. Henson (Eds.), *Music and the brain.* London: Willen Heinemann.

Benton, A. L., & Fogel, M. L. (1962). Three-dimensional constructional praxis: A clinical test. *Archives of Neurology, 7,* 347–354.

Benton, A. L., & Hamsher, K. deS. (1976). *Multilingual Aphasia Examination.* Iowa City: University of Iowa. (*Manual,* revised, 1978).

Benton, A. L., Hamsher, K. deS., Varney, N. R., & Spreen, O. (1983). *Contributions to neuropsychological assessment.* New York: Oxford University Press.

Benton, A. L., Levin, H. S., & Van Allen, M. W. (1974). Geographic orientation in patients with unilateral cerebral disease. *Neuropsychologia, 12,* 183–191.

Benton, A. L., & Van Allen, M. W. (1968). Impairment in facial recognition in patients with cerebral disease. *Cortex, 4,* 344–358.

Benton, A. L., Van Allen, M. W., & Fogel, M. L. (1964). Temporal orientation in cerebral disease. *Journal of Nervous and Mental Disease, 139,* 110–119.

Bihrle, A.M., Brownell, H.H., & Gardner, H. (1988). Humor and the right hemisphere: A narrative perspective. In H. A. Whitaker (Ed.), *Contemporary reviews in neuropsychology* (pp. 109–126). New York: Springer-Verlag.

Birren, J. E., & Dieckmann, L. (1991). Concepts and content of Quality of Life in the later years: An overview. In J. E. Birren, J. E. Lubben, J. C. Rowe, & D. E. Deutchman (Eds.), *The concept and measurement of quality of life in the frail elderly* (pp. 344–360). New York: Academic Press.

Birren, J. E., Lubben, J. E., Rowe, J. C., & Deutchman, D. E. (Eds.). (1991). *The concept and measurement of quality of life in the frail elderly.* New York: Academic Press.

Bloise, C. G. R., & Tompkins, C. A. (1993). Right brain damage and inference revision revisited. *Clinical Aphasiology, 21,* 145–153.

Blonder, L. X., Bowers, D., & Heilman, K. M. (1991). The role of the right hemisphere in emotional communication. *Brain, 114,* 1115–1127.

Blonder, L. X., Burns, A. F., Bowers, D., Moore, R. W., & Heilman, K. M. (1993). Right hemisphere facial expressivity during natural conversation. *Brain and Cognition, 21,* 44–56.

Bloom, R. L., Ferrand, C. T., & Paternostro, P. (1993, November). *Discourse monitoring by left brain-damaged and right brain-damaged adults.* Paper presented at American Speech-Language-Hearing Association Annual Convention, Anaheim, CA.

Boake, C. (1991). Social skills training following head injury. In J. S. Kreutzer & P. H. Wehman (Eds.), *Cognitive rehabilitation for persons with traumatic brain injury: A functional approach* (pp. 181–189). Baltimore: Paul H. Brookes.

Boning, R. A. (1976). *Specific Skills Series.* Baldwin, NY: Barnell-Loft.

Bourgeois, M.S. (1991). Communication treatment for adults with dementia. *Journal of Speech and Hearing Research, 34,* 831–844.

Boyd, T. M., Sautter, S., Bailey, M. B., Echols, L. D., & Douglas, J. W. (1987, February). *Reliability and validity of a measure of everyday problem solving.* Paper presented at the annual meeting of the International Neuropsychological Society, Washington, DC.

Braden, J. P. (1992). Review of the Rivermead Perceptual Assessment Battery. In J. J. Kramer & J. C. Conoley (Eds.), *The Eleventh Mental Measurements Yearbook* (pp. 773–775). Lincoln, NE: The Buros Institute of Mental Measurements of the University of Nebraska-Lincoln.

Bradshaw, J. L., Pierson-Savage, J. M., & Nettleton, N. C. (1988). Hemispace asymmetries. In H. A. Whitaker (Ed.), *Contemporary reviews in neuropsychology* (pp. 1–35). New York: Springer-Verlag.

Bransford, J. D., & Johnson, M. K. (1973). Considerations of some problems of comprehension. In W. G. Chase (Ed.), *Visual information processing.* New York: Academic Press.

Brickenkamp, R. (1981). *Test d2: Aufmerksamkeits-Belastungs-Test Handanweisung* (7th ed.) [*Test d2: Concentration-Endurance Test: Manual,* 5th ed.]. Gottingen: Verlag fur Psychologie Dr. C.J. Hogrefe.

Brinton, B., & Fujiki, M. (1989). *Conversational management with language-impaired children.* Rockville, MD: Aspen Publishers.

Britton, B. K., Van Dusen, L., Glynn, S. M., & Hemphill, D. (1990). The impact of inferences on instructional text. In A. C. Grasser & G. H. Bower (Eds.), *Inferences and text comprehension* (pp. 53–70). San Diego: Academic Press.

Brookshire, R. H. (1972). Effects of task difficulty on naming by aphasic subjects. *Journal of Speech and Hearing Research, 15,* 551–558.

Brookshire, R. H. (1976). Effects of task difficulty on sentence comprehension performance of aphasic subjects. *Journal of Communication Disorders, 9,* 167–173.

Brookshire, R. H. (1992). *An introduction to neurogenic communication disorders* (4th ed). St. Louis: Mosby-Year Book.

Brookshire, R. H. & Nicholas, L. E. (1984). Comprehension of directly and indirectly stated main ideas and details in discourse by brain-damaged and non-brain-damaged listeners. *Brain and Language, 21,* 21–36.

Brookshire, R. H., & Nicholas, L. E. (1993a). Influence of aphasic adults' connected speech abnormalities on listener judgments of communicative success. Research proposal funded by Department of Veteran's Affairs Rehabilitation Research program.

Brookshire, R. H., & Nicholas, L. E. (1993b). *Discourse Comprehension Test.* Tucson, AZ: Communication Skill Builders.

Brookshire, R. H., & Nicholas, L. E. (1994). Test-retest stability of measures of connected speech in aphasia. *Clinical Aphasiology, 22,* 119–133.

Brown, L., Sherbenou, R. J., & Johnsen, S. K. (1990). *Test of Nonverbal Intelligence* (TONI-2). Austin, TX: PRO-ED.

Brownell, H. H. (1988). The neuropsychology of narrative comprehension. *Aphasiology, 2,* 247–250.

Brownell, H. H., Carroll, J. J., Rehak, A., & Wingfield, A. (1992). The use of pronoun anaphora and speaker mood in the interpretation of conversational utterances by right-hemisphere brain-damaged patients. *Brain and Language, 43,* 121–147.

Brownell, H. H., Potter, H. H., Bihrle, A. M., & Gardner, H. (1986). Inference deficits in right brain-damaged patients. *Brain and Language, 227,* 310–321.

Brunn, J. L., & Farah, M. J. (1991). The relation between spatial attention and reading: Evidence from the neglect syndrome. *Cognitive Neuropsychology, 8,* 59–75.

Bryan, K. L. (1989). *The Right Hemisphere Language Battery.* Kibworth, England: Far Communications.

Buck, R. (1976). A test of nonverbal receiving abilities: Preliminary studies. *Human Communication Research, 2,* 162–171.

Buck, R. (1978). The slide-viewing technique for measuring nonverbal sending accuracy: A guide for replication. (Abstract). *Catalog of Selected Documents in Psychology, 8,* 63.

Buck, R. (1984). *The communication of emotion.* New York: The Guilford Press.

Buck, R., & Duffy, R. J. (1980). Nonverbal communication of affect in brain-damaged patients. *Cortex, 16,* 351–362.

Burns, M. S., Halper, A. S., & Mogil, S. I. (1983). *Communication problems in right hemispheric brain damage: Diagnostic and treatment approaches.* Chicago: Rehabilitation Institute of Chicago.

Burns, M. S., Halper, A. S., & Mogil, S. I. (1985). *Rehabilitation Institute of Chicago Evaluation of Communication Problems in Right Hemisphere Dysfunction (RICE)*. Rockville, MD: Aspen.

Butter, C. M., Kirsch, N. L., & Reeves, G. (1990). The effect of lateralized dynamic stimuli on unilateral spatial neglect following right-hemisphere lesions. *Restorative Neural Neuroscience, 2,* 39–46.

Campbell, T. F., & Bain, B. (1991). How long to treat: A multiple outcome approach. *Language, Speech, and Hearing Services in Schools, 22,* 271–276.

Cannito, M. P., Hayashi, M. M., & Ulatowska, H. K. (1988). Discourse in normal and pathologic aging: Background and assessment strategies. *Seminars in Speech and Language, 9,* 117–133.

Caplan, B. (1987). Assessment of unilateral neglect: A new reading test. *Journal of Clinical and Experimental Neuropsychology, 9,* 359–364.

Caplan, B. (1988). Nonstandard neuropsychological assessment: An illustration. *Neuropsychology, 2,* 12–17.

Caramazza, A. (1989). Cognitive neuropsychology and rehabilitation: An unfulfilled promise? In X. Seron & G. Deloche (Eds.), *Cognitive approaches in neuropsychological rehabilitation* (pp. 383–398). Hillsdale, NJ: Lawrence Erlbaum.

Chapman, L. J., & Chapman, J. P. (1973). Problems in the measurement of cognitive deficit. *Psychological Bulletin, 79,* 380–385.

Chapman, L. J., & Chapman, J. P. (1978). The measurement of differential deficit. *Journal of Psychiatric Research, 14,* 303–311.

Cherney, L. R., & Canter, G. J. (1993). Informational content in the discourse of patients with probable Alzheimer's Disease and patients with right brain damage. *Clinical Aphasiology, 21,* 123–134.

Cicone, M., Wapner, W., & Gardner, H. (1980). Sensitivity to emotional expressions and situations in organic patients. *Cortex, 16,* 145–158.

Cockburn, J., & Smith, P. T. (1991). The relative influence of intelligence and age on everyday memory. *Journal of Gerontology, 46,* 31–36.

Colsher, P. L., Cooper, W. E., & Graff-Radford, N. (1987). Intonational variability in the speech of right-hemisphere damaged patients. *Brain and Language, 32,* 379–383.

Cooper, W. E., & Klouda, G. V. (1987). Intonation in aphasic and right-hemisphere-damaged patients. In J. H. Ryalls (Ed.), *Phonetic approaches to speech production in aphasia and related disorders* (pp. 59–77). Boston: Little, Brown.

Corey, M., & Sprunk, H. S. (1987). *Social comprehension and reasoning.* Puyallup, WA: Good Samaritan Hospital Center for Cognitive Rehabilitation.

Coslett, H. B., Bowers, D., & Heilman, K. H. (1987). Reduction in cerebral activation after right hemisphere stroke. *Neurology, 37,* 957–962.

Davies, A. (1968). The influence of age on Trail Making test performance. *Journal of Clinical Psychology, 24,* 96–98.

Davis, G. A. (1983). *A survey of adult aphasia.* Englewood Cliffs, NJ: Prentice–Hall.

Davis, G. A. (1986). Questions of efficacy in clinical aphasiology. In R.H. Brookshire (Ed.), *Clinical aphasiology* (Vol. 16, pp. 154–162). Minneapolis: BRK Publishers.

Davis, G. A. (1993). *A survey of adult aphasia and related language disorders.* Englewood Cliffs, NJ: Prentice-Hall.

Davis, G. A., & Wilcox, M. J. (1985). *Adult aphasia rehabilitation: Language pragmatics.* San Diego: College-Hill Press.

Delis, D., Kramer, J., & Kaplan, E. (1984). *The California proverb test*. Unpublished protocol. Copyright.

Diller, L., & Weinberg, J. (1977). Hemi-inattention in rehabilitation: The evolution of a rational remediation program. In E. A. Weinstein & R. P. Friedland (Eds.), *Advances in neurology* (Vol. 18, pp. 63–82). New York: Raven Press.

Dodd, D., & White, R. M., Jr. (1980). *Cognition: Mental structures and processes*. Boston, MA: Allyn & Bacon.

Doyle, P. J., Goldstein, H., & Bourgeois, M. S. (1987). Experimental analysis of syntax training in Broca's aphasia: A generalization and social validation study. *Journal of Speech and Hearing Disorders, 52*, 143–155.

Doyle, P. J., Goldstein, H., Bourgeois, M. S., & Nakles, K. O. (1989). Facilitating generalized requesting behavior in Broca's aphasia: An experimental analysis of a generalization training procedure. *Journal of Applied Behavior Analysis, 22*, 157–170.

Dunn, L. M., & Markwardt, F. C., Jr. (1970). *Peabody Individual Achievement Test*. Minneapolis: American Guidance Service.

Ehrlich, J. S., & Sipes, A. L. (1985). Group treatment of communication skills for head trauma patients. *Cognitive Rehabilitation, 3*, 32–37.

Eysenck, M. W., & Keane, M. T. (1990). *Cognitive psychology: A student's handbook*. Hillsdale, N.J.: Lawrence Erlbaum Associates.

Farah, M. J., Brunn, J. L., Wallace, M. A., & Madigan, N. (1989). Structure of objects in central vision affects the distribution of visual attention in neglect. *Society for Neuroscience Abstracts, 15*, 481.

Fey, M. E., & Cleave, P. L. (1990). Early language intervention. *Seminars in Speech and Language, 11*, 165–181.

Fleet, W. S., Watson, R. T., Valenstein, E., & Heilman, K. (1986). Dopamine agonist therapy for neglect in humans. (Abstract). *Neurology, 36*(Suppl. 1), 347.

Foxx, R. M., & Bittle, R. (1989). *Thinking it through: Teaching a problem-solving strategy for community living*. Champaign, IL: Research Press.

Fratalli, C. (1991). *Functional communication scales for adults*. Rockville, MD: American Speech-Language-Hearing Association.

Frederiksen, C. H., Bracewell, R. J., Breuleux, A., & Renaud, A. (1990). The cognitive representation and processing of discourse: Function and dysfunction. In Y. Joanette & H. H. Brownell (Eds.), *Discourse ability and brain damage: Theoretical and empirical perspectives* (pp. 69–110). New York: Springer-Verlag.

Frederiksen, C. H., & Stemmer, B. (1993). Conceptual processing of discourse by a right hemisphere brain-damaged patient. In H. H. Brownell & Y. Joanette (Eds.), *Narrative discourse in neurologically impaired and normal aging adults* (pp. 239–278). San Diego: Singular Publishing Group.

Friedman, R. B., Ween, J. E., & Albert, M. L. (1993). Alexia. In K. Heilman & E. Valenstein (Eds.), *Clinical neuropsychology, 3rd ed.* New York: Oxford University Press.

Fry, E. B. (1978). *Fry Readability Scale*. Providence, RI: Jamestown Publishers.

Gajar, A., Schloss, P.J., Schloss, C.N., & Thompson, C.K. (1984). Effects of feedback and self-monitoring on head trauma youths' conversational skills. *Journal of Applied Behavior Analysis, 17*, 353–358.

Gates, A., & McGinitie, W. (1978). *Gates-McGinitie Reading Tests*. New York: Teachers College Press.

Gauthier, L., Dehaut, F., & Joanette, Y. (1989). The Bells Test: A quantitative and qualitative test for visual neglect. *International Journal of Clinical Neuropsychology, 11*, 49–54.

Gerber, S., & Gurland, G. (1989). Applied pragmatics in the assessment of aphasia. *Seminars in Speech and Language: Aphasia and Pragmatics, 10,* 263–281.

German, D. J. (1990). *Test of Adolescent/Adult Word Finding.* Allen, TX: DLM Teaching Resources.

German, D. J. (1991). *Test of Word Finding in Discouse.* Allen TX: DLM Teaching Resources.

Gernsbacher, M. A., & Faust, M. E. (1991). The mechanism of suppression: A component of general comprehension skill. *Journal of Experimental Psychology: Learning, Memory, and Cognition, 17,* 245–262.

Gernsbacher, M. A., Varner, K. R., & Faust, M.E. (1990). Investigating differences in general comprehension skill. *Journal of Experimental Psychology: Learning, Memory, and Cognition, 16,* 430–445.

Getzels, J. W., & Jackson, P. W. (1962). *Creativity and intelligence.* New York: Wiley.

Gilewski, M. J., Zelinski, E. M., & Schaie, K. W. (1990). The Memory Functioning Questionnaire for assessment of memory complaints in adulthood and old age. *Psychology and Aging, 5,* 482–490.

Goldman, R., Fristoe, M., & Woodcock, R. W. (1970). *Goldman-Fristoe-Woodcock Test of Auditory Discrimination.* Circle Pines, MN: American Guidance Service.

Goldstein, H. (1990). Assessing clinical significance. In L. B. Olswang, S. F. Warren, & N. J. Minghetti (Eds.), *Treatment efficacy research in communication disorders* (pp. 91–98). Rockville, MD: American Speech-Language-Hearing Foundation.

Goldstein, K. H., & Scheerer, M. (1953). Tests of abstract and concrete behavior. In A. Weider (Ed.), *Contributions toward medical psychology: Theory and psychodiagnostic methods* (Vol. 2, pp. 702–730). New York: Ronald Press.

Gollin, E. S. (1960). Developmental studies of visual recognition of incomplete objects. *Perceptual and Motor Skills, 11,* 289–298.

Golper, L. A. C., Gordon, M. E., & Rau, M. T. (1984). Coverbal behavior and perceptions of organicity. *Clinical aphasiology* (Vol. 14, pp. 94–105). Minneapolis: BRK Publishers.

Goodglass, H., & Kaplan, E. (1983). *The Boston Diagnostic Aphasia Examination.* Philadelphia: Lea and Febiger.

Gordon, W. A., Hibbard, M. R., Egelko, S., Diller, L., Simmens, S., Langer, K., Sano, M., Orazem, J., & Weinberg, J. (1984). *Evaluation of the deficits associated with right brain damage: Normative data on the Institute of Rehabilitation Test Battery.* New York: Department of Behavioral Sciences, Rusk Institute of Rehabilitation Medicine, New York University Medical Center.

Gordon, W. A., Hibbard, M. R., Egelko, S., Diller, L., Shaver, M. S., Lieberman, A., & Ragnarsson, K. (1985). Perceptual remediation in patients with right brain damage: A comprehensive program. *Archives of Physical Medicine and Rehabilitation, 66,* 353–359.

Gordon, W. A., Ruckdeschel-Hibbard, M., Egelko, S., Weinberg, J., Diller, L., Scotzin Shaver, M., & Piasetsky, E. (1986). *Techniques for the treatment of visual neglect and spatial inattention in right brain damaged individuals.* New York: Department of Rehabilitation Medicine Rusk, Institute of Rehabilitation Medicine, New York University Medical Center.

Gorham, D. R. (1956). *Proverbs Test.* Louisville, KY: Psychological Test Specialists.

Gottschaldt, K. (1928). Uber den Einfluss der Erfahrung auf die Wahrnehmung von Figuren. *Psychologische Forschung, 8,* 18–317.

Graesser, A. C., & Bower, G. H. (Eds.). (1990). *Inferences and text comprehension.* San Diego: Academic Press.

Grant, D. A., & Berg, E. A. (1948). A behavioral analysis of degree of reinforcement and ease of shifting to new responses in a Weigl-type card-sorting problem. *Journal of Experimental Psychology, 38,* 404–411.

Grice, H. (1975). Logic and conversation. In P. Cole & J. Morgan (Eds.), *Syntax and semantics: Speech acts* (pp. 41–58). New York: Academic Press.

Gronwall, D. M. A. (1977). Paced auditory serial-addition task: A measure of recovery from concussion. *Perceptual and Motor Skills, 44,* 367–373.

Gur, R. C., Packer, I. K., Hungerbuhler, I. P., Reivich, M., Obrist, W. D., Amarnek, W. S., & Sackeim, H. A. (1980). Differences in the distribution of gray and white matter in human cerebral hemispheres. *Science, 207,* 1226–1228.

Halligan, P. W., & Marshall, J. C. (1989a). Laterality of motor response in visuo-spatial neglect: A case study. *Neuropsychologia, 27,* 1301–1307.

Halligan, P. W., & Marshall, J. C. (1989b). Two techniques for the assessment of line bisection in visuo-spatial neglect: A single case study. *Journal of Neurology, Neurosurgery, and Psychiatry, 52,* 1300–1302.

Halper, A. S., & Cherney, L. R. (1991, November). *Establishing internal consistency of a test for right brain damage.* Paper presented at the American Speech-Language-Hearing Association Annual Convention, Atlanta, GA.

Halper, A. S., Burns, M. S., Cherney, L. R., & Mogil, S. I. (1991). *RIC Evaluation of Communication Problems in Right Hemisphere Dysfunction-2 (RICE-2).* Rockville, MD: Aspen.

Hammill, D. D. (1985). *Detroit Tests of Learning Aptitude (DTLA-2).* Austin, TX: PRO-ED.

Hanna, G., Schell, L. M., & Schreiner, R. (1977). *The Nelson Reading Skills Test.* Chicago: Riverside Publishing.

Harris, J. E., & Morris, P. E. (1984). *Everyday memory, actions and absent-mindedness.* London: Academic Press.

Heaton, R. K. (1981). *Wisconsin Card Sorting Test. Manual.* Odessa, FL: Psychological Assessment Resources.

Hebb, D. O., & Morton, N. W. (1943). The McGill Adult Comprehension Examination: "Verbal Situation" and "Picture Anomaly" series. *Journal of Educational Psychology, 34,* 16–25.

Heilman, K. M., Watson, R. T., & Valenstein, E. (1985). Neglect and related disorders. In K. M. Heilman & E. Valenstein (Eds.), *Clinical Neuropsychology* (2nd ed., pp. 243–293). New York: Oxford University Press.

Henley, S., Pettit, S., Todd-Pokropek, A., & Tupper, A. (1985). Who goes home? Predictive factors in stroke recovery. *Journal of Neurology, Neurosurgery, and Psychiatry, 48,* 1–6.

Hier, D.B., Mondlock, J., & Caplan, L.R. (1983a). Behavioral abnormalities after right hemisphere stroke. *Neurology, 33,* 337–344.

Hier, D.B., Mondlock, J., & Caplan, L.R. (1983b). Recovery of behavioral abnormalities after right hemisphere stroke. *Neurology, 33,* 345–350.

Hillis Trupe, E., & Hillis, A. (1985). Paucity vs. verbosity: Another analysis of right hemisphere communication deficits. *Clinical aphasiology* (Vol. 15, pp. 83–96). Minneapolis: BRK Publishers.

Hirst, W., & Kalmar, D. (1987). Characterizing attentional resources. *Journal of Experimental Psychology: General, 116,* 68–81.

Hirst, W., LeDoux, J., & Stein, S. (1984). Constraints on the processing of indirect speech acts: Evidence from aphasiology. *Brain and Language, 23,* 26–33.

Holland, A. L. (1980). *Communicative Abilities in Daily Living (CADL).* Baltimore: University Park Press.

Holland, A. L. (1994). Cognitive neuropsychological theory and treatment for aphasia: Exploring the strengths and limitations. *Clinical Aphasiology, 22,* 275–282.

Hooper, H. E. (1958). *The Hooper Visual Organization Test.* Los Angeles: Western Psychological Services.

Hooper Visual Organization Test (VOT). (1983). Manual. Los Angeles: Western Psychological Services.

Horner, J. (1980). Visual agnosic misnaming: Treatment of a right CVA patient one year post onset. In R. H. Brookshire (Ed.), *Clinical aphasiology: Conference proceedings* (pp. 316–330). Minneapolis: BRK Publishers.

Horner, J., Lathrop, D. L., Fish, A. M., & Dawson, D. (1987). Agraphia in left and right hemisphere stroke and Alzheimer dementia patients. In R. H. Brookshire (Ed.), *Clinical aphasiology* (Vol. 17, pp. 73–83). Minneapolis: BRK Publishers.

Horner, J., & Nailling, K. (1980). Raven's *Coloured Progressive Matrices:* Interpreting results through analysis of problem-type and error-type. In R. H. Brookshire (Ed.), *Clinical aphasiology: Conference proceedings* (pp. 226–239). Minneapolis: BRK Publishers.

Hough, M. S. (1990). Narrative comprehension in adults with right and left hemisphere brain-damage: Theme organization. *Brain and Language, 38,* 253–277.

Hough, M. S., DeMarco, S., Bedsole, J. K., Fox, B. O., & Pabst, M. (1993, November). *Word finding errors in four groups of brain-damaged adults.* Paper presented at the American Speech-Language-Hearing Association Annual Convention, Anaheim, CA.

Hough, M. S., & Pierce, R. S. (1994). Pragmatics and treatment. In R. Chapey (Ed.), *Language intervention strategies in adult aphasia* (3rd ed., pp. 246–268). Baltimore: Williams & Wilkins.

House, A., Rowe, D., & Standen, P. J. (1987). Affective prosody in the reading voice of stroke patients. *Journal of Neurology, Neurosurgery, and Psychiatry, 50,* 910–912.

Huber, W. (1990). Text comprehension and production in aphasia: analysis in terms of micro- and macroprocessing. In Y. Joanette & H. H. Brownell (Eds.), *Discourse ability and brain damage: Theoretical and empirical perspectives* (pp. 154–179). New York: Springer-Verlag.

Joanette, Y., Brouchon, M., Gauthier, L., & Samson, M. (1986). Pointing with left vs. right hand in left visual field neglect. *Neuropsychologia, 24,* 391–396.

Joanette, Y., & Brownell, H. H. (Eds.). (1990). *Discourse ability and brain damage: Theoretical and empirical perspectives.* New York: Springer-Verlag.

Joanette, Y., & Goulet, P. (1990). Narrative discourse in right-brain-damaged right-handers. In Y. Joanette & H. H. Brownell (Eds.), *Discourse ability and brain damage: Theoretical and empirical perspectives* (pp. 131–153). New York: Springer-Verlag.

Joanette, Y., & Goulet, P. (1994). Right hemisphere and verbal communication: Conceptual, methodological, and clinical issues. *Clinical Aphasiology, 22,* 1–23.

Joanette, Y., Goulet, P., & Hannequin, D. (1990). *Right hemisphere and verbal communication.* New York: Springer-Verlag.

Jones-Gotman, M., & Milner, B. (1977). Design fluency: The invention of nonsense drawings after focal cortical lesions. *Neuropsychologia, 15,* 653–674.

Just, M. A., & Carpenter, P. A. (1992). A capacity theory of comprehension: Individual differences in working memory. *Psychological Review, 99,* 122–149.

Kaplan, J. A., Brownell, H. H., Jacobs, J. R., & Gardner, H. (1990). The effects of right hemisphere damage on the pragmatic interpretation of conversational remarks. *Brain and Language, 38,* 315–333.

Kaplan, E., Goodglass, H., & Weintraub, S. (1983). *Boston Naming Test.* Philadelphia: Lea & Febiger.

Karnath, H. O., Schenkel, P., & Fischer, B. (1991). Trunk orientation as the determining factor of the contralateral deficit in the neglect syndrome and as the physical anchor of the internal representation of body orientation in space. *Brain, 114,* 1997–2014.

Kartsounis, L. D., & Warrington, E. K. (1989). Unilateral visual neglect overcome by cues implicit in stimulus arrays. *Journal of Neurology, Neurosurgery, and Psychiatry, 52,* 1253–1259.

Kearns, K. P. (1993). Functional outcome: Methodological considerations. *Clinical Aphasiology, 21,* 67–72.

Kearns, K. P., & Potechin Scher, G. (1989). The generalization of response elaboration training effects. *Clinical Aphasiology, 18,* 223–245.

Kellermann, K. (1991). The conversation MOP: II. Progression through scenes in discourse. *Human Communication Research, 17,* 385–414.

Kellermann, K., Broetzmann, S., Tae-Seop, L., & Kitao, K. (1989). The conversation MOP: Scenes in the stream of discourse. *Discourse Processes, 12,* 27–61.

Kempler, D., & Van Lancker, D. (1986). *The Familiar and Novel Language Comprehension Test (FANL-C).* Unpublished protocol (Copyright, 1986).

Kennedy, M., & Perez, W. (1993, November). *Managing conversational deficits in cognitively impaired adults: A cognitive perspective.* Paper presented at the American Speech-Language-Hearing Association Annual Convention, Anaheim, CA.

Kennedy, M., Strand, E., Burton, W., & Peterson, C. (1994). Analysis of first-encounter conversations of right-hemisphere-damaged adults. *Clinical Aphasiology, 22,* 67–80.

Kent, R. D. (1985). Science and the clinician: The practice of science and the science of practice. *Seminars in Speech and Language, 6,* 1–12.

Kent, R. D., & Rosenbek, J. C. (1982). Prosodic disturbance and neurologic lesion. *Brain and Language, 15,* 259–291.

Kimberg, D. Y., & Farah, M. J. (1993). A unified account of cognitive impairments following frontal lobe damage: The role of working memory in complex, organized behavior. *Journal of Experimental Psychology: General, 122,* 411–428.

Kinsella, G., Olver, J., Ng, K., Packer, S., & Stark, R. (1993). Analysis of the syndrome of unilateral neglect. *Cortex, 29,* 135–140.

Kintsch, W., & van Dijk, T. A. (1978). Toward a model of text comprehension and production. *Psychological Review, 85,* 363–394.

Kirk, S. A., McCarthy, J. J., & Kirk, W. D. (1968). *Illinois Test of Psycholinguistic Abilities.* Urbana, IL: University of Illinois Press.

Klonoff, P. S., Sheperd, J. C., O'Brien, K. P., Chiapello, D. A., & Hodak, J. A. (1990). Rehabilitation and outcome of right-hemisphere stroke patients: Challenges to traditional diagnostic and treatment methods. *Neuropsychology, 4,* 147–163.

Koike, K. J. M., & Asp, C. W. (1981). Tennessee test of rhythm and intonation patterns. *Journal of Speech and Hearing Disorders, 46,* 81–87.

Kolb, B., & Whishaw, I. Q. (1990). *Fundamentals of neuropsychology.* New York: W. H. Freeman.

Kosslyn, S. M., Chabris, C. F., Marsolek, C. J., & Koenig, O. (1991). Categorical versus coordinate spatial relations: Computational analyses and computer simulations. *Journal of Experimental Psychology: Human Perception and Performance, 18,* 562-577.

Ladavas, E., Menghini, G., & Umilta, C. (1994). A rehabilitation study of hemispatial neglect. *Cognitive Neuropsychology, 11,* 75-95.

LaPointe, L. (1991). *Base-10 Response Form.* San Diego: Singular Publishing Group.

LaPointe, L., & Horner, J. (1979). *Reading Comprehension Battery for Aphasia.* Tigard, OR: CC Publications.

Lemieux, S., Goulet, P., & Joanette, Y. (1993, October). *Interpretation of speech acts by right-brain-damaged patients: The effect of ecological context.* Paper presented at the Academy of Aphasia, Tuscon, AZ.

Levin, H. S., Benton, A. L., & Grossman, R. G. (1982). *Neurobehavioral consequences of closed head injury.* New York: Oxford University Press.

Levin, H. S., O'Donnell, V. M., & Grossman, R. G. (1979). The Galveston orientation and amnesia test: A practical scale to assess cognition after head injury. *Journal of Nervous and Mental Disease, 167,* 675-684.

Lezak, M. D. (1983). *Neuropsychological assessment* (2nd ed.). New York: Oxford University Press.

Liotti, M., & Tucker, D. M. (1992). Right hemisphere sensitivity to arousal and depression. *Brain and Cognition, 18,* 138-151.

Lodge-Miller, K. A., Robin, D. A., & Schum, R. L. (1993). Attentional impairments following closed head injury. *Journal of Medical Speech-Language Pathology, 1,* 133-146.

Lomas, J., Pickard, L., Bester, S., Elbard, H., Finlayson, A., & Zoghaib, C. (1989). The Communicative Effectiveness Index: Development and psychometric evaluation of a functional communication measure for adult aphasia. *Journal of Speech and Hearing Disorders, 54,* 113-124.

Lubinski, R. (1991). Environmental considerations for elderly patients. In R. Lubinski (Ed.), *Dementia and communication* (pp. 257-278). Philadelphia: B. C. Decker.

Lundgren, K., Moya, K. L., & Benowitz, L. I. (1984). Perception of nonverbal cues after right brain damage. (Abstract). In R. H. Brookshire (Ed.), *Clinical aphasiology: Conference proceedings* (p. 282). Minneapolis: BRK Publishers.

Mackisack, E. L., Myers, P. S., & Duffy, J. R. (1987). Verbosity and labeling behavior: The performance of right hemisphere and non-brain-damaged adults on an inferential picture description task. In R. H. Brookshire (Ed.), *Clinical aphasiology,* (Vol. 17, pp. 143-151). Minneapolis: BRK Publishers.

Marquardsen, J. (1969). The natural history of acute cerebrovascular disease. *Acta Neurologica Scandinavia, 45*(Suppl. 38), 1-192.

Massaro, M., & Tompkins, C. A. (1994). Feature Analysis for treatment of communication disorders in traumatically brain-injured patients: An efficacy study. *Clinical Aphasiology, 22,* 245-256.

McCarthy, R. A. & Warrington, E. K. (1990). *Cognitive neuropsychology: A clinical introduction.* San Diego: Academic Press.

McKoon, G., & Ratcliff, R. (1992). Inference during reading. *Psychological Review, 99,* 440-466.

McLeod, C. M. (1991). Half a century of research on the Stroop effect: An integrative review. *Psychological Bulletin, 109,* 163-203.

McNeil, M. R., Odell, K., & Campbell, T. F. (1982). The frequency and amplitude of fluctuating auditory processing in aphasic and non-aphasic brain-damaged persons. In R. H. Brookshire (Ed.), *Clinical aphasiology: Conference proceedings* (pp. 220–229). Minneapolis: BRK Publishers.

McNeil, M. R., & Prescott, T. E. (1978). *Revised Token Test.* Austin, TX: PRO-ED.

McReynolds, L., & Kearns, K. P. (1983). *Single-subject experimental design in communicative disorders.* Baltimore: University Park Press.

McShane, J. (1980). *Learning to talk.* Cambridge, MA: Cambridge University Press.

Meeker, M., Meeker, R., & Royd, G. H. (1985). *Structure of Intellect Learning Abilities Test (SOI-LA).* Los Angeles: Western Psychological Services.

Mentis, M., & Prutting, C. (1991). Analysis of topic as illustrated in a head-injured and normal adult. *Journal of Speech and Hearing Research, 34,* 583–595.

Milner, B. (1971). Interhemispheric differences in the localization of psychological processes in man. *British Medical Bulletin, 27,* 272–277.

Mlcoch, A. G., & Metter, E. J. (1994). Medical aspects of stroke rehabilitation. In R. Chapey (Ed.), *Language intervention strategies in adult aphasia* (3rd ed., pp. 27–46). Baltimore: Williams & Wilkins.

Molloy, R., Brownell, H. H., & Gardner, H. (1990). Discourse comprehension by right hemisphere stroke patients: Deficits of production and revision. In Y. Joanette & H. H. Brownell (Eds.), *Discourse ability and brain damage: Theoretical and empirical perspectives* (pp. 113–130). New York: Springer-Verlag.

Mooney, C. M., & Ferguson, G. A. (1951). A new closure test. *Canadian Journal of Psychology, 5,* 129–133.

Morrow, L. A., & Ratcliff, G. (1988). The disengagement of covert attention and the neglect syndrome. *Psychobiology, 16*(3), 261–269.

Morrow, L. A., Vrtunski, P. B., Kim, Y., & Boller, F. (1981). Arousal responses to emotional stimuli and laterality of lesion. *Neuropsychologia, 19,* 65–72.

Mross, E. (1990). Text analysis: Macro- and microstructural aspects of discourse processing. In Y. Joanette & H. H. Brownell (Eds.), *Discourse ability and brain damage: Theoretical and empirical perspectives* (pp. 50–68). New York: Springer-Verlag.

Murphy, G. L. (1990). The psycholinguistics of discourse comprehension. In Y. Joanette & H. H. Brownell (Eds.), *Discourse ability and brain damage: Theoretical and empirical perspectives* (pp. 28–49). New York: Springer-Verlag.

Myers, P. S. (1979). Profiles of communication deficits in patients with right cerebral hemisphere damage. In R. H. Brookshire (Ed.), *Clinical aphasiology: Conference proceedings* (pp. 38–46). Minneapolis: BRK Publishers.

Myers, P. S. (1981). Treatment of right hemisphere damaged patients: A panel discussion. In R. H. Brookshire (Ed.), *Clinical aphasiology: Conference proceedings* (pp. 272–276). Minneapolis: BRK Publishers.

Myers, P. S. (1986). Right hemisphere communication impairment. In R. Chapey (Ed.), *Language intervention strategies in adult aphasia* (2nd ed., pp. 444–461). Baltimore: Williams & Wilkins.

Myers, P. S. (1991). Inference failure: The underlying impairment in right-hemisphere communication disorders. *Clinical Aphasiology, 20,* 167–180.

Myers, P. S. (1994). Communication disorders associated with right-hemisphere brain damage. In R. Chapey (Ed.), *Language intervention strategies in adult aphasia* (3rd ed., pp. 514–534). Baltimore: Williams & Wilkins.

Myers, P. S., & Brookshire, R. H. (in press). Effects of noun type on naming performance of right-hemisphere-damaged and non-brain-damaged adults. *Clinical Aphasiology.*

Myers, P. S., Linebaugh, C. W., & Mackisack-Morin, L. (1985). Extracting implicit meaning: Right versus left hemisphere damage. *Clinical aphasiology* (Vol. 15, pp. 72–82). Minneapolis: BRK Publishers.

Myers, P. S., & Mackisack, E. L. (1990). Right hemisphere syndrome. In L. L. LaPointe (Ed.), *Aphasia and related neurogenic language disorders* (pp. 177–195). New York: Thieme Medical Publishers.

National Center for Health Statistics. (1991). *National health discharge survey* [DHHD Publication No. PHS 92-1509]. Hyattsville, MD: U.S. Department of Health and Human Resources.

Nelson, H. E. (1976). A modified card sorting test sensitive to frontal lobe defects. *Cortex, 12,* 313–324.

Nelson, H. E. (1982). *The Nelson Adult Reading Test (NART).* Windsor, England: NFER-Nelson.

Newhoff, M., & Apel, K. (1990). Impairments in pragmatics. In L. L. LaPointe (Ed.), *Aphasia and related neurogenic language disorders* (pp. 221–233). New York: Thieme Medical Publishers.

Nicholas, L. E., & Brookshire, R. H. (1993a). A system for scoring main concepts in the connected speech of non-brain-damaged and aphasic speakers. *Clinical Aphasiology, 21,* 87–99.

Nicholas, L. E., & Brookshire, R. H. (1993b). A system for quantifying the informativeness and efficiency of the connected speech of adults with aphasia. *Journal of Speech and Hearing Research, 36,* 338–350.

Nicholas, L. E., Brookshire, R. H., MacLennan, D. L., Schumacher, J. G., & Porrazzo, S. A. (1989). Revised administration and scoring procedures for the Boston Naming Test and norms for non-brain-damaged adults. *Aphasiology, 3,* 569–580.

Nunnally, J. C. (1978). *Psychometric theory* (2nd ed.). New York: McGraw-Hill.

Odell, K., Collins, M., Dirkx, T., & Kelso, D. (1985). A computerized version of the Coloured Progressive Matrices. In R. H. Brookshire (Ed.), *Clinical aphasiology* (Vol. 15, pp. 47–56). Minneapolis: BRK Publishers.

Odell, K., McNeil, M., Collins, M., & Rosenbek, J. (1984). Some comparison between auditory and reading comprehension in aphasic adults. (Abstract) In R. H. Brookshire (Ed.), *Clinical aphasiology: Conference proceedings* (p. 276). Minneapolis: BRK Publishers.

Pardo, J. V., Fox, P. T., & Reichle, M. E. (1991). Localization of a human system for sustained attention by positron emission tomography. *Nature, 349,* 61–64.

Parente, R., & Anderson-Parente, J. K. (1990). Vocational memory training. In J. S. Kreutzer & P. Wehman (Eds.), *Community intergration following traumatic brain injury* (pp. 157–168). Baltimore: Paul H. Brookes.

Patel, V. L., & Groen, G. J. (1986). Knowledge based solution strategies in medical reasoning. *Cognitive Science, 10,* 91–116.

Patry, R., & Nespoulous, J.-L. (1990). Discourse analysis in linguistics: Historical and theoretical background. In Y. Joanette & H. H. Brownell (Eds.), *Discourse ability and brain damage: Theoretical and empirical perspectives* (pp. 3–27). New York: Springer-Verlag.

Penn, C. (1988). The profiling of syntax and pragmatics in aphasia. *Clinical Linguistics and Phonetics, 2,* 179–207.

Phelps, M. E., Mazziotta, J. C., & Huang, S.-C., (1982). Study of cerebral blood function with positron computed tomography. *Journal of Cerebral Blood Flow Metabolism, 2,* 113–162.

Pimental, P. A., & Kingsbury, N. A. (1989). *Mini Inventory of Right Brain Injury.* Austin, TX: PRO-ED.

Pizzamiglio, L., Antonucci, G., Judica, G., Montenero, P., Razzano, C., & Zoccolotti, P. (1992). Cognitive rehabilitation of the hemineglect disorder in chronic patients with unilateral right brain damage. *Journal of Clinical and Experimental Neuropsychology, 14,* 901–923.

Porch, B. E. (1981). *Porch Index of Communicative Ability.* Palo Alto, CA: Consulting Psychologists Press.

Porteus, S. D. (1965). *Porteus Maze Test. Fifty years' application.* New York: Psychological Corporation.

Posner, M. I., & Driver, J. (1992). The neurobiology of selective attention. *Current Opinion in Neurobiology, 2,* 165–169.

Posner, M. I., Inhoff, A. W., & Friedrich, F. J. (1987). Isolating attentional systems: A cognitive-anatomical analysis. *Psychobiology, 15,* 107–121.

Posner, M. I., & Petersen, S. E. (1990). The attention system of the human brain. *Annual Review of Neuroscience, 13,* 25–42.

Posner, M. I., Walker, J. A., Friedrich, F. A., & Rafal, R. D. (1984). Effects of parietal injury on covert orienting of attention. *The Journal of Neuroscience, 4,* 1863–1874.

Posner, M. I., Walker, J. A., Friedrich, F. A., & Rafal, R. D. (1987). How do the parietal lobes direct covert attention? *Neuropsychologia, 25,* 135–145.

Prutting, C. A., & Kirchner, D. M. (1987). A clinical appraisal of the pragmatic aspects of language. *Journal of Speech and Hearing Disorders, 52,* 105–119.

Radloff, L. S. (1977). The CES-D Scale: A self-report depression scale for research in the general population. *Applied Psychological Measurement, 1,* 385–401.

Ratcliff, G. (1982). Disturbances of spatial orientation associated with cerebral lesions. In M. Potegal (Ed.), *Spatial abilities: Development and physiological functions* (pp. 301–333). New York: Academic Press.

Ratliffe, S. A., & Hudson, D. D. (1988). *Skill building for interpersonal competence.* New York: Holt, Rinehart, and Winston.

Raven, J. C. (1965). *The Coloured Progressive Matrices.* New York: The Psychological Corporation.

Rehak, A., Kaplan, J. A., & Gardner, H. (1992). Sensitivity to conversational deviance in right-hemisphere-damaged patients. *Brain and Language, 42,* 203–217.

Reitan, R. M. (1958). Validity of the Trail Making Test as an indicator of organic brain damage. *Perceptual and Motor Skills, 8,* 271–276.

Reitan, R. M., & Wolfson, D. (1985). *The Halstead-Reitan Neuropsychological Test Battery.* Tucson, AZ: Neuropsychology Press.

Reuter-Lorenz, P. A., & Posner, M. I. (1990). Components of neglect from right-hemisphere damage: An analysis of line bisection. *Neuropsychologia, 28,* 327–333.

Rey, A. (1941). L'examen psychologique dans les cas d'encephalopathie traumatique. *Archives de Psychologie, 28*(112), 286–340.

Rey, A. (1964). *L'examen clinique en psychologie.* Paris: Presses Universitaires de France.

Riddoch, M. J., & Humphreys, G. W. (1983). The effect of cuing on unilateral neglect. *Neuropsychologia, 21,* 589–599.

Rizzo, M., & Robin, D. A. (1990). Simultanagnosia: A defect of sustained attention yields insights on visual information processing. *Neurology, 40,* 447–455.

Robertson, I. (1990). Does computerized cognitive rehabilitation work? *Aphasiology, 4,* 381–405.

Robertson, I. H., Gray, J. M., & McKenzie, S. (1988). Microcomputer-based cognitive rehabilitation of visual neglect: Three multiple baseline single-case studies. *Brain Injury, 2,* 151–163.

Robertson, I. H., Gray, J. M., Pentland, B., & Waite, L. J. (1990). Microcomputer-based rehabilitation for unilateral left visual neglect: A randomized controlled trial. *Archives of Physical Medicine and Rehabilitation, 71,* 663–668.

Robin, D. A., & Rizzo, M. (1989). The effect of focal cerebral lesions on intramodal and cross-modal orienting of attention. *Clinical Aphasiology, 18,* 61–74.

Robin, D. A., Tranel, D., & Damasio, H. (1990). Auditory perception of temporal and spectral events in patients with focal left and right cerebral lesions. *Brain and Language, 39,* 539–555.

Roman, M., Brownell, H. H., Potter, H. H., Seibold, M. S., & Gardner, H. (1987). Script knowledge in right hemisphere-damaged and in normal elderly adults. *Brain and Language, 31,* 151–170.

Rosenbek, J. C., & LaPointe, L. L. (1985). The dysarthrias: Description, diagnosis, and treatment. In D. F. Johns (Ed.), *Clinical management of neurogenic communicative disorders* (2nd ed., pp. 97–152). Needham, MA: Allyn & Bacon.

Rosenbek, J. C., LaPointe, L. L., & Wertz, R. T. (1989). *Aphasia: A clinical approach.* Austin, TX: PRO-ED.

Rosenthal, R., Hall, J. A., DiMatteo, M. R., Rogers, P. L., & Archer, D. (1979). *Sensitivity to nonverbal communication: The PONS test.* Baltimore: The Johns Hopkins University Press.

Ross, D. G. (1986). *Ross Information Processing Assessment.* Austin, TX: PRO-ED.

Ross, E. (1981). The aprosodias: Functional-anatomical organization of the affective components of language in the right hemisphere. *Archives of Neurology, 38,* 561–569.

Ross, E. (1984a). Disturbances of emotional language with right hemisphere lesions. In A. Ardila & F. Ostrosky-Solis (Eds.), *The right hemisphere: Neurology and neuropsychology* (pp. 109–123). London: Gordon and Breach.

Ross, E. (1984b). Right hemisphere's role in language, affective behavior and emotion. *Trends in Neuroscience, 7,* 342–346.

Ross, E., Harney, J. H., de Lacoste-Utamsing, C., & Purdy, P. D. (1981). How the brain integrates affective and propositional language: A unified behavioral function. *Archives of Neurology, 38,* 745–748.

Salthouse, T. (1988). The role of processing resources in cognitive aging. In M. L. Howe & C. J. Brainerd (Eds.), *Cognitive development in adulthood* (pp. 185–239). New York: Springer-Verlag.

Sandson, J., & Albert, M. L. (1984). Varieties of perseveration. *Neuropsychologia, 22,* 715–732.

Schank, R. C. (1982). *Dynamic memory.* Cambridge: Cambridge University Press.

Schneiderman, E. I., Murasugi, K. G., & Saddy, J. D. (1992). Story arrangement ability in right brain-damaged patients. *Brain and Language, 43,* 107–120.

Schneiderman, E. I., & Saddy, J. D. (1988). A linguistic deficit resulting from right-hemisphere damage. Brain and Language, 34, 38–53.

Schwartz, M. F., & Whyte, J. (1992). Methodological issues in aphasia treatment research: The big picture. In J. E. Cooper (Ed.), *Aphasia treatment: Current approaches and research opportunities* (pp. 17–23). Washington, DC: National Institute on Deafness and Other Communication Disorders.

Seashore, C., Lewis, D., & Saetveit, J. (1960). *Seashore measures of musical talents*. New York: Psychological Corporation.

Seron, X., Coyette, F., & Bruyer, R. (1989). Ipsilateral influences on contralateral processing in neglect patients. *Cognitive Neuropsychology, 6,* 475–498.

Shallice, T. (1982). Specific impairments of planning. In P. Broadbent & & L. Weisknartz (Eds.), *The neuropsychology of cognitive function* (pp. 199–209). London: The Royal Society.

Shallice, T. (1988). *From neuropsychology to mental structure*. Cambridge, England: Cambridge University Press.

Shallice, T., & Burgess, P. (1991a). Higher-order cognitive impairments and frontal lobe lesions in man. In H. S. Levin, H. M. Eisenberg, & A. L. Benton (Eds.), *Frontal lobe function and dysfunction* (pp. 125–138). New York: Oxford University Press.

Shallice, T., & Burgess, P. (1991b). Deficits in strategy application following frontal lobe damage in man. *Brain, 114,* 727–741.

Shallice, T., & Evans, M. E. (1978). The involvement of the frontal lobes in cognitive estimation. *Cortex, 4,* 294–303.

Sherratt, S. M., & Penn, C. (1990). Discourse in a right–hemisphere brain-damaged subject. *Aphasiology, 4,* 539–560.

Silverman, F. H. (1985). *Research design and evaluation in speech-language pathology and audiology* (2nd ed.). Englewood Cliffs, NJ: Prentice-Hall.

Simmons-Mackie, N. N., & Damico, J. S. (1993, June). *Communicative competence in aphasia: Evidence for compensatory strategies*. Paper presented at the Clinical Aphasiology Conference, Sedona, AZ.

Smith, A. (1973). *Symbol Digit Modalities Test*. Los Angeles: Western Psychological Services.

Smith, M. L., & Milner, B. (1984). Differential effects of frontal-lobe lesions on cognitive estimation and spatial memory. *Neuropsychologia, 22,* 697–705.

Sohlberg, M. M., & Mateer, C. A. (1986). *Attention process training (APT)*. Puyallup, WA: Association for Neuropsychological Research and Development.

Sohlberg, M. M., & Mateer, C. A. (1989a). *Introduction to cognitive rehabilitation: Theory and practice*. New York: Guilford Press.

Sohlberg, M. M., & Mateer, C. A. (1989b). *Assessing and training prospective memory using the PROMS (Prospective memory screening) and PROMT (Prospective Memory Training)*. Puyallup, WA: Association for Neuropsychological Research and Development.

Solomon, P. R., Goethals, G. R., Kelley, C. M., & Stephens, B. R. (1989). *Memory: Interdisciplinary approaches*. New York: Springer-Verlag.

Somodi, L., Robin, D. A., & Luschei, E. (in press). A model of sense of effort of the tongue. *Brain and Language*.

Spector, C. C. (1990). Linguistic humor comprehension of normal and language-impaired adolescents. *Journal of Speech and Hearing Disorders, 55,* 533–541.

Spector, C. C. (1992). Remediating humor comprehension deficits in language-impaired students. *Language, Speech, and Hearing Services in Schools, 23,* 20–27.

Spencer, K. A., Tompkins, C. A., & Schulz, R. (submitted). *Post-stroke depression: A review and critical analysis*.

Spencer, K. A., Tompkins, C. A., Schulz, R., & Rau, M. T. (in press). The psychosocial outcomes of stroke: A longitudinal study of depression risk. *Clinical Aphasiology*.

Spilker, B. (1990). Introduction. In B. Spilker (Ed.), *Quality of life assessment in clinical trials* (pp. 3–9). New York: Raven Press.

Spreen, O., & Strauss, E. (1991). *A compendium of neuropsychological tests.* New York: Oxford University Press.

Squire, L. R. (1987). *Memory and brain.* New York: Oxford University Press.

Stankov, L. (1988). Aging, attention, and intelligence. *Psychology and Aging, 3,* 59–74.

Stanton, K., Yorkston, K. M., Kenyon, V. T., & Beukelman, D. R. (1981). Language utilization in teaching reading to left neglect patients. In R. H. Brookshire (Ed.), *Clinical aphasiology: Conference proceedings* (pp. 262–271). Minneapolis: BRK Publishers.

Stemmer, B., Giroux, F., & Joanette, Y. (1994). Production and evaluation of requests by right-hemisphere brain-damaged individuals. *Brain and Language, 47,* 1–31.

Stokes, T., & Baer, D. M. (1977). An implicit technology of generalization. *Journal of Applied Behavior Analysis, 10,* 349–367.

Stone, S. P., Halligan, P. W., Wilson, B., Greenwood, R. J., & Marshall, J. C. (1991). Performance of age-matched controls on a battery of visuo-spatial neglect tests. *Journal of Neurology, Neurosurgery, and Psychiatry, 54,* 341–344.

Stone, S. P., Patel, P., Greenwood, R. J., & Halligan, P. W. (1992). Measuring visual neglect in acute stroke and predicting its recovery: The Visual Neglect Recovery Index. *Journal of Neurology, Neurosurgery, and Psychiatry, 55,* 431–436.

Stone, S. P., Wilson, B., Wroot, A., Halligan, P. W., Lange, L. S., Marshall, J. C., & Greenwood, R. J. (1991). The assessment of visuo-spatial neglect after acute stroke. *Journal of Neurology, Neurosurgery, and Psychiatry, 54,* 345–350.

Stroop, J. R. (1935). Studies of interference in serial verbal reactions. *Journal of Experimental Psychology, 18,* 643–662.

Swinney, D. A. (1979). Lexical access during sentence comprehension: (Re)consideration of context effects. *Journal of Verbal Learning and Verbal Behavior, 20,* 645–660.

Swinney, D. A., & Osterhout, L. (1990). Inference generation during auditory language comprehension. In A. C. Graesser & G. H. Bower (Eds.), *Inferences and text comprehension* (pp. 17–33). San Diego: Academic Press.

Terman, L. M., & Merrill, M. A. (1973). *Stanford-Binet Intelligence Scale. Manual for the Third Revision, Form L-M.* Boston: Houghton Mifflin.

Thompson, C. K. (1989). Generalization research in aphasia: A review of the literature. *Clinical aphasiology, 18* (pp. 195–222). Boston, MA: College-Hill.

Thompson, C. K., & Byrne, M. E. (1984). Across setting generalization of social conventions in aphasia: An experimental analysis of "loose training." In R. H. Brookshire (Ed.), *Clinical aphasiology: Conference proceedings, 1984* (pp. 132–144). Minneapolis: BRK Publishers.

Tompkins, C. A. (1990). Knowledge and strategies for processing lexical metaphor after right or left hemisphere brain damage. *Journal of Speech and Hearing Research, 33,* 307–316.

Tompkins, C. A. (1991a). Automatic and effortful processing of emotional intonation after right or left hemisphere brain damage. *Journal of Speech and Hearing Research, 34,* 820–830.

Tompkins, C. A. (1991b). Redundancy enhances emotional inferencing by right- and left-hemisphere-damaged adults. *Journal of Speech and Hearing Research, 34,* 1142–1149.

Tompkins, C. A. (1993, April). *Mechanisms of discourse comprehension impairment in right hemisphere damaged adults.* Paper presented at the Midwest Aphasiology Conference, Iowa City, IA.

Tompkins, C. A. (1994). Applying research principles to language intervention. In R. Chapey (Ed.), *Language intervention strategies in adult aphasia* (3rd ed., pp. 571–583). Baltimore: Williams & Wilkins.

Tompkins, C. A., Bloise, C. G. R., Timko, M. L., & Baumgaertner, A. (1994). Working memory and inference revision in brain-damaged and normally aging adults. *Journal of Speech and Hearing Research, 37,* 896–912.

Tompkins, C. A., Boada, R., & McGarry, K. (1992). The access and processing of familiar idioms by brain-damaged and normally aging adults. *Journal of Speech and Hearing Research, 35,* 626–637.

Tompkins, C. A., Boada, R., McGarry, K., Jones, J., Rahn, A. E., & Ranier, S. (1993). Connected speech characteristics of right-hemisphere-damaged adults: A re-examination. *Clinical Aphasiology, 21,* 113–122.

Tompkins, C. A., & Flowers, C. R. (1985). Perception of emotional intonation by brain-damaged adults: The influence of task processing levels. *Journal of Speech and Hearing Research, 28,* 527–538.

Tompkins, C. A., & Mateer, C. A. (1985). Right hemisphere appreciation of prosodic and linguistic indications of implicit attitude. *Brain and Language, 24,* 185–203.

Tompkins, C. A., Spencer, K. A., & Boada, R. (1994). Contextual influences on judgments of emotionally ambiguous stimuli by brain-damaged and normally aging adults. *Clinical Aphasiology, 22,* 325–333.

Treisman, A. M., & Gelade, G. (1980). A feature-integration theory of attention. *Cognitive Psychology, 12,* 97–136.

Trope, I., Rozin, P., Nelson, D. K., & Gur, R. C. (1992). Information processing in the separated hemispheres of callosotomy patients: Does the analytic-holistic dichotomy hold? *Brain and Cognition, 19,* 123–147.

Tucker, D. M., & Frederick, S. L. (1989). Emotion and brain lateralization. In H. Wagner & A. Manstead (Eds.), *Handbook of social psychophysiology* (pp. 27–70). New York: Wiley.

Tucker, F. M., & Hamby, E. I. (1987, November). *Prosodic imitation in right hemisphere damage.* Paper presented at the American Speech-Language-Hearing Association Annual Convention, New Orleans, LA.

Ulatowska, H. K., Allard, L., & Chapman, S. B. (1990). Narrative and procedural discourse in aphasia. In Y. Joanette & H. H. Brownell (Eds.), *Discourse ability and brain damage: Theoretical and empirical perspectives* (pp. 180–198). New York: Springer-Verlag.

van Dijk, T. A., & Kintsch, W. (1983). *Strategies of discourse comprehension.* New York: Academic Press.

Van Lancker, D. (1990). The neurology of proverbs. *Behavioural Neurology, 3,* 169–187.

Vanier, M., Gauthier, L., Lambert, J., Pepin, E. P., Robillard, A., Dubouloz, C. J., Gagnon, R., & Joanette, Y. (1990). Evaluation of left visuospatial neglect: Norms and discrimination of two tests. *Neuropsychology, 4,* 87–96.

Wambaugh, J. L., Thompson, C. K., Doyle, P. J., & Camarata, S. (1991). Conversational discourse of aphasic and normal adults: An analysis of communicative functions. *Clinical Aphasiology, 20,* 343–353.

Wapner, W., Hamby, S., & Gardner, H. (1981). The role of the right hemisphere in the apprehension of complex linguistic materials. *Brain and Language, 14,* 15–32.

Warren, R. L., Gabriel, C., Johnston, A., & Gaddie, A. (1987). Efficacy during acute rehabilitation. In R. H. Brookshire (Ed.), *Clinical aphasiology* (Vol. 17, pp. 1–11). Minneapolis: BRK Publishers.

Warren, R. L., Loverso, F. L., & DePiero, J. (1991). The relationships among level of measurement, generalization, and reimbursement. *Clinical Aphasiology, 19,* 163–170.

Warrington, E. K. (1984). *Recognition Memory Test.* Windsor, England: NFER-Nelson.

Weber, A. M. (1986). *Measuring attentional capacity.* Unpublished doctoral dissertation,
University of Victoria, Victoria, Canada.

Weber, A. M. (1988). *Attentional Capacity Test.* Paper presented at the International
Neuropsychology Society Meeting, New Orleans, LA.

Webster, J. S., Cottam, G., Gouvier, W. D., Blanton, P., Beissel, G. F., & Wofford, J. (1988).
Wheelchair obstacle course performance in right cerebral vascular accident victims.
Journal of Clinical and Experimental Neuropsychology, 11, 295–310.

Webster, J. S., Godlewski, M. C., Hanley, G. L., & Sowa, M. V. (1992). A scoring method
for logical memory that is sensitive to right-hemsiphere dysfunction. *Journal of
Clinical and Experimental Neuropsychology, 14,* 222–238.

Webster, J. S., Jones, S., Blanton, P., Gross, R., Beissel, G. F., & Wofford, J. (1984). Visual
scanning training with stroke patients. *Behavior Therapy, 15,* 129–143.

Wechsler, D. (1955). *Wechsler Adult Intelligence Scale.* New York: Psychological Corporation.

Wechsler, D. (1981). *Wechsler Adult Intelligence Scale-Revised.* New York: Psychological
Corporation.

Wechsler, D. (1945). A standardized memory scale for clinical use. *Journal of Psychology,
19,* 87–95.

Wechsler, D. (1987). *Wechler Memory Scale-Revised.* New York: Psychological
Corporation.

Weinberg, J., Diller, L., Gordon, W. A., Gerstman, L. J., Lieberman, A., Lakin, P., Hodges,
G., & Ezrachi, O. (1977). Visual scanning training effect on reading-related tasks in
acquired right brain damage. *Archives of Physical Medicine and Rehabilitation, 58,*
479–486.

Weinberg, J., Diller, L., Gordon, W. A., Gerstman, L. J., Lieberman, A., Lakin, P., Hodges,
G., & Ezrachi, O. (1979). Training sensory awareness and spatial organization in
people with right brain damage. *Archives of Physical Medicine and Rehabilitation,
60,* 491–496.

Weinberg, J., Piasetsky, E., Diller, L., & Gordon, W. (1982). Treating perceptual organization deficits in nonneglecting right brain damaged stroke patients. *Journal of Clinical
Neuropsychology, 4,* 59–75.

Wertz, R. T. (1985). Neuropathologies of speech and language: An introduction to patient
management. In D. F. Johns (Ed.), *Clinical management of neurogenic communication disorders* (2nd ed., pp. 1–96). Needham, MA: Allyn & Bacon.

Wertz, R. T. (1986). Specialty recognition in neurogenic speech, language, and cognitive
disorders: Clinical competence in aphasia and apraxia of speech. In R. H. Brookshire
(Ed.), *Clinical aphasiology* (Vol. 16, pp. 319–324). Minneapolis: BRK Publishers.

Weylman, S., Brownell, H.H., Roman, M., & Gardner, H. (1989). Appreciation of indirect
requests by left- and right-brain-damaged patients: The effects of verbal context and
conventionality of wording. *Brain and Language, 36,* 580–591.

Whitehead, R. (1991). Right hemisphere processing superiority during sustained visual
attention. *Journal of Cognitive Neuroscience, 3,* 329–334.

Whiting, S., Lincoln, N. B., Bhavnani, G., & Cockburn, J. (1985). *The Rivermead
Perceptual Assessment Battery.* Windsor, England: NFER-Nelson.

Whitney, J. L., & Goldstein, H. (1989). Using self-monitoring to reduce disfluencies in
speakers with mild aphasia. *Journal of Speech and Hearing Disorders, 54,* 576–586.

Whyte, J. (1992). Attention and arousal: Basic science aspects. *Archives of Physical Medicine and Rehabilitation, 73*, 940–949.

Wilkins, A. J., Shallice, T., & McCarthy, R. (1987). Frontal lesions and sustained attention. *Neuropsycyhologia, 25*, 359–365.

Wilson, B. A. (1992). Memory therapy in practice. In B. A. Wilson & N. Moffat (Eds.), *Clinical management of memory problems* (2nd ed., pp. 120– 153). San Diego: Singular Publishing Group.

Wilson, B. A., Cockburn, J., & Baddeley, A. D. (1985). *The Rivermead Behavioural Memory Test.* Bury St. Edmunds, Suffolk, England: Thames Valley Test Company.

Wilson, B. A., Cockburn, J., & Halligan, P. (1987). *Behavioural Inattention Test.* Bury St. Edmunds, Suffolk, England: Thames Valley Test Company.

Wilson, R. S., Rosenbaum, G., & Brown, G. (1979). The problem of premorbid intelligence in neuropsychological assessment. *Journal of Clinical Neuropsychology, 1*, 49–53.

Winterling, D., Crook, T., Salama, M., & Gobert, J. (1986). A self-rating scale for assessing memory loss. In A. Bes, J. Cahn, S. Hoyer, J. P. Marc-Vergnes, & H. M. Wisniewski (Eds.), *Senile dementias: Early detection* (pp. 482–486). London: John Libbey Eurotext.

Woodcock, R. L., & Johnson, B. (1977). *Woodcock-Johnson Psychoeducational Battery.* Boston: Teaching Resources Corporation.

World Health Organization. (1980). *International classification of impairments, disabilities, and handicaps.* Geneva: WHO.

Ylvisaker, M. S., & Holland, A. L. (1985). Coaching, self-coaching, and rehabilitation of head injury. In D. F. Johns (Ed.), *Clinical management of neurogenic communication disorders* (2nd ed., pp. 243–257). Needham, MA: Allyn & Bacon.

Ylvisaker, M. S., & Szekeres, S. F. (1994). Communication disorders associated with closed head injury. In R. Chapey (Ed.), *Language intervention strategies in adult aphasia* (3rd ed., pp. 546–567). Baltimore: Williams & Wilkins.

Yokoyama, K., Jennings, R., Ackles, P., Hood, P., & Boller, F. (1987). Lack of heart rate changes duing an attention demanding task after right hemisphere lesions. *Neurology, 37*, 624–630.

Yorkston, K. M., & Beukelman, D. R., & Bell, K. R. (1988). *Clinical management of dysarthric speakers.* Boston: College-Hill Press.

Zoccolotti, P., Scabini, D., & Violani, C. (1982). Electrodermal responses in patients with unilateral brain damage. *Journal of Clinical Neuropsychology, 4*, 143–150.

INDEX